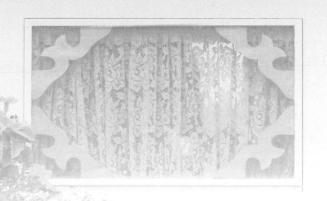

Homemaker Home Health Aide

Seventh Edition

Homemaker Home Health Aide

Seventh Edition

Suzann Balduzzi
RN, BSN, M.S of Ed.

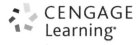
CENGAGE
Learning®

Singapore • United Kingdom • United States

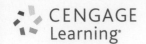

**Homemaker Home Health Aide,
Seventh Edition
Suzann Balduzzi**

SVP, GM Skills & Global Product
Management: **Dawn Gerrain**

Product Director: **Matt Seeley**

Associate Product Manager: **Laura Stewart**

Senior Director, Development: **Marah
Bellegarde**

Product Development Manager:
Juliet Steiner

Content Developer: **Deborah Bordeaux**

Product Assistant: **Hannah Kinisky**

Vice President, Marketing Services: **Jennifer
Ann Baker**

Marketing Manager: **Jon Sheehan**

Senior Production Director: **Wendy Troeger**

Production Director: **Andrew Crouth**

Senior Content Project Manager: **Kenneth
McGrath**

Managing Art Director: **Jack Pendleton**

Cover image(s): **©Westhoff/iStock.com**

For product information and technology assistance, contact us at
Cengage Learning Customer & Sales Support, 1-800-354-9706

For permission to use material from this text or product,
submit all requests online at **www.cengage.com/permissions**
Further permissions questions can be emailed to
permissionrequest@cengage.com

Library of Congress Control Number: 2014947680

ISBN-13: 978-1-133-69150-1

Cengage Learning
20 Channel Center Street
Boston, MA 02210
USA

Cengage Learning is a leading provider of customized learning solutions with office
locations around the globe, including Singapore, the United Kingdom, Australia, Mexico,
Brazil, and Japan. Locate your local office at:
www.cengage.com/global

Cengage Learning products are represented in Canada by Nelson Education, Ltd.

To learn more about Cengage Learning, visit **www.cengage.com**

Purchase any of our products at your local college store or at our preferred online store
www.cengagebrain.com

Notice to the Reader
Publisher does not warrant or guarantee any of the products described herein or perform any
independent analysis in connection with any of the product information contained herein.
Publisher does not assume, and expressly disclaims, any obligation to obtain and include
information other than that provided to it by the manufacturer. The reader is expressly warned
to consider and adopt all safety precautions that might be indicated by the activities described
herein and to avoid all potential hazards. By following the instructions contained herein, the
reader willingly assumes all risks in connection with such instructions. The publisher
makes no representations or warranties of any kind, including but not limited to, the warranties
of fitness for particular purpose or merchantability, nor are any such representations implied
with respect to the material set forth herein, and the publisher takes no responsibility with
respect to such material. The publisher shall not be liable for any special, consequential, or
exemplary damages resulting, in whole or part, from the readers' use of, or reliance upon, this
material.

Printed in United States of America
Print Number: 01   Print Year: 2014

Dedication

Suzann Balduzzi would like to dedicate this book and special thanks to her husband Bob, to her sons Dave and Dan who exhibited patience and understanding during this project.

Summary Contents

Contents

UNIT 3   Developing Effective Communication Skills and Documentation   29

UNIT 4   Safety   47

UNIT 5   Homemaking Service   59

Unit 15	**Musculoskeletal System: Arthritis, Body Mechanics, and Restorative Care**	**257**

UNIT 16   Nervous System   303

UNIT 17   Circulatory System   315

UNIT 18   Respiratory System   325

UNIT 19   Reproductive System   333

UNIT 20   Endocrine System and Diabetes   339

List of Procedures

Preface

The latest employment surveys list the career of home health aide as one of the fastest growing jobs in the United States. The increasing demand for home health aides is due to several factors, such as early discharge of clients from acute care facilities, individuals living longer, and the availability of home health aides with a higher level of skill to perform more routine and complex tasks. *Homemaker/Home Health Aide,* seventh edition, is a comprehensive textbook designed for use in initial training programs for home health aides and as a reference in required continuing education courses.

The book is divided into eight sections: Section 1, Becoming a Home Health Aide; Section 2, Stages of Human Development; Section 3, Preventing the Spread of Infectious Disease; Section 4, Understanding Health; Section 5, Body Systems and Common Disorders; Section 6, Clients Requiring Special Care; Section 7, Maternal/Infant Care; and Section 8, Employment. The practical applications of procedures required by the Omnibus Reconciliation Act (OBRA) are included in each unit. The procedures are presented in a step-by-step format and are illustrated with photographs to assist the learner in understanding the various steps. Note: Agencies and states differ in what procedures they allow home health aides to perform. Always check with your agency for which procedures you are allowed to perform in your state.

Changes to the Seventh Edition

The seventh edition is organized into 26 units plus a Glossary, Appendix A: Emergency Procedures Guidelines, and Appendix B: Prefixes and Suffixes Commonly Used in Medical Terminology. Major changes by unit include the following:

Unit 1 Home Health Services

- Added physician assistant and chaplain to the health team

- Updated statistics on reasons for increase employment of home health aides
- Updated information on Medicare
- Information on the Affordable Care Act
- Updated photos

Unit 2 Home Health Aide Responsibilities and Legal Rights

- Additional terms, such as corporal punishment, ethical standards, legal standards, and personal history information (PHI), were added
- Information on PHI in computerized records
- Updated photos
- Added information on assistive living facilities

Unit 3 Developing Effective Communication Skills and Documentation

- Added information and procedure on documenting on a computer
- Updated abbreviations
- Added use of a cell phone

Unit 4 Safety

- Updated tips on home safety for the client with dementia
- Updated do's and don'ts

Unit 5 Homemaking Service

- Updated guidelines for making an occupied bed
- Updated guidelines for making an unoccupied bed

Unit 6 Infancy to Adolescence

- Updated information on common infant and childhood diseases
- Updated and more detailed information on infant and child car seat requirements

- Revised information on autism spectrum disorder
- Added information on whooping cough

Unit 7 Early and Middle Adulthood

- Information on lesbian and homosexual couples
- Updated information on the importance of exercise
- Integrated use of computers and electronic media throughout the unit

Unit 8 Older Adulthood

- Updated information on hearing aids
- Updated terminology
- Expanded information on pain management, such as rating pain and other measures other than medication to assist in the relief of pain
- Greatly expanded discussion of the role of the home health aide in medication administration
- Added the five rights in giving medications
- Revised information on communicating with a client who has hearing loss
- Revised the procedure for caring for a client with an artificial eye
- Updated statistics
- Added information on working with a client with low vision
- Added new photos

Unit 9 Infection Control

- New diagram on the chain of infection
- Updated information on HIV/AIDS
- Updated all procedures including hand hygiene
- Added information on use of alcohol hand rubs
- New terminology, such as ELISA, Clostridium *difficile* (C-*diff*), and immunization
- Added information and photos on bed bugs
- Expanded information on hepatitis

Unit 10 From Wellness to Illness

- New procedure for taking a temporal artery temperature
- Revised information on types of thermometers used to measure a client's temperature
- Added new photos
- Improved sequencing of unit

Unit 11 Mental Health

- Expanded information on delirium
- Information on signs of depression and suicide
- Updated information on post-traumatic stress disorder

Unit 12 Digestion and Nutrition

- Replaced the Food Pyramid with the MyPlate
- New information on cardiac, renal, and gluten-free diet
- New information on alternative nutrition
- Added information on tips for feeding the client
- Updated heartburn/acid reflux information
- Added Smart Choices
- Updated Dietary Guidelines for Americans
- New discussion of bariatric clients and obesity
- Expanded information of foods containing potassium

Unit 13 Elimination

- Updated information on urinary tract infections
- Updated information on kidney dialysis, peritoneal dialysis, and hemodialysis
- Expanded information on types of incontinence
- Replaced cubic centimeter measurements with millimeter measurements
- Added information on hernias and gall bladder disorder
- Expanded information on constipation
- Improved sequencing of information within all procedures

Unit 14 Integumentary System

- Explanation of the terms *shearing* and *friction*
- Revised information on care of pressure sores
- Added information on denture care
- Discussion of bathing options in an assistive living facility
- Added new photos

Unit 15 Musculoskeletal System: Arthritis, Body Mechanics, and Restorative Care

- Updated terminology
- Added information on safe patient handling and mobility (SPHM) programs and standards

- Added information on musculoskeletal disorders (MSDs)
- Added procedures on pivot disc and sliding board transfers
- Added information on nursing care for hip and knee replacements
- Expanded information on drugs used to treat arthritis
- Expanded explanation of cartilage, joint capsule, and synovium
- Expanded information on lift belts
- Revised procedure on dangling
- Updated warning signs for arthritis
- Revised the procedures on using the mechanical and stand lift and added photos to explain the steps
- Updated cast care and procedure on caring for a cast
- Discussion of drugs used in the treatment of bones and muscle conditions
- Added new photos

Unit 16 Nervous System

- Updated information on Parkinson's disease and multiple sclerosis
- Updated information on risk factors for strokes
- Added information on transient ischemic attacks (TIAs)
- Added names of medications used to treat common nervous disorders
- Added diagnostic tests for strokes
- Added discussion of immediate treatment after a client has had a stroke -BEFAST
- Updated vocabulary list
- Revised discussion of care for a client having a seizure

Unit 17 Circulatory System

- Updated terminology
- Updated discussion of risk factors for cardiac diseases
- Explanation of cardiovascular diseases
- Expanded discussion of tests used for diagnosing heart conditions
- Added information on signs and symptoms to watch for
- Added discussion of treatment for cardiac disorders
- Expanded information on elastic support hose

- Added discussion of diagnostic tests for blood disorders
- Additional information on leukemia

Unit 18 Respiratory System

- Updated information on nebulizers
- Added information on diagnostic tests for respiratory disorders
- Updated information on emphysema
- Updated information on use of oxygen in the home
- Added discussion of treatments for respiratory disorders
- Added new photos
- Added information on chronic obstructive pulmonary disease (COPD)
- Updated safety precautions with use of oxygen

Unit 19 Reproductive System

- Added information on preventing sexually transmitted diseases

Unit 20 Endocrine System and Diabetes

- Revised section on hypothyroidism and hyperthyroidism
- New discussion of oral drugs used for treatment of type II diabetes
- Updated discussion of risk factors for the disease
- Updated information on tests used to diagnose diabetes
- Revised discussion of nutrition and diet therapy
- Updated information on finger-stick blood testing
- Added information on possible kidney damage with diabetes
- Updated discussion of signs and symptoms of hyperglycemia and hypoglycemia
- Added new photos

Unit 21 Caring for the Client Who Is Terminally Ill

- Added information on mental health directives
- Expanded information on pain control, hospice, advance directives, living will, and durable power of attorney
- Discussion of palliative care
- Added new photos

Unit 22 Caring for the Client with Alzheimer's Disease

- Updated statistics
- List of new drugs used in treatment of Alzheimer's disease
- Added discussion of warning signs of the disease
- Added information on caregiver support
- Added information on home environment, dressing of client, and incontinence
- Updated discussion of care for wandering and sundowning
- Added coverage of communication and sexuality changes
- Updated photos

Unit 23 Caring for the Client with Cancer

- Added new cancer terminology
- Expanded information on nursing care for clients receiving adjuvant therapy, chemotherapy, hormone therapy, targeted biologic therapy, and radiation
- Added discussion of short-term side effects of each type of cancer therapy
- Updated information on cancer of the larynx
- Updated information on colorectal cancer
- Discussion of the ABCDs of melanoma

Unit 24 Maternal Care

- Updated photos
- Updated information on care of an infant penis and umbilical cord
- Updated information on nutrition and breast-feeding
- Added information on toxemia of pregnancy

Unit 25 Infant Care

- Expanded information on breast-feeding positions
- Added information on birth control measures for mothers who are breast-feeding or not breast-feeding

Unit 26 Job-Seeking Skills

- Updated information on résumés and felonies
- Added information on the services available from Workforce Connections Career Exploration Agency
- Discussion of how to prepare for a group interview
- Added information on online job applications

Comprehensive Teaching and Learning Resources

Workbook to Accompany *Homemaker Home Health Aide*, Seventh Edition

The workbook was written to assist the learner to become part of the home care team as a homemaker home health aide. Each chapter of the workbook is correlated to a unit in the textbook and includes the following features:

- Learning Objectives remind you of important concepts covered in the text.
- Terms to Define emphasize the essential terms you should be familiar with in each unit.
- Application Exercises reinforce your knowledge through a variety of question types related to the chapter content. Communication and documentation exercises and practice situations provide you with practice in applying the concepts learned in the text.
- Crossword puzzles give you practice learning important vocabulary.
- Chapter quizzes allow you to test your knowledge of the material in each unit.

ISBN   978-1-133-69152-5

Instructor's Companion Website

The Instructor's Manual includes several features to assist you in instructing home health aides, including teaching tips and strategies, course syllabus, unit lesson plans, class activities, additional review questions, case studies with questions for discussion, quizzes and a final examination, answers to the textbook review questions and case studies, and answers to the review questions in the workbook.

Cengage Learning Testing Powered by Cognero is a flexible, online system that allows you to:

- author, edit, and manage test bank content from multiple Cengage Learning solutions
- create multiple test versions in an instant
- deliver tests from your learning management system (LMS), your classroom, or wherever you want

Start right away!
Cengage Learning Testing Powered by Cognero works on any operating system or browser.

- No special installs or downloads needed
- Create tests from school, home, the coffee shop—anywhere with Internet access

What will you find?

- *Simplicity at every step*. A desktop-inspired interface features drop-down menus and familiar, intuitive tools that take you through content creation and management with ease.
- *Full-featured test generator*. Create ideal assessments with your choice of 15 question types (including true/false, multiple choice, opinion scale/Likert, and essay). Multi-language support, an equation editor, and unlimited metadata help ensure your tests are complete and compliant.
- *Cross-compatible capability*. Import and export content into other systems.

Basic Skills for Home Care Aides DVD Series

The *Basic Skills for Home Care Aides DVD Series* presents those procedures required by OBRA for home care aides in an easy-to-follow, step-by-step format. By allowing learners to observe the skills from start to finish, they will have a better understanding of everything they'll need to know for each skill, including all of the necessary equipment. By concentrating on the core skills required to pass the national home care certification exam, learners will be able to

view all the steps needed to complete each skill on which they will be tested. Refer to the DVD Menu on page xxxiii in this book for a listing of key concepts for each segment.

ISBN   978-1-4018-3182-0

Reviewers

We would like to acknowledge the following individuals for their valuable suggestions and comments during the revision process.

Sheila R. Adams, RN, MSN
Program Coordinator, Department Chair, Assistant Professor,
Richmonds Community College, Hamlet, NC

Michele F. Emond
Department Head, Allied Health Worcester Technical High School

Tanya Gwin
Nursing Assisting Instructor
Copper Mountain Community College

Bob Hagberg, RN
Allied Health Instructor
Fort Scott Community College

Georgette Howard, RN, MSN
Nursing Assistant Program Coordinator
Glendale Community College, Glendale, AZ

FEATURES

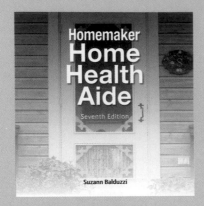

The seventh edition of *Homemaker/Home Health Aide* has been completely revised and updated and is designed to train new individuals entering the field for the first time, and practicing home health aides to be caring, dedicated, and skilled para-professionals. This book emphasizes the role of the home health aide as a valuable member of the health care team. The following features are intended to help you master the content as you prepare for your role on the health care team as a home health aide.

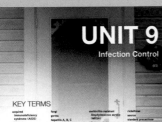

Unit Opening Page

Each unit opening page contains key terms and learning objectives.

The **key terms** list alerts you to important terms to become familiar with in each unit. When each term is first introduced in the unit, it is highlighted in bold-face and color. Each term is defined at this point. Read the definition of the term and note how it is used so you will be comfortable using the term. Note that each term and definition is also included in the Glossary at the back of the book.

The **learning objectives** let you know what is expected of you as you read the text. The review questions at the end of each unit measure your success in mastering each objective.

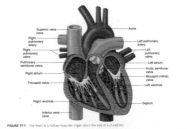

Photographs and Line Drawings

We listened! All of the photos involving home health aides were replaced in this edition. The new photos more positively reflect the role of the home health aide as a valuable member of the health care team. These photos and the line drawings help clarify and reinforce the unit content. Full-color anatomy drawings help you locate body components and understand body organization.

Procedures

The practical applications of procedures required by OBRA are included in each unit. Procedures are presented in an easy-to-learn, step-by-step format, and are enhanced with photographs to help you understand the various steps of each skill. Each procedure includes a purpose to reinforce the importance of the skill being performed.

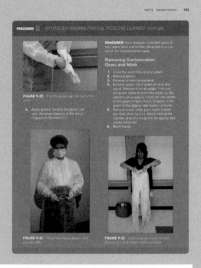

Workbook Review

The workbook review serves as a reminder to take advantage of additional practice in mastering the content of each unit by completing the review exercises in the workbook, and reviewing key information for each unit.

Review

A variety of review questions at the end of each unit test your understanding of the unit content. Each review includes two case studies with related questions that provide you with an opportunity to apply what you have learned to a clinical scenario.

Basic Skills for Home Care Aides DVD Series

An excellent supplement to your text, the *Basic Skills for Home Care Aides DVD Series* demonstrates the skills required of home care aides by OBRA. The learner can observe 80 core skills from start to finish in order to ensure a thorough understanding of everything they will need to know to be a successful home care aide.

Available at CengageBrain.com
ISBN: 978-1-4018-3182-0

DVD Menu of Content Segments

Segment 1 Orientation to Home Health Care and Communication

- Where to work
- Reimbursement
- Clients
- Home health team
- Care plan
- Good work practices
- Observation skills
- Documenting client care
- Legal protections
- Communication
- Common communication problems

Segment 2 Infection Control and Safety

- Infection control
- Biohazardwaste disposal
- Hand hygiene
- Gloving
- Putting on and removing personal protective equipment
- Blood spills
- Safety
- Dementia
- Risks for burns
- Fire safety
- Falling
- Choking

Segment 3 Body Mechanics

- Body mechanics
- Positioning the client
- Moving the client up in bed using the lift sheet
- Turning the client toward you
- Log rolling the client
- Dangling a client
- Transfer belt
- Postural supports
- Transferring from/to wheelchair, bed, and toilet
- Transferring the client using a mechanical lift

Segment 4 Rehabilitation Skills

- Exercising clients
- Active range-of-motion exercises with isometric movements
- Passive range-of-motion exercises
- Exercising guidelines
- Walking with crutches, walkers, or a cane
- Joint conditions
- Bone fractures
- Cold applications

- Dressing/undressing the client
- Adaptive devices

Segment 5 Personal Hygiene and Grooming

- Skin
- Pressure sores
- Back rubs
- Changing bed linens
- Applying ointments
- Changing dressings
- Oral care

Segment 6 Personal Care

- Bed bath
- Tub bath or shower
- Shampooing hair in bed
- Bag bath
- Nail care
- Warm foot soak
- Shaving a male client

Segment 7 Nutrition and Fluid Balance

- Nutrition
- The digestive system
- Digestive problems/diseases
- Planning meals
- Tips for preparing meals
- Feeding the client
- Fluid balance
- Measuring/recording fluid intake/output
- Alternative nutrition delivery

Segment 8 Elimination

- The urinary system
- Urinary conditions
- Collecting a clean-catch urine sample
- Giving and emptying a bedpan
- Giving and emptying a urinal
- Assisting the client in using a commode

- Caring for a urinary catheter
- Applying a condom catheter
- Connecting a urinary leg bag
- Emptying a urinary drainage bag
- Retraining the bladder
- Regulating the bowels
- Applying adult briefs
- Bowel movements
- Giving a commercial enema
- Inserting a rectal suppository
- Collecting a stool specimen
- Colostomies

Segment 9 Vital Signs, Pain, and Medication

- Vital signs
- Temperature
- Pulse
- Respiration
- Blood pressure
- Measuring weight and height
- Stages of consciousness
- Pain
- Assisting the client with self-administered medication

Segment 10 Special Treatments and Caring for the Dying

- Collecting a sputum specimen
- Cough and deep-breathing exercises
- Oxygen therapy
- Caring for a hearing aid
- Seizures
- Finger-stick blood testing
- Applying elastic stockings
- Assisting with breast-feeding
- Bottle-feeding an infant
- Burping an infant
- Bathing an infant
- Death and dying

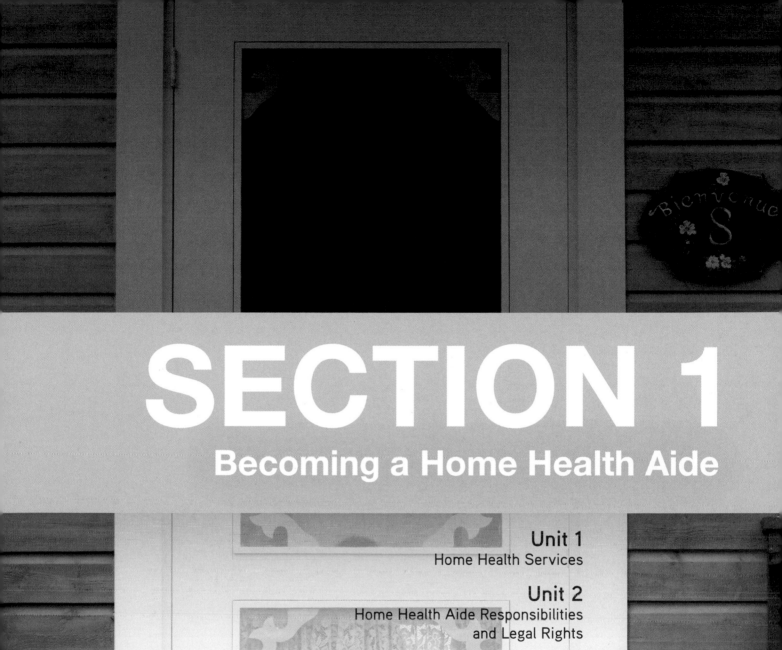

SECTION 1
Becoming a Home Health Aide

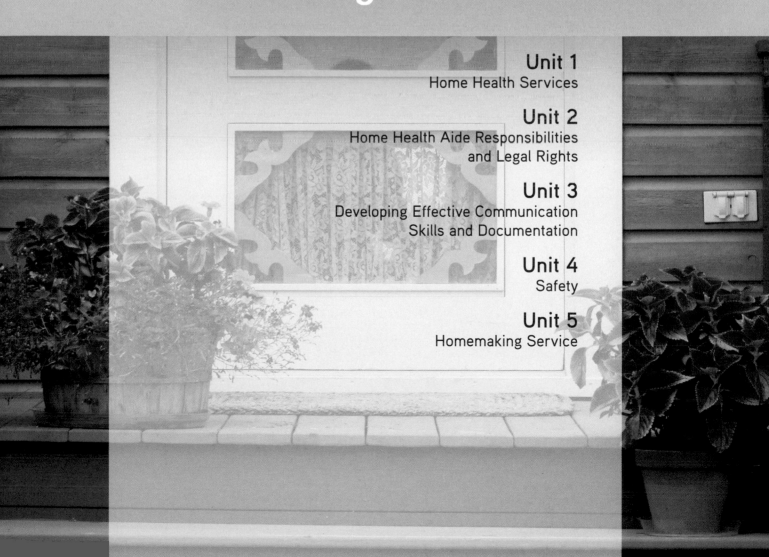

UNIT 1
Home Health Services

KEY TERMS

activities of daily living (ADL)

acute illness

adult day-care center

Affordable Care Act

assisted-living center

Background Information Disclosure Form

case manager (CM)

certified home health aide

certified nursing assistant (CNA)

chaplain

chronic illness

companion

culture

developmentally disabled

diversity

enterostomal therapist (RN, ET) or Wound, Ostomy, Continent Nurse (WOCN)

health care provider

home care aide

home health aide

home health care agencies

homemaker

homemaker/home health aide

hospice

licensed practical nurse (LPN) or licensed vocational nurse (LVN)

long-term care insurance

managed care

Medicaid

Medicare

Nurse Aide Registry

nurse practitioner (RN, NP)

occupational therapist (OT)

Omnibus Budget Reconciliation Act (OBRA)

Outcome and Assessment Information Set (OASIS)

personal care worker

physical therapist (PT)

physician assistant (PA)

Prospective Payment System (PPS)

registered dietitian (RD)

registered nurse (RN)

respiratory therapist (RRT)

respite care

skilled long-term care facility

social worker (BSW, MSW)

speech therapist (ST)

terminal illness

LEARNING OBJECTIVES

After studying this unit, you should be able to:

- Name six reasons why the need for home care is increasing

- Discuss the role of a home health aide

- List five nursing procedures provided by the home health aide

- Name members and functions of various members of the home care team

- Name four health care workplaces outside of the hospital setting

- Give an example of a managed care organization

- Explain the Affordable Care Act

- List four different types of illnesses or disabilities a client might have

- List three programs that assist in paying for health care costs

- List two requirements of the Omnibus Budget Reconciliation Act (OBRA) that affect you as a home health aide

The Development of Home Health Services

In the early years of our society, a majority of the population lived on farms in rural areas. The family unit was often an extended family, with different generations living together and sharing responsibilities. Family members cared for each other. Women were typically not employed outside of the home. It was their responsibility to care for the children and for family members with disabilities. If the mother could not care for the child, the grandmother or aunt did the caregiving. A member of the community who was trained in medicine or health care may have come to the home for emergencies or, in the case of midwives, for labor and delivery. But, there were few, if any, hospitals and nursing homes. Home care agencies did not exist.

The Industrial Revolution of the 20th and 21st centuries created sweeping economic and social changes in our society. It created jobs in the city and automobiles to get there. Children began to move away from their parents' homes, finding employment in a variety of places throughout the world. Currently, there has been an increase in single parents attempting to raise their children on their own.

The first homemaker service was established by a social service agency in the United States in 1903. Its main purpose was to provide child care. In the early 1920s employment agencies advertised for mature, practical women experienced in child care and household management. During the Depression of the 1930s the Work Projects Administration funded a program to train the unemployed as "housekeeping aides." They received formal training and some on-the-job training as well. In 1959, the National Conference on Homemaker Service met in Chicago. It was decided that homemaker service should be given to families with children, chronically ill persons, or senior adults. It was advised that these individuals should receive care in the home whenever possible, without regard to family income. In 1960, at another conference, personal care and health care were seen as added duties of a homemaker's job; the term **home health aide** came into use. Home health aides were expected to work only under direct nursing supervision.

Today, all states have guidelines and laws setting minimum standards for certified nursing assistants and certified home health aides training programs and testing. State guidelines and standards vary from state to state. In Maine the nursing assistant programs are a minimum of 180 hours, in California 160 hours, in Alaska 140 hours, and in Wisconsin 120 hours. In California, the home health aide must be a **certified nursing assistant (CNA)** before coming into a home health aide program, and given a state certification upon completion of the program. In Wisconsin, a home health aide does not need to be certified or have extra training unless he or she works for a Medicare-approved home care agency. The majority of home care agencies—private and public—require a minimum of a basic nursing assistant certification for employment. Additional training in home care is either obtained through the home health care agency itself or through a state-approved agency.

The **Omnibus Budget Reconciliation Act**, known as **OBRA** and passed in 1987, mandates national standards for federally funded nursing homes and home health agencies. This act was created as a result of the outcry from people disgusted with the poor care being given in long-term care facilities and in the client's own home. Included in this act is the requirement of a minimum of 75 hours of training for nursing assistants. The training program and instructors must meet the specific guidelines defined under this act. After an individual completes this program, she or he is eligible to take a competency test based on OBRA requirements. This test consists of both a written test and demonstration of minimum competency in performing required procedures. If the individual does not pass the competency test the first time, he or she is given two more opportunities to retake the test. Once an individual completes both the training program and competency test, she or he is placed on the state **Nurse Aide Registry** for the state in which the individual resides. The state in which the test was administered will issue this individual a card stating that he or she is listed on that state's registry.

The home health aide programs will require basic nursing assistant education and additional education in home health care. Samples of additional topics covered in the program include an introduction to home care, tasks in the home, medical/social needs, personal care, and nutrition. Each state is somewhat different in its work and education requirements (cnatips.com/registry/nurse-aide-tx.php). If you have any questions on your state's requirements, you need to talk with someone from your state nursing assistant/home health registry office. Another excellent resource is your instructor for the home health aide training program. The home health worker must also complete a Background Information Disclosure Form and show no evidence of caregiver abuse after the age of 18, if she or he decides to be employed in an agency that receives federal or state funding. The primary goal of OBRA regulations is to improve care both for individuals in long-term care facilities and for those in their own homes.

Increase in Need for Home Care Services

Home care is now one of the fastest growing businesses in this country. There are a number of reasons for the increase in the need for home care. One of the main reasons is that older adults, the main recipients of home care, are the fastest growing population in the country. The nation's over-65 population is projected to grow from 40 million to 72 million by 2030; 27 million will need home care by 2050, the government estimates.

People are living longer due to advances in health care and modern technology. Approximately 23% of older adults need assistance with personal care activities and 27% have difficulty in home management activities.

A second reason for the increased need for home care services is the high cost of hospital care and the trend on the part of providers and payers to keep costs down. As a result of this trend, clients are often sent home from the hospital as soon as medically possible. Many of these clients still need follow-up care, which can be provided by a home health agency. This trend has led to the tremendous growth in the field of home health care.

A third reason for the increase in home care is that most individuals prefer to remain in their own homes when they become ill or frail, rather than moving to an unfamiliar setting, such as a nursing home. They wish to sleep in their own beds, eat at their own kitchen tables, and talk on their own phones. They want to have control over their own lifestyles—when they get up in the morning and go to bed at night, what they have for dinner, and who they let into their homes. They want to be near their loved ones, friends, and neighbors.

As a result, there has been a move away from long-term care placement, now that home care services are more readily available. It is sometime necessary, however, to make that move to a skilled long-term care facility (residential home for individuals who need 24-hour skilled care). In many areas of the country, there is a shortage of nursing home beds due to a lack of government funding.

The fourth reason for the increase in home health services is the dramatic growth in assistive living facilities throughout the states. Most of the individuals who live in these type of facilities need minor assistance in their activities of daily living (ADLs) plus meals, laundry service, and cleaning services. These complexes offer great employment opportunities for the home health aide.

A fifth reason for the steady increase in home care services is the growing acceptance of the home as a place to die. Hospice services make this possible by offering services to the terminally ill in their homes. Medicare and many other insurance providers pay for hospice care, in which health care providers work as a team to allow clients to die with dignity in their own homes.

A sixth reason for the steady increase in demand is that more insurance providers and agencies are covering the cost of home care. The Veteran Administration, for example, is now paying for equipment and care given by the veteran's spouse.

Types of Home Care Workers

Home care workers play key roles in their clients' lives. They perform many of the duties that are necessary for their clients to remain at home. Their duties may fall into two main categories: care of the person and care of the home. Care of the person includes assistance with ADLs, such as bathing, dressing, and toileting, and simple nursing tasks, such as taking blood pressure or assisting with exercises (Figure 1-1). Care of the home includes light housekeeping, cooking, shopping, and other homemaking duties (Figure 1-2).

Care of the person requires more training than care of the home. Some workers do all of the tasks just mentioned; others may have more limited roles. The role depends on the amount of training that the worker has had and how the person is classified on the state registry (Figure 1-3). The case manager designs a separate care plan to be followed for each client. The care plan specifically outlines the home care worker's responsibilities.

The following are some of the more commonly used titles for home care workers:

Companion—Keeps the client company or maintains safety; usually does not provide personal or home-making services.

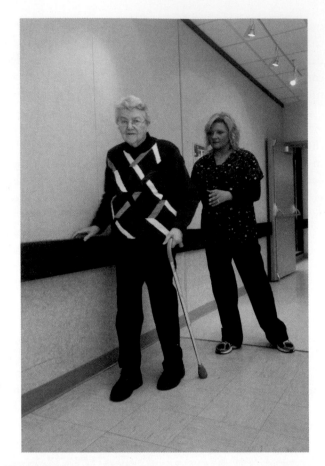

FIGURE 1-1 A home health aide assisting a client with ambulating.

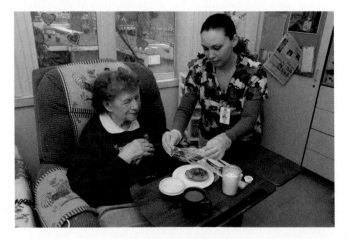

FIGURE 1-2 A home health aide prepares a client for a meal.

Homemaker—Performs household duties, such as laundry and cooking, as well as light housecleaning.

Personal care worker—Assists with a minimal level of daily living activities, such as meal preparation and companionship, as well as minimal assistance with personal care.

Certified home health aide—Provides substantial assistance with personal care, such as bathing and dressing, care of client's immediate environmental surroundings, and assistance with rehabilitation activities and self-administered medication.

Homemaker/home health aide—Assists in general household tasks, as well as those listed for the home health aide.

Home care aide—Works with the client with the goal of assisting the client with independent living under professional supervision.

The Health Care Team

Home health care can be defined as all those services that promote, maintain, and/or restore physical, social, or emotional health to clients in the home setting. The home health aide is one member of the health care team who sees the client more frequently than other members of the team. Many agencies have team conferences where all members of the health care team meet to discuss the client and identify any problems or needs. The home health aide provides critical information to the team regarding the client. Teamwork, observation skills, and communication are essential. The entire health care team relies on the home health aide to provide vital observations, documentation, and communication. Other health care personnel who are part of the health care team include the following:

Case manager (CM)—Assesses the overall needs of the client and decides what services should be provided; usually performed by a nurse or social worker; may supervise the home care worker. (Many home care agencies combine the role of the case manager and the registered nurse.)

Chaplain—Provides help with the spiritual needs of the client.

Health care provider—A general term for an agency, institution, or member of the health care team who provides medical care for the consumer.

Enterostomal therapist (RN, ET) or **Wound, Ostomy, Continent Nurse (WOCN)**—A specialist who works with clients who have ostomies or clients who require special skin or wound care.

Licensed practical nurse (LPN) or licensed vocational nurse (LVN)—Provides direct care to the client, such as treatments and medication; may supervise home care workers.

A. Routine homemaker functions or tasks include the following:

1. Washing dishes
2. Doing light housekeeping, i.e., dusting, scrubbing floors, vacuuming rooms that the client uses
3. Maintaining needed supplies
4. Preparing and serving meals
5. Doing laundry
6. Shopping for client if no other arrangements can be made
7. Accompanying client to medical clinic or other activity

B. Routine home health aide functions done for the client:

1. Under the supervision of a registered nurse or case manager, arranging the schedule so that the client follows the care plan, such as increased physical activity or other activity of daily living
2. Recording care and observations on client's record
3. Measuring vital signs and weight
4. Assisting with toileting needs
5. Assisting with oral care
6. Assisting with dressing and undressing
7. Assisting with eating
8. Assisting with transfer of client from bed to chair and vice versa
9. Assisting with repositioning a client
10. Reminding clients to take medications on schedule
11. Reinforcing or changing unsterile simple dressings
12. Caring for ostomy bags or urinary drainage bags
13. Measuring and recording intake and output
14. Assisting with grooming—including shampooing, shaving, and nail care
15. Making and changing bed linens
16. Assisting client with walking and other prescribed exercises
17. Assisting with applications of prosthetic devices, i.e., hearing aids and braces
18. Assisting with rehabilitation measures
19. Assisting with skin care
20. Applying elastic support hose
21. Notifying case manager of any notable change in the client's condition

FIGURE 1-3   Home health functions approved by most states.

Nurse practitioner (RN, NP)—Specializes in additional training in physical examination and assessment, and works under a health care provider's supervision. The nurse practitioner may work with children, infants, clients who are pregnant, older adults, and clients with cancer.

Occupational therapist (OT)—Evaluates the client's ability to perform skills necessary for independent daily living, such as bathing, dressing, and cooking; works with the client to improve abilities; and develops a plan of care. The family and home health aide assist in the plan of care.

Physical therapist (PT)—Evaluates the home environment in preparation of the client's return, assists with safety adaptations, and instructs the client on an appropriate exercise program and usage of special equipment.

Physician assistant (PA)—A health care professional licensed to practice medicine with physician supervision. PAs conduct physical exams and diagnose and treat illnesses.

Registered dietitian (RD)—Provides information regarding the prescribed dietary needs of the client. Assists in meal planning adjustment according to the medical condition of the client.

Registered nurse (RN)—Initiates the plan of care ordered by the health care provider; performs assessment, planning, and interventions for the necessary home care skills and teaching; and evaluates the effectiveness of the plan. Acts as the case manager for the client.

Respiratory therapist (RRT)—Assists the client with any breathing problems. Works with the client with breathing equipment and checks the equipment to see if it is functioning properly.

Social worker (BSW, MSW)—Provides information about community services, financial resources, long-term planning, and respite care. Helps the client and family with psychosocial (emotional, social, and financial) problems.

Speech therapist (ST)—Assesses the client's ability to communicate—hear, speak, understand, and write; works with the client to improve abilities. Also assesses swallowing difficulties and works with the client to improve swallowing functions.

Registered nurses monitor the client on a continuous basis. Nursing visits are planned according to the level of care and education needed for the client and family members. Emergency support nursing care is available 24 hours a day, 7 days a week through a certified home health care agency. The frequency of social worker visits ranges from once a week to once a month. The social worker role is to assist the client and the family with their financial, legal, and funeral needs. The social worker uses skill as a clinician for problem solving and crisis intervention. A vital part of a home health aide's responsibility is to be an active participant of the health care team. The case manager assesses the client and develops a plan of care, which the home health aide follows. All members of the health care team rely on the home health aide for keeping them informed on day-to-day changes occurring with the client (Figure 1-4).

Health Care Workplaces Outside the Hospital or Long-Term Care Facility

Home care agencies differ in many ways: types of service provided, fees for services, policies and procedures, and administrative structures. They can be large or small; non-profit or for-profit; Medicare certified or non-Medicare certified; and private, religiously affiliated, or publicly operated.

Adult Day-Care Centers

Adult day-care centers provide care for adults who need minimal care or supervision during the day. The health care worker in this setting will assist the client in eating, bathing, and recreational activities. The client might come every day or only once a week to the center. These centers are great for a spouse who is a primary caregiver and needs a break for a day from the stress of constant caregiving. These types of centers often are equipped with specialized bathing equipment to bathe a client, if the client's primary caregiver is unable to do this task or the client's home does not have the proper equipment to do it.

Assisted-Living Facility

Assisted-living centers vary from a two-bedroom condominium with kitchen to a private room with a shared dining room and central dayroom (Figure 1-5). Individuals can elect to have all meals prepared or eat one meal a day in the central dining area. Generally, these facilities offer a supervised medication program, cleaning and laundry services, and minor assistance in ADLs. The client pays according to the services requested.

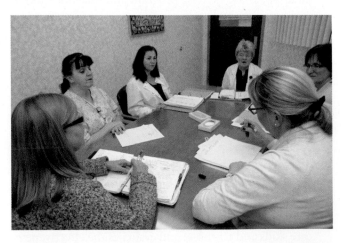

FIGURE 1-4 Health care professionals working as a team in deciding the best care plan for the client.

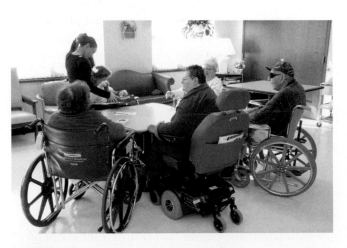

FIGURE 1-5 An assisted-living complex.

Homemaker/Home Care Agencies

These agencies provide a variety of nonmedical home support services. They provide companions, homemakers, and personal care workers for the client. These workers are employed to help the client with cleaning, cooking, minimal personal care, shopping, and companionship.

Home Health Care Agencies

Home health care agencies, some of which are affiliated with hospitals, focus on the medical or nursing aspect of care. Their professionally trained personnel (e.g., registered nurses, speech therapist, physical therapist, etc.) can perform dressing changes, monitor vital signs, and complete other tasks ordered by the health care provider. The majority of them offer services provided by the certified home health aide. Their services may be paid for by the client, private insurance, Medicaid, or Medicare.

Self-Employment

Self-employed workers have the benefit of working independently, but face some challenges as well. They must find their own clients. If their clients are temporarily hospitalized or placed in a long-term care facility, they are out of work. Unless these workers obtain a private professional liability insurance policy at their own expense, they will not be financially protected from claims and lawsuits if their clients are injured while under their care. Additionally, they will be responsible for filing federal and state estimated income tax returns as well as their year-end returns. They will be responsible for the payment of 100% of their Social Security taxes unless advance arrangements are made with their clients to pay the employer's portion of the tax.

Reimbursement Issues Influencing Health Care

Reimbursement from insurance and Medicare has gone through different models in the last few years. In 2000, the **Prospective Payment System (PPS)** was implemented in home care, and it has great influence on how home health agencies are paid. This system is based on the **Outcome and Assessment Information Set (OASIS)**. The objective of this tool is to standardize assessment data collection throughout the country, with the aim of improving the quality of home health care. Today, a registered nurse performs an assessment of the client and then completes the OASIS form and enters data into the computer for transmission to each state. In 2000, these assessments became the basis of payment and are required in order to bill for services. The information on the admission/OASIS form will determine how much the insurance company or Medicare will pay for care of the client within a 60-day period. *In order for an agency to receive adequate reimbursement for care of its clients, it is crucial that the home health aide report and document any change in the condition of each individual client.*

Affordable Care Act

The **Affordable Care Act** puts consumers in charge of their health care. Under this law, a new "Patient's Bill of Rights" gives the American people stability as well as flexibility in making choices concerning their health. This law requires that nearly everyone have health insurance by January 1, 2014. See http://HHS.gov/Health Care for more information.

Medicare

Currently, all individuals in the United States who have paid into Social Security are entitled to apply for **Medicare** insurance once they are disabled or when they turn 65. Medicare Part A (Hospital Insurance) covers inpatient care in hospitals and skilled nursing facilities. It covers hospice care and some home health care. There is no charge for Part A. Medical Insurance (Part B) helps cover health care provider services and outpatient hospital care (e.g., diagnostic tests, durable medical equipment, and diabetic supplies). In 2014, if you enrolled in Part B when you were first eligible, the premium for Part B was $104 per month. Medicare Part C offer health plan options run by Medicare-approved private insurance companies. Medicare Part D covers the cost of prescription drugs. Medicare also covers individuals with end-stage renal disease requiring dialysis or a kidney transplant. Medicare insurance pays for part of the cost of health care, but certainly not all. The new "Medicare & You" (see MyMedicare .gov) helps a person to narrow down the supplemental Medicare health plans available and provides important information about special programs that might help pay for health care costs that Medicare does not pay for.

Hospice Medicare Benefits (HMB) are available for clients who have Medicare Part A and have been certified by a physician as having a terminal illness and a life expectancy of 6 months or less. Medicare will pay hospice for home health aide services, supplies, equipment, and medications, as well as medical, spiritual, and social services.

To qualify for Medicare reimbursement for home health services, an individual must:

- Be under the care of a doctor who certifies the need for care
- Have a skilled need requiring intermittent, skilled nursing care or therapy.
- Be receiving services from a Medicare-certified home health agency as provided by a registered nurse

Medicaid

Medicaid is a federally and state-funded program that pays for health care services for persons whose income is below a certain amount. The coverage provided to recipients and the minimum income level that makes one eligible varies from state to state. Some states also have programs that allow them to provide services to seniors living in the community whose income is above the Medicaid level. These seniors usually pay according to their income. A person can qualify for both Medicare and Medicaid or other community support programs. Medicare and Medicaid offerings vary from state to state, as no two states offer the same coverage.

Whenever government funding is involved, the federal or state government can regulate the health care industry and demand that certain standards be maintained with regard to health care facilities, health care workers, and educational requirements. The home health aide must be aware of these standards.

Long-Term Care Insurance

Long-term care insurance provides help in paying for long-term care. This type of insurance covers some of the costs for home health care, respite care, adult day-care services, assisted-living facilities, and long-term care facilities. In order to qualify, a client must be unable to perform some ADLs (bathing, eating, toileting, walking, or dressing, for example). The coverage will vary according to the policy. The premium cost increases with increasing age. This type of insurance could keep one's estate from being financially exhausted.

Managed Care

Health maintenance organizations (HMOs) are examples of **managed care**. This is a method of health care delivery that attempts to cut costs through providing gatekeepers to control access to and use of health care providers, hospitals, nursing facilities, and other forms of care. The goal of this gatekeeper, whether it be a nurse case manager or a health care provider, is to provide the best quality care for the lowest cost. Home care, for example, may be a less costly and more appealing alternative in certain situations. Managed care companies usually offer their patients fewer choices of hospitals, nursing homes, and health care providers. The out-of-pocket cost to the patient, however, is usually lower than with traditional insurance.

The Client

Home care clients are of all ages, from birth to more than 100 years old. They are typically affected by one or more illnesses or disabilities. An **acute illness** is one that arises quickly, requires immediate care, and can be expected to go away, such as a cold, flu, or appendicitis. A **chronic illness** is a long-standing health problem, such as Alzheimer's disease, Parkinson's disease, or arthritis. Many individuals over the age of 70 are affected by one or more of these chronic illnesses. **Developmentally disabled** means the person has a severe chronic emotional or physical disability that occurs before the age of 22, such as cerebral palsy or Down syndrome. A **terminal illness** is one that is expected to result in death within a limited time period.

Home care clients are truly diverse. **Diversity** is the differences, such as race, religion, and culture, that you will see in your clients. They represent different cultures and ethnic groups—Hispanics, Asians, Eastern Europeans, and so forth. They are different races, including African Americans, Caucasians, and Native Americans. They practice different religions such, as Protestantism, Catholicism, Judaism, Islam, or Buddhism.

The ethnic makeup of our senior population is rapidly changing. The U.S. Census Bureau expects there will be a large increase in seniors in the Asian and Hispanic populations as compared to the African American and Caucasian populations.

Home health workers cannot expect to know everything about every different culture, race, or religion. It is important, however, to realize that there are differences, to be accepting of them, and to be willing to learn about them. Home health aides may learn, for example, that Native American medicine and religion cannot be separated and that these clients will turn to traditional healing practices from time to time. A home health aide may observe the strength of family ties in the Hispanic and Asian cultures or learn about the dietary practices of the Orthodox Jewish faith. In addition, the home health aide may be called to do **respite care** work for the family of a child with developmental disabilities, an adult with disabilities, or a terminally ill person. This means taking care of the client when the main caregiver needs a break to go shopping, visit with friends, or even rest a bit.

Religious practices, traditions, types of food, and the manner in which food is prepared are very often determined by the culture and religion of the individual (Figure 1-6). The home health aide must (1) accept the practices of others, (2) be sensitive to the client's needs, and (3) follow the instructions given by the case manager in meeting the needs of the client, regardless of religion, color, or belief. An aide must not judge clients, but must allow them the freedom to follow their own practices and beliefs while providing safe and proper care. It is important that these practices be communicated to the health care team.

In each unit of this text, you will find new words to master and new techniques to learn. As your knowledge grows, so does your confidence as an individual. In becoming a home health aide, you can be proud of your newly acquired skills. Satisfaction comes from being able to use your new knowledge and skills in caring for clients who need your care.

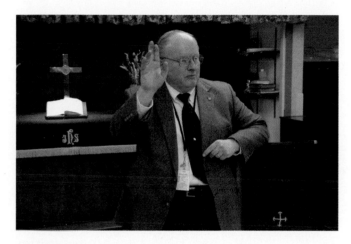

FIGURE 1-6   Religious practices can vary.

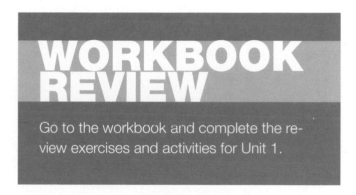

WORKBOOK REVIEW

Go to the workbook and complete the review exercises and activities for Unit 1.

REVIEW

1. List four reasons for the increasing trend toward home care.

   _____

   _____

   _____

   _____

2. List two main services provided by the home health aide.

   _____

   _____

3. Name two differences between Medicare and Medicaid.

   _____

   _____

4. A(n) ___ helps clients to improve their abilities to perform the skills necessary for independent daily living, such as bathing, dressing, and cooking.
   a. physical therapist
   b. speech therapist
   c. health care provider
   d. occupational therapist

5. A ___ agency focuses on the medical aspects of home care, many of which are reimbursed by Medicare.
   a. homemaker/home care agency
   b. home health care agency
   c. skilled nursing facility
   d. hospital

6. Which of the following is one example of a managed care organization?
   a. Nursing home
   b. HMO (health maintenance organization)
   c. Department store
   d. School

7. Payment for home health aide services is collected by the agency that assumes responsibility for your client. These payments may come from
   a. Medicare.
   b. Medicaid.
   c. the client.
   d. any of the above.

8. Home health aide care involves which of the following?
   a. Client care and housekeeping activities
   b. Supervising the client's care
   c. Laundry and wallpapering
   d. Client care and giving injections

9. A hospice cares for clients who
   a. are chronically ill.
   b. are acutely ill.
   c. are terminally ill.
   d. have a developmental disability.

10. A home health aide needs to be aware of the client's
    a. cultural differences.
    b. physical needs.
    c. family situation.
    d. all of the above.

11. Your mother, who is 80 years old, has cancer and needs home care. Her only income is from Social Security, which is $800 a month. She has no other income or assets. What is the name of the federal and state program that will help pay for her care at home? _____

12. Name the act, passed in 1987, that mandates training guidelines for home health aides. _____
    _____

13. A(n) _____ is a health care specialist who works with a client to improve the client's ability to hear and speak.

14. T   F   Adrian Z has just been placed on kidney dialysis and is waiting for a kidney transplant. The home health aide drives him to the local hospital for kidney dialysis three times a week. He is 68 years of age and is on Medicare Part A and Part B. Medicare will assist in paying for the cost of his kidney dialysis.

15. T   F   An example of an acute illness is Alzheimer's disease.

16. T   F   An important duty of a home health aide is to report and document changes in client behavior.

UNIT 2

Home Health Aide Responsibilities and Legal Rights

KEY TERMS

abandonment
abuse
aiding and abetting
assault
battery
career
confidentiality
corporal punishment
defamation
ethical standards

ethics
evaluation
false imprisonment
flexible
Health Insurance
    Portability and
    Accountability Act
    (HIPAA)
hygiene
interaction

interpersonal
    relationships
invasion of privacy
legal standards
liability
libel
malpractice
neglect
negligence
ombudsman

personal health
    information (PHI)
procedure
punctuality
reliability
slander
theory

LEARNING OBJECTIVES

After studying this unit, you should be able to:

- List three important qualities of the home health aide

- Give five examples of actions to avoid that can lead to liability

- Give examples of good personal hygiene

- Define ethics, and identify two examples of ethical practice

- Define the following legal terms—aiding and abetting, defamation, assault, battery, and malpractice

- Describe eight "rights of clients"

- Describe eight "rights of home health aides"

- Explain the purpose of the Health Insurance Portability and Accountability Act

- Define client abuse

- List four types of client abuse and give an example of each

- Discuss what to do if you suspect client abuse

Skills and Qualities of the Home Health Aide

A **career** is an occupation or profession for which one has been specially educated. Teacher, lawyer, electrician, and home health aide are examples of careers. In addition to the training and education that are required for each career, certain personal qualities or characteristics make people good at what they do. It is important for a teacher to like children, for a lawyer to be a good communicator, and for an electrician to be cautious and not take risks. Likewise, a number of special qualities make for a good home health aide.

An ad in the newspaper for a home health aide may read something like what is shown in Figure 2-1.

Responsibilities of the Home Health Aide

Punctuality and **reliability** are very important characteristics for the home health aide. Your client depends on you. If you will be riding the bus, for example, it would be wise to study the bus schedule ahead of time to ensure proper location of the closest bus stop, and to allow adequate time to arrive at the client's home. If you use your own car, as the majority of home health aides do, be sure to check the location of your client's home and the route to take ahead of time. Due to the irregularity of assignments, a home health aide must be **flexible** and have access to reliable transportation. A global positioning system (GPS) is great to use to plan your route. Check with your agency for its reimbursement policy for mileage to your client's home. The majority of agencies will pay mileage plus salary for travel between clients' homes.

WANTED:

Home health aides to care for persons in their own homes. Applicants must have the following qualities:

- Flexible
- Willing and able to follow instructions
- Well-organized
- Dependable
- Good interpersonal skills
- Observant
- Ethical
- Good personal hygiene
- Punctual

FIGURE 2-1   Sample ad in newspaper.

This is a good question to ask, once you become employed with an agency, as driving from one home to another can become quite costly and also time consuming.

It is your responsibility to inform the agency and the client if you cannot report to work as scheduled. Remember that your client is dependent on you, and the agency depends on you to show up for work as scheduled. Check with your agency regarding its policy for being absent or taking time off and whom to contact if you need to miss work.

Working Hours. Working hours may be irregular. Primarily the working hours are during the day, but occasionally a home health aide may be required to work during the evening and night shifts or on weekends. It is the home health aide's responsibility to notify the client of his or her approximate arrival time. One or more clients might be visited in one day or on different days during the week. This means the home health aide must be able to quickly adjust from one type of situation to another and be able to feel comfortable meeting new people. A time sheet needs to be completed every day and returned to your agency either every week or every month depending on the agency's policy (Figure 2-2).

Variety of Assignments. The aide must adjust to the different family situations and varied health care needs of the clients. In one home, the aide might be expected to care for infants, preschool children, and teenagers. In another home, there may be only people with disabilities or elderly people. No two home situations are the same. Thus, the aide will have to establish new interpersonal relationships in each case. Some clients are angry, abusive, depressed, or otherwise difficult; others are pleasant and cooperative.

Variety of Settings and Equipment. The aide must adapt to homes that are not as well equipped as others. Surroundings differ from case to case. Some homes are neat and pleasant, whereas others are untidy and depressing. Some homes have modern equipment and beautiful furnishings. Other homes offer the bare necessities of life. Some homes have great and new equipment to work with and others do not. The home health aide will be expected to treat all clients with dignity regardless of their financial position. Each human being is entitled to respectful and dignified care.

If you arrive at the client's home to find the door locked and no one seems to be home, you should call your case manager or inform the agency of the situation.

	Time Start	Time Finish	*Travel Time	Total Hours	Client Miles	Employee Miles
Date						
SUN						
MON						
TUE						
WED						
THU						
FRI						
SAT						

```
┌─────────────┐
│             │  Home Health
└─────────────┘
- - - - - - - - - - - - - - - - - - - - - -
     Timeslips due in the office by Monday 9:00 a.m.

Client _____

Address _____

Employee Signature x _____

Office _____ Saturday's Date _____
```

Please specify AM or PM on times.   Total   Total

*Extend TT into far right Total Hours Column   Misc. Expense

Client Signature x _____

For Office Use Only:

BILLED HHA PCW HCA RN LPN SUP MMV
(HOUR/VSIT)

PAID   HHA PCW HCA RN LPN SUP MMV
(HOUR/VSIT)

Fee Source: MA INS MC PP COUNTY _____

CHC

White-Payroll   Yellow-Billing   Pink-Client   Gold-Employee

FIGURE 2-2   Sample of a time sheet that a home health aide needs to complete.

They will give you directions for additional action. It may be that the client needed to be hospitalized or has gone away with his or her family and the agency forgot to notify you.

Ability to Follow Instructions

Home health aides generally work on their own, with periodic visits by their case managers. They receive detailed instructions explaining when to visit clients and what services to perform, which is usually on the written care plan. At first glance, the role of the home health aide may appear to be simple. It is made up of everyday tasks: keeping a house in order, preparing and cleaning up after meals, and providing personal care of the client. Home health aides may feel that they know how to take care of a house and have been doing housekeeping tasks since early childhood. Their clients, however, may differ in how they want their homes cleaned. Clients have the right to have their homes cleaned in the method they desire. In addition, the aide may benefit by learning new ways to do certain jobs. Once a new method is learned, the aide can compare it with the old way and perhaps discover a more efficient technique.

By learning to focus on the components of a task, the aide will find that understanding comes more easily. Components are the separate parts that make up a whole. Learning how to do something, when to do it, and what should be done first will add up to a more complete understanding.

There are many ways to do some tasks, for example, preparing a meal. Certain essential components of the task if not completed correctly and in the right order will mean the task has been done wrong. You need to follow the client's dietary requirements and prepare food accordingly, for example. You can toast the bread before or after you slice a tomato, but you must put ingredients away and clean up after preparing food. Other tasks, however, have rigid procedures and only one way to proceed, such as washing hands before taking a temperature. A **procedure** is a list of steps used to complete a task.

There are usually two parts to the instructions given to the home health aide. The first is called theory. **Theory** is the information that forms a basis for action. In classroom lectures and in the assigned readings, the student learns theory. The second component is devoted to practice. Practice is the actual performance of the procedures. Practice is combined with the theory to enable the student to build skills in both areas at the same time.

The student will need to demonstrate a designated list of procedures satisfactorily in front of an instructor. Each procedure will be demonstrated by the instructor before the student performs the procedure. The instructor will give the student a copy of the procedure with all the required steps listed. Use these procedural guidelines in practicing each procedure in the laboratory. Your instructor will determine if you have learned the procedure correctly by giving you an evaluation. An **evaluation** may consist of written tests or demonstrations where you actually perform the procedure. Evaluation helps the student know which areas require extra study or practice.

Willingness to Follow Instructions

As important as being able to understand the instructions of your case manager is being willing to follow them. Before caring for a client, the home health aide should be sure to ask for all essential information. The case manager will provide a home care plan for the client, outlining the specific care to be provided and the aide's responsibilities. This includes household duties, client needs, and the name and telephone number of the case manager. If the home health aide has any questions or concerns about the client's care plan, be sure to ask for clarification.

Both ability and willingness to follow instructions affect the home health aide's liability when things go wrong.

Constructive Criticism

The home health aide should develop a nondefensive attitude toward criticism by the professional staff at the agency where he or she is employed. Constructive criticism is a way of achieving additional skills or upgrading present techniques. The aide must be open to new suggestions. Recognizing one's ability to adapt to new ideas presented by more experienced staff members will result in the improvement of your own professional skills. Look kindly on and accept the guidance of your case manager, as this will only benefit your clients as well as yourself. Your goal must be to move in a positive direction toward optimum client care.

Legal Terms

The home health aide should be familiar with the following legal terms:

Abandonment is being left without care or support by family or agency.

Aiding and abetting is not reporting dishonest acts that one observed.

Assault is an intentional attempt or threat to touch a person without the person's consent.

Battery is the actual touching of a person's body without the person's consent.

Corporal punishment is use of painful treatment to change or correct behavior.

Defamation is stating untrue statements about a person, which would injure this person's name and reputation.

False imprisonment is the unlawful restriction of a person's freedom of movement.

Invasion of privacy is exposing or making public a person's name, photograph, or private information without the consent of the person.

Liability refers to the degree to which you will be held financially responsible for the damages resulting from your negligence.

Libel is a false written statement about another person.

Malpractice is the failure to exercise reasonable judgment in the application of professional knowledge.

Negligence is an action on your part or your failure to act that either causes or contributes to the cause of a personal injury or property damage to others.

Slander is making a false oral statement about another person.

Health Insurance Portability and Accountability Act of 1996

The **Health Insurance Portability and Accountability Act (HIPAA)** was created to develop guidelines for maintaining and transmitting health information that identifies individual clients. HIPAA went into effect in April 2003. This act mandates that your entire client's health information—oral, paper, or electronic—be protected and confidential. This includes any medical information used to make a decision about the client's health care coverage, as well as the client's name, address, and telephone number. HIPAA was developed to allow the flow of health information needed to provide and promote quality health care while assuring proper protection of individual **personal health information (PHI)**. See Figure 2-3 for an example policy covering PHI.

The law describes certain individual rights. Upon written request, an individual may view or make copies of his or her protected health information, which is in a designated record set defined by the plan. Individuals may also make a written request to receive an accounting disclosure of their health information on payment of their care (what charges were for health

---

COMPONENTS OF A POLICY TO PROTECT AND SECURE PHI IN COMPUTERIZED RECORDS

- Computer access is governed by user password that should not be shared with anyone.
- Once the user is logged on to the computer, the computer screen should not be left unattended or accessible for public viewing.
- All unnecessary computer-generated paper must be shredded.
- Users must know how to correct an entry error.
- Users must know how to chart client-sensitive materials such as the results of blood tests.

FIGURE 2-3 Components of a policy to protect and secure PHI in computerized records.

care and what costs were paid for by Medicare or private insurance).

You might ask, how does this act affect a home health aide? As you work as a home health aide, you have an opportunity to read the client's chart, interact with the family members, know if this client's health care is being paid for by Medicaid, and know the health condition of the client. You must keep all of this information confidential. You are allowed to discuss information about your client with other members of the home health care team, and it must be limited to the team members only (Figure 2-4). Do not discuss your client with your friends or family.

The ethical duty of confidentiality requires that information shared during the course of a professional relationship be kept secure and confidential from others. The

home health aide must protect all documentation so that others cannot read it. If aides are caring for multiple clients, they cannot take any of their paper documents into another client's home. They must turn papers face down in the home, so no one can read them. If they are doing their documentation electronically, they must never give their password out to anyone.

A few of your clients might live in a senior high-rise mobile park, and often clients are curious about who else in the complex has a home health aide, or what is wrong with that person. You are not allowed to tell another client who else you are caring for.

The Security Rule of 2005 mandates that a health care agency must have policies and procedures to ensure the privacy and confidentiality of PHI stored in computers.

Situations for Home Health Aides to Avoid

Do only and exactly what your case manager instructs you to do. There are some situations you should recognize and avoid:

1. *Doing more than is assigned.* Practice saying "no" in a tactful way, encouraging the client to contact the case manager if more services are wanted. When you do something that was not assigned, you are assuming responsibility (liability) for these acts, and your agency is no longer responsible.

2. *Doing less than is assigned.* This may put the client in danger and lead to a charge of negligence, which means "an action or lack of action that leads to an accident or injury."

3. *Doing hasty, careless, or poor-quality work.* You have received training in the proper way to carry out your work activities. It is your responsibility to work carefully. Sometimes, even with the greatest amount of care being taken, accidents happen: a valuable vase breaks while you are dusting it or a client falls. If you have been carrying out your assigned duties and exercising a reasonable amount of care, you usually are not held liable for the damage or injury that results; agencies carry liability insurance to cover these types of accidents.

4. *Using your car for work activities.* This applies to transporting a client in your car, even when you

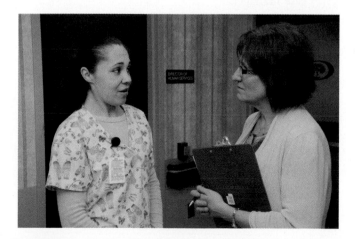

FIGURE 2-4 An aide interacting with a case manager.

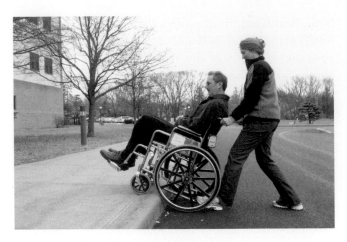

FIGURE 2-5 An aide taking the client to an appointment.

are taking the client to the doctor's office or just out for a ride, without letting your auto insurance agency know (Figure 2-5). If an accident occurs, you might be liable for the resulting damages and you may be required to personally pay for those damages if you do not have proper coverage. Be sure your driver's license is current and in good standing, ensure that your car is in good repair, and have the approval of your agency to take the client in your car. Also, check to make sure you will be paid mileage for use of your car by your agency. Before employing an individual, some agencies will require that the home health aide has a valid driver's license, car, and proper automobile insurance.

5. *Failing to do accurate and daily reporting and documentation.* Always document your care as soon as completed. This will help you remember important details that, if you waited, you might forget. If you are in a hurry and decide not to chart, but plan to do it the next day when you will have more time, the following scenario might occur: The client's daughter comes to visit her mother and sees that nothing is written on the chart that day and immediately assumes that no one was there to care for her mother. The daughter becomes quite upset over this incident, which could have easily been avoided, and calls the home health agency.

6. *Failing to act in an emergency.* You should know what the emergency plan is for each client you care for, and you should be prepared to follow it. In a life-threatening situation, call 911 if available in your area. If 911 service is not available, call for an ambulance before calling your case manager. There are a few exceptions before calling an ambulance in an emergency. In some cases the family wants to

be notified before calling an ambulance; or, some agencies want to be notified first before calling an ambulance. This information should be clearly stated in the client's care plan. Some agencies may require you to be certified in cardiopulmonary resuscitation (CPR) and first aid before you are hired. Do not try to perform first aid or CPR if you have not been trained to do so.

7. *Attempting to do things that are beyond your abilities.* It is okay to say, "I don't know how to do that. Let's see if we can get someone who does." You are not employed as a nurse, a plumber, an electrician, or a counselor—do not try to be one.

8. *Injuring yourself or the client by doing something you are not assigned or adequately trained to do.* If you have been assigned to do something you do not feel comfortable doing, ask for more training. Trying to do something without assignment and adequate training, such as moving a client with a Stand lift, can leave you liable for injury that results.

9. *Failing to report unsafe working conditions that later cause injury to you or another home health aide.* Do not take unnecessary risks. Immediately report your concerns to the agency per protocol.

10. *Doing a client's banking is not a normal duty of a home health aide.* If a client wants you to purchase personal items, be sure you save all receipts and have the approval of your agency to do it.

11. *Performing tasks that you are legally not permitted to perform by state regulations.* "Scope of practice" refers to staying within the boundaries of what you are able to do. If you are not sure, check with your case manager.

Organizational Skills

A successful aide possesses good organizational skills (Figure 2-6). An aide must manage time well to be able to complete all the tasks required in the allotted time. The instructions may include light housekeeping, laundry and ironing, meal preparation, shopping, and personal care of the client. The aide will have to decide the best way to plan each day's activities. This will require flexibility, practical judgment, and time organization. Some pitfalls to avoid are:

- Not replacing or ordering supplies when needed
- Watching television

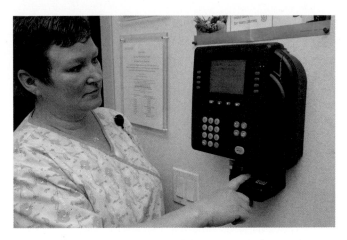

FIGURE 2-6   A home care aide checking in for work at an assistive living facility.

- Not setting priorities and jumping from one task to another
- Putting off unpleasant tasks because they are disagreeable
- Talking to friends on your cell phone or doing personal business
- Stopping frequently for a cup of coffee

Prior to starting your work, it is a good idea to make a list of tasks that need to be done for your client that day. If you are responsible for the client's personal care, that must be your first priority. Next is your homemaking tasks. Check, also, to see if you have all the supplies you need to accomplish all necessary tasks. As you work, you can check off the list as you go; this will lessen your chance of forgetting some tasks. After all of the routine tasks are completed and the client care procedures are done, then you might start the less important tasks. Each plan should be flexible enough to allow for the unexpected.

A home health aide may be scheduled to work with several clients during a week. It is not unusual to stay with one client for only two hours and then be on your way to another client's home for another two hours. It is a good idea to write your own personal notes on each assignment so as not to forget something or some peculiarity of the client. Another suggestion as you work is to record in your notepad or on your electronic device any supplies that are getting low and any observations about your client, so once you are ready to chart, you will remember to write this down. You may want to leave a note for family members or other care providers to provide better continuity of care.

When beginning a new job, the aide must adjust to the client's or family's routine. Aides should not reorganize the entire house or daily schedule to suit themselves. An aide's job is to make the client comfortable and to assist the family, not to change their lifestyle. Remember, as a home health aide, you are a guest in the client's home.

Interpersonal Skills

When people live, work, or play together, one person acts and the other reacts or responds to the act. This process is called an **interaction** (Figure 2-7).

People are expected to handle interactions as a part of everyday life. The feelings and understandings that result from the interactions between two or more persons form what are called **interpersonal relationships**. To the person entering a service occupation, such as a home health aide, interpersonal relationships and compassion can determine success or failure. Each of the persons involved in these relationships is entitled to be treated with dignity. Everyone should follow the golden rule—treat others as you would like to be treated. This helps to establish good interpersonal relationships (Figure 2-8).

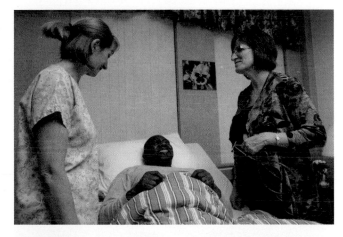

FIGURE 2-7   A home health aide needs to interact with clients and family members.

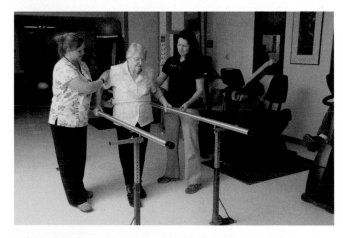

FIGURE 2-8   A home health aide interacting with a physical therapist and client.

Home health aides must remember that they are entering a home where an illness or problem already exists, which might cause the family members and client to be unhappy or bitter. Anger, fear, and other emotional reactions may be obvious. The client might be in pain or be cranky, sad, or depressed. The home health aide who is aware of the source of the problem often finds it easier to accept the behavior of clients and family members. As a result, awkward interpersonal relationships often can be avoided.

Good Personal Health and Hygiene

A home health aide must observe the personal **hygiene** standards expected of any health team member (Figure 2-9). When working in other people's homes, the aide should reflect the highest standards. This means being clean and well groomed each workday. The person who goes on a job

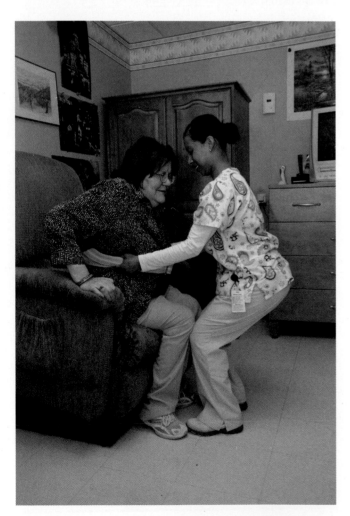

FIGURE 2-9 A neatly dressed aide assisting a client out of a chair.

unbathed, with dirty hair and nails, and wearing wrinkled, stained clothes makes a bad impression. A sloppy appearance implies that the person also has a poor self-image and sloppy working habits. Remember, too, that how you look reflects the pride you have in yourself and in your work.

An aide who is appropriately dressed or in the proper uniform projects a more professional appearance and makes the client feel more comfortable. Home care agencies vary greatly in their dress codes. A few agencies require a designated uniform and name badge, whereas others may allow the aide to wear comfortable, clean, casual clothing. Most agencies do not allow their home health aides to wear blue jeans or shorts and often have policies regarding tattoos and body piercings.

Guidelines for Personal Appearance of the Home Health Aide

Following are guidelines the home health aide should follow:

- Bathe daily and use deodorant.
- Do not wear strong perfumes or strong aftershave lotion.
- Brush your teeth regularly and use mouthwash if necessary.
- Do not smoke while on duty in the client's home; if need be you can smoke on your break outside the client's home. Clients with lung disease, allergies, respiratory illness, or personal distaste for the smell of cigarettes may have an adverse reaction to cigarette smoke.
- Wear makeup moderately; if you have tattoos, cover them with clothing; body piercing jewelry such as in the nose, tongue, and eyebrows should be removed while on duty.
- For men, shave daily and keep beard or mustache neat and clean.
- Shampoo your hair often; if you have long hair, pull it back so it is off your collar.
- Fingernails are to be clean and short.
- Jewelry should be limited. Small post earrings for pierced ears are usually acceptable.
- Bracelets, dangling earrings and necklaces, and large stone rings are not acceptable, as clients who are confused might grab them and a large ring can tear a client's skin.

- Shoes should be clean and in good repair.
- Wear a watch with a second hand and your name badge from your agency. Your name badge may have a photo of you and your first name.

Ethical Behavior

Ethics refers to a standard or code of behavior concerned with what is "right" and what is "wrong." Health care providers take an oath when they are licensed in which they promise to help and care for clients without causing unnecessary pain or suffering. Although there is no written code for home health aides, they are expected to uphold a definite set of standards as they practice their profession.

Ethical Standards

Ethical standards for home health aides include the following:

- Be honest in your dealings with clients and coworkers. Stealing involves not only the taking of objects or money, but also the falsifying of reports recording time and activities.
- Never discuss the financial, emotional, family, medical, or other problems of the client with outsiders. **Confidentiality** is a commitment to keep your client's affairs private. The home health aide must not discuss the client's health, family situation, finances, or any other personal matter with anyone except the case manager or other agency staff directly involved in the client's care. This includes the worker's family and friends.
- Respect the cultural and religious practices of the client and family.
- Never walk out in the middle of an assignment. Some people may be more pleasant to work with than others. If a personality conflict or the work load is impossible to deal with, the aide should try to finish the shift, then call the case manager and explain the problem. If the aide is working a private case or did not get the job through an agency, the problem should be discussed directly with the person who employed the aide. Having accepted the duties as an employee, a home health aide is ethically bound to give service for the wages paid.
- Do not accept money or gifts. This is a policy of most agencies.
- Report possible cases of abuse to your case manager.

- Do not have any sexual contact with a client or family member.
- Safeguard the confidential information you acquired from any source concerning the client.
- Do not adjust the client's care plan without consulting the case manager.

Professional Standards

Professional standards for home health aides include the following:

- Maintain high standards of personal health and appearance.
- Be dependable and reliable.
- Carry out the responsibilities of the job in the best way you possibly can.
- Show respect for the client's privacy and modesty.
- Recognize and respect the right of clients to determine their lifestyle. Ask the client how they would like to be addressed.
- Keep your professional life separate from your personal life. If the client asks you for information about your family, you can respond, but try to refocus the conversation around the client's interests.
- Control any negative reactions to chronic disability or the living conditions of the client.
- Maintain safe conditions in the working environment.
- Do not use the client's medications for your own health problems.
- Do not give your home or cell phone number to the client unless the case manager instructs you to do so. Occasionally, a client may become lonesome and call you continuously just to talk. Do not use your personal cell phone for texting or personal calls while you are working.

Client's Rights

The home health aide must respect the rights of the clients. The following is a list of common client rights that are mandated by Omnibus Budget Reconciliation Act (OBRA) regulations:

1. Every client shall be treated with consideration, respect, and full recognition of the client's dignity and individuality.

2. Every client shall receive care, treatment, and services that are adequate, appropriate, and in compliance with relevant federal and state law.

3. Every client has the right to be free from mental and physical abuse.

4. Every client shall be informed of these rights in writing and in the language the client can understand.

5. Every client who is responsible for a fee for service shall be given a statement of the services available from the agency and related charges.

6. Every client shall participate in the development of the plan of care and discharge plan and be informed of all treatments, when and how services will be provided, and the name and functions of any person and affiliated agency providing care and services.

7. Every client has the right to refuse treatment after being fully informed of and understanding the consequence of such actions.

8. Every client shall be informed of the procedure for submitting complaints to the agency. If the client is not satisfied by the agency response, the client may complain to the state Department of Health and Social Services.

9. Every client shall have the right to recommend changes in policies and services to agency staff, the area office representatives of the department, or any outside representative of the client's choice free from restraints, interference, coercion, discrimination, or reprisal.

10. Every client shall receive respect and privacy, including confidential treatment of client records, and the right to refuse release of records to any individuals outside the agency.

11. Every client has the right to privacy.

12. Every client has the right to request change of caregiver.

13. Every client has the right to be informed of the state consumer hotline number.

Home Health Aide's Rights

As an employee of an agency or your client, you also have rights. Examples of your rights are:

1. The right to take pride in a job well done

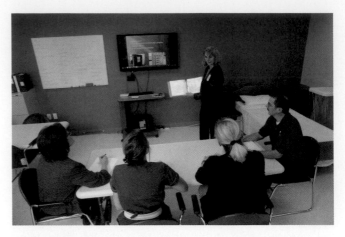

FIGURE 2-10   An aide attending an inservice as part of her job.

2. The right to make suggestions and complaints within designated channels without fear of retaliation

3. The right not to be abused physically, verbally, or sexually by clients

4. The right to recommend care plan changes designed to facilitate care delivery and reduce caregiver stress

5. The right to be informed when complaints concerning client treatment are alleged against you

6. The right to a fair hearing with your case manager

7. The right to a confidential investigation

8. The right to be informed of the investigation's outcome

9. The right to be paid for your services by your agency for a predetermined salary and mileage for travel

10. The right to attend continuing education programs offered by your agency at no cost to you (Figure 2-10)

11. The right to work in a safe environment

Client Abuse

Abuse of a client violates ethical standards and makes you liable for legal prosecution. Ethical standards (guides to moral behavior) require that you do no harm to clients. **Legal standards** (guides to lawful behavior) enforce this through laws, with penalties if you are found guilty. **Abuse** is defined as the willful infliction of physical pain, injury, mental anguish or fear, unreasonable confinement, or the willful deprivation by a caretaker of services that are necessary to maintain mental and physical health. Abuse may be emotional, financial, involuntary seclusion, mental, physical, or sexual, as follows:

- *Emotional or psychological abuse* is defined as the infliction of anguish, pain, or distress through verbal or nonverbal acts. Examples include using profanity or obscene words, shouting, teasing, or other methods to humiliate the client. Obvious signs might be passive, withdrawn, and emotionless behavior of the client and lack of reaction to pain.

- *Financial abuse* is using the client's money inappropriately or stealing money or other valuables. The client might mention that money is missing or state that he or she was forced to sign checks for services the client never received.

- **Neglect** is defined as refusal or failure to fulfill any person's obligations or duties for an individual.

- *Physical abuse* is hitting, burning, or pinching another person. Another example is forcing a treatment on a client that the client has requested not to be done. Signs of abuse include frequent, unexplained injuries; complaints of pain without obvious injuries; and burns or bruises suggesting the use of a cigarette, curling iron, or other object.

- *Sexual abuse* is making sexual advances to someone or touching a person in inappropriate places. Signs of sexual abuse include injury to genital areas, difficulty in sitting or walking, and fear of being alone with caregivers.

Every state now mandates reporting to the state Department of Health if a person has reasonable cause to believe that a child or an adult who is receiving care is being abused. If a home health aide knows or has a reasonable belief that a client is being abused by the client's family, another caregiver, or anyone else, the aide **must report** the abuse to the client's case manager. It is a law that home health aides must report any suspicions of abuse. It is important that you document what you saw or heard and other pertinent observations, not your opinion about the abuse. There are criminal penalties imposed by the state if a person fails to make a report. Every state gives legal immunity from civil or criminal liability to the reporting person unless that person acted in bad faith or with a malicious purpose. If the home health aide is self-employed, he or she must report directly to the state Department of Health in the state where the abused person resides. In response to a report, the state sends out

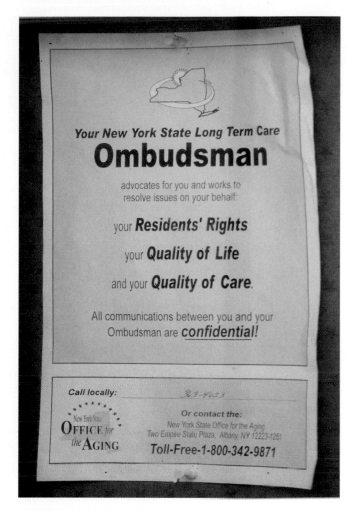

FIGURE 2-11   An ombudsman sign in an assistive living facility.

an **ombudsman** who investigates and mediates problems regarding the complaint (Figure 2-11).

Although it is known that in 90% of all reported elder abuse cases the abuser is a family member, it is not known how many of these abusive family members are also caregivers. Researchers have estimated that anywhere from 5% to 23% of all caregivers are physically abusive. Most agree that abuse is related to the stresses associated with providing care.

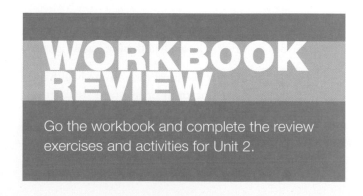

WORKBOOK REVIEW

Go the workbook and complete the review exercises and activities for Unit 2.

REVIEW

1. The home health aide will be expected to adapt to which of the following?
    a. Irregular hours
    b. A variety of assignments and settings
    c. A variety of different types of equipment
    d. All of the above

2. The home health aide should watch for which of the following changes in a client because it may be a sign that there is physical abuse?
    a. Enlarged pupils
    b. Bruises on both arms
    c. Bluish lip color
    d. Increasing "forgetfulness"

3. The case manager asks the aide to do something for a client but the aide does not know how to do it. The aide should do which of the following?
    a. Ask a family member in the home to do it.
    b. Call the agency and ask for another worker to help.
    c. Look in her pocket manual and try to find out how to do it.
    d. Tell the case manager immediately that she does not know how to do it.

4. Ethical conduct for a home health aide involves which of the following?
    a. Doing everything the client asks you to do
    b. Discussing your personal problems with the client to relieve the client's boredom
    c. Carrying out the responsibilities of your job in the best way you can
    d. All of the above

5. Which of the following is a form of abuse?
    a. Following prescribed nursing care
    b. Making sexual advances toward your client
    c. Preparing special diets according to instructions
    d. Bathing the client and observing skin integrity

6. T   F   HIPAA is an act that prohibits a home care agency from releasing the client's health information to a drug company without the client's permission.

7. T   F   A client has a right to refuse to take medication.

8. T   F   A home health aide has a right to work in a safe environment.

9. T   F   It is ethical for a home health aide to discuss a client's health or lifestyle with friends if they do not know or live near the client.

10. Match each of the following terms with the correct example.
    a. libel   d. procedure
    b. slander   e. battery
    c. abandonment   f. negligence

1. _____ false written statement about another
2. _____ making an oral false statement about another
3. _____ a client being left without care
4. _____ touching a person without that person's consent
5. _____ failure to act; forgetting to do a task
6. _____ a list of steps used to complete a task

11. List five actions that could lead to liability and should be avoided.

_____

_____

_____

_____

_____

12. List five rights of clients.

_____

_____

_____

_____

_____

13. List three rights of home health aides.

_____

_____

_____

14. Give four examples of good personal hygiene.

_____

_____

_____

Case Studies

15. Mrs. Stanley, 85 years old, lives with her 50-year-old son, Harold, who is struggling with an alcohol problem. While bathing her, you observe a number of unexplainable bruises on Mrs. Stanley's arms. You also notice that Harold is short-tempered with his mother. You are suspicious that Harold is abusing Mrs. Stanley. What should you do in this situation? What should you do if Mrs. Stanley admits the abuse but asks you not to tell anyone? What are other possible signs of abuse that a home health aide could observe?

16. Agency Care Well does not provide transportation services for its clients. Mr. Baxter, a 78-year-old client, realizes that this is the case but needs a ride to the grocery store. He asks you to drive him there after your regular work hours. He offers to pay you twice your normal hourly wage. Should you provide the ride for Mr. Baxter? If not, why not? What other solutions might there be to Mr. Baxter's problem?

UNIT 3

Developing Effective Communication Skills and Documentation

KEY TERMS

active listening
body language
clichés
communication
cultural diversity

documentation
Health Insurance
   Portability and
   Accountability Act
   (HIPAA)
invalidate

listening
nonjudgmental
nonverbal
   communication
objective

observation
paraphrasing
passive listening
report
subjective

LEARNING OBJECTIVES

After studying this unit, you should be able to:

- Explain why health care team members need to communicate

- Describe guidelines for effective communication

- Explain the importance of positive feedback

- List barriers to communication

- Acquaint oneself with methods to communicate with clients from a different culture, clients who are hard-of-hearing, or clients who have limited vision

- List basic rules for charting

- Interpret medical abbreviations and vocabulary words

- Explain the meaning of the "24-hour clock"

- Explain the contents of the client plan of care

- Identify information that can be collected about a client using sight, hearing, touch, smell, and taste

- Explain how you would answer the client's phone

The ability to communicate effectively may be the most important skill that a care provider can learn. **Communication** is the successful transmission of information from one person to another. A care provider's work with people consists primarily of performing tasks, but it also includes establishing positive relationships. The care provider often must communicate why a certain task needs to be done or perhaps coax the person to help with the task. The care provider may also communicate concern—or frustration—in nonverbal ways. Communication with the client's family may involve explaining the reasons why the care provider cannot do certain tasks the family wants, or the need to encourage the family to offer more assistance.

Cultural Diversity

Culture is defined as the behaviors, values, beliefs, habits, and customs of a group of people, which have been passed on from one generation to another. In the United States, we have **cultural diversity**, which is a mixture of individuals from different cultures. Different cultures require slightly different approaches in their personal care and in communication. It would be ideal if all the caregivers could be of the same culture as their clients, but that is not possible. However, many Native Americans request that only individuals from their own tribe be their caregivers; they do not like caregivers of another culture performing their personal care. In addition, Native Americans often prefer nontraditional medicines and cultural healers (medicine men) in treating illnesses rather than health care providers and prescription drugs. In some cultures, it is considered very disrespectful to have the caregiver look the client directly in the eyes. Another difference among individuals of different cultures is how they deal with pain—Asians, Russians, and women in certain cultures are taught from early years not to complain about pain. Some cultures believe that if an individual is sick, it is due to supernatural powers or evil spirits, not from the disease process. In some cultures, it is disrespectful for a woman to start the conversation because the male needs to be the first one to speak, or it may be disrespectful to ask the client a question. Other cultural differences deal with personal approach: two people may need to shake hands or embrace one another before talking. This is their right and we need to adjust care according to their beliefs. If any of these cultural differences do exist, they should be in the client's care plan and explained to you by your case manager. Take time to learn about your clients and their beliefs. Always be respectful of and interested in other cultures without being judgmental.

To enhance the communication process with a client who does not speak or understand English, the case manager may make arrangements for an interpreter to visit the client when you are there and assist you with fundamental communication needs.

In summary, when caring for a client of another culture:

- Avoid body language that may be offensive or misunderstood.
- Plan your care based on the communication needs and cultural background of the client.
- Adopt special approaches when the client speaks another language.
- Do not judge your client in any way.
- Communicate with the client in a nonthreatening way.
- Research cultural information as necessary.

Stressful Conditions in the Home

Family can be defined as a group of people living in the same household and usually under one head—including parents, children, relatives, and friends. As a home health aide, you must remember that every family operates differently and no two families are alike. It is wise not to take sides with family members in caring for your client. Often the stress of illness and disability brings changes in the behavior of family members. All family members may not agree on the medical care and treatment provided by the health care team. Some family members live in another part of the country and do not realize the care required for their relative who is dependent on a caregiver 24 hours a day, 7 days a week. The financial aspect of care can also become a heavy stressor on families, especially in a chronic long-term illness. Sons or daughters might ask clients for money that they may use to pay bills or, unfortunately, for their drug problem. The home health aide may witness family members spending the client's money on their own addictions, but must maintain confidentiality, sharing concerns only with the proper health care team members.

Communication in the Workplace

Good communication is essential in the worker-supervisor relationship. A worker who knows what, how, and to whom he or she should report is an effective team member. The end result of good communication is great patient care.

Communicating, something that we all do every day, seems easy, but it is actually a complicated process. There are three key aspects of communication: how messages are sent and received, active listening, and nonverbal communication.

Send a Clear Message

Communication is a two-way process. The sender must send a message and the receiver must receive it for communication to occur. However, the communication is not successful unless the meaning of the message sent and the one received are the same. This is not easy to accomplish. At many points something can go wrong. Figure 3-1 is a graphic description of the communication process.

Problems in communication can begin before words are even spoken. We have all experienced times when our thoughts are unclear. Although we are not sure what we want to say, we say it anyway. The resulting confusion is no surprise. In Figure 3-1 we see that "thoughts" are the actual beginning of the communication process. Taking the time to organize our thoughts before speaking is the basis for all clear communication.

We run into quite a few problems putting our thoughts into words. One major problem is that we often neglect to communicate at all. For many different reasons, we do not talk to each other, and the result is rarely good. When clear communication of expectations has not taken place, mistakes happen that could have been avoided. Care providers often have thoughts, feelings, and information that the case manager should know about. When the care providers do not communicate clearly with the case manager, problems can occur. For example, a worker may feel angry because the case manager has given her a very difficult client when she is feeling work-related stress or "burned out." The case manager will not know how the worker is

feeling unless she mentions it. Only then can she get the support she needs.

Putting the thoughts into words and actually delivering the message are also important steps. Often we have organized our thoughts and rehearsed how we want to say them, but we find it hard to deliver the message. If the worker who is feeling work-related stress is afraid the case manager will not receive the message well or will "interpret" the message in the wrong way, she will find it very hard to deliver the message.

Good communication involves two people. Thinking of our example and looking at Figure 3-1, the worker feels work-related stress and thinks about how to talk to the case manager ("thoughts"). She tells the case manager how she is feeling ("puts into words" and "delivers message"). The case manager listens to the worker ("receives message"), thinks about all of the complex cases the worker is carrying right now ("interprets the message"), and tells the worker that she understands the worker's complex caseload right now and it is no wonder that the worker is feeling some stress ("gives feedback").

Observation

The home health aide is in a unique position to observe client needs in the home environment. Through frequent observation and interaction with the client, the aide will see changes in the client's behavior and the environment. In this role the aide has two responsibilities: to orient the client and to provide observations to other members of the care team.

Orientation to place, day, and time as a part of the daily routine with the client may be helpful to some clients, for example: "Good morning, Mrs. Jones. It's 9 o'clock, time for your breakfast. You know, this is the coldest January 5th I can remember." For many homebound ill people, one day is similar to another. Reminders of the day, the time, the season, and life outside the home are helpful. If a client seems unable to remember even after this orientation, the home health aide will report this to other health care team members or the family.

For the work team to be effective, the home health aide must make sure that she is providing as much detail as possible about the client to other members of the health care team. Observing and reporting are key aspects of the care provider's work. She is the eyes and ears of the family and of the employer. Good case notes can help keep families and others updated and informed about the client. Figure 3-2 includes some commonly used abbreviations that may be encountered and used in clients' care plans. Figure 3-3 includes a list of abbreviations used in

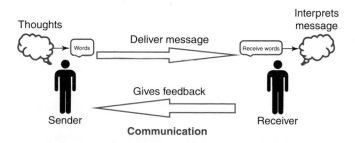

FIGURE 3-1 The communication process.

ā–before
ad lib–as desired
ac–before meals
ADLs–activities of daily living
Amb–ambulatory
bid–twice a day
BM–bowel movement
BP–blood pressure
BRP–bathroom privileges
C–Celsius
c̄–with
CBR–complete bed rest
c/o–complains of
CPR–cardiopulmonary resuscitation
DOE–dyspnea on exertion
dsg–dressing
F–Fahrenheit
Fe–iron
gtt–drop
H_2O–water
HOB–head of bed
HOH–hard of hearing
HS–hour of sleep
Ht–height
I & O–intake and output
IV–intravenous
K–potassium
Lab–laboratory
lb–pound
mg–milligram
mL–milliliter
Na–sodium salt
noc–night
NPO–nothing by mouth

O_2–oxygen
OD–right eye
OS–left eye
OT–occupational therapy
OU–both eyes
oz–ounce
p̄–after
pc–after meals
PO–by mouth
prep–prepare for
prn–when needed or necessary
pt–patient
PT–physiotherapy, physical therapy
q2h–every 2 hours
q3h–every 3 hours
q4h–every 4 hours
qd–every day
qid–four times a day
qod–every other day
ROM–range of motion exercises
s̄–without
Spec–specimen
SSE–soap solution enema
ST–speech therapy
stat–immediately
Temp–(T)–temperature
tid–three times a day
TLC–tender loving care
TPR–temperature, pulse, respiration
U/A–urinalysis
VS–vital signs: TPR and BP
w/c–wheelchair
Wt–weight

FIGURE 3-2   Standard medical abbreviations must be learned and understood to correctly chart for the client.

the diagnosis of a condition or disease of a client. Accurate and clear communication is important to give the best care possible for your client. If the care is shared by family caregivers, these abbreviations will be helpful only if they are understood by everyone who needs to use them. Figure 3-4 lists vocabulary words used to describe colors, Figure 3-5 lists vocabulary words used to describe behaviors, and Figure 3-6 lists common vocabulary words used in clients' documentation.

Positive Feedback

For some reason, many of us have difficulty complimenting others and receiving compliments. We may be thinking a kind thought, but we do not put it into words. Unless the other person is a mind reader, it means nothing. One should always state the positive action that a person is doing first, rather than saying a negative statement. We all like "warm fuzzies," and such compliments will help the client's self-esteem. For example, the client, Mr. Keane, has just progressed from a walker to a cane. He was able to walk from his kitchen to the bathroom with little difficulty, but very slowly. The aide states, "Mr. Keane, you are doing great without your walker. It is good you are not walking fast the first time, as you may lose your balance." A negative approach for the aide would be, "Mr. Keane, you should be able to walk faster now that you have a cane." Remember that compliments and praise are comforting to a client and also for the home health aide.

Do you know how much a family caregiver or client appreciates a compliment? For example, you might say to your client, "Mr. Jones, you are walking better and better each day! Today you walked 10 feet, twice as far as last week. It won't be long before you are walking without my help. Congratulations!"

Putting Thoughts into Words

The message being sent often has more than one meaning, and the receiver must try to figure out what the sender really means. There are many common phrases and words that have a wide range of meanings. Consider the following words and phrases: *often, occasionally, always, almost always, sometimes, seldom, never.* Misunderstanding simple words like these can cause problems. A client may want her bathroom cleaned "often." To her this means daily, but to the worker it means once per week. In this example, the client's anger and the worker's frustration may be avoided if the meaning of the word is clarified.

There is not likely to be total agreement on many terms that we commonly use. We must be very careful that the understanding of the sender and the receiver is the same. Communication can be difficult when the message is not clear enough and when the person who receives the message does not ask for clarification. To clarify what is meant, you can ask a series of questions to make sure you understand. This is doubly important to do if your client is from another culture.

Message Delivery

Any message can be delivered in a variety of ways. Comedians say that the success of a joke depends on delivery. Tone of voice, facial expressions, body language, and gestures all affect how a message is delivered. For example, tone of voice can make a profound difference in the way a message is sent. Nonverbal communication also may include eye contact, posture, and the distance between people. Try repeating the following messages using different tones of voice:

> *"That's OK, I'm not angry."*
>
> *"I'm glad my mother-in-law is coming to dinner."*
>
> *"No, I'm not busy."*
>
> *"You were sick yesterday."*
>
> *"That is not my job."*

Ad–Alzheimer's disease	HPV–human papillomavirus
AIDS–acquired immunodeficiency syndrome	MI–myocardial infarction (heart attack)
Alz–Alzheimer	MRSA–methicillin-resistant *Staphylococcus aureus* infection
ARC–AIDS-related complex	
ASHD–arteriosclerosis (hardening of the arteries)	MS–multiple sclerosis
CA–cancer	PID–pelvic inflammatory disease
CHF–congestive heart failure	PVD–peripheral vascular disease
COPD–chronic obstructive pulmonary disease	STD–sexually transmitted disease
CVA–cerebral vascular accident (stroke)	TB–tuberculosis
DJD–degenerative joint disease	TIA–transient ischemic attack (small stroke)
DM–diabetes mellitus	URI–upper respiratory infection
Fx–fracture	UTI–urinary tract infection
HIV–human immunodeficiency virus	VD–venereal disease

FIGURE 3-3 Abbreviations used in the diagnosis of a condition or disease. Many times more than one diagnosis will be listed for a client.

Ashen	gray
Bile	greenish
Cyanotic	bluish
Jaundice	yellow
Necrotic	black
Pale	white

FIGURE 3-4 Vocabulary words used to describe colors.

Comatose	responds only if stimulated–deep sleep
Combative	strikes out
Incoherent	responds wrongly to questions
Lethargic	tired
Tremors	fine, quick movements of hands
Withdrawn	retreats into oneself

FIGURE 3-5 Vocabulary words used to describe behaviors.

Abrasions	scrapes
Anorexia	no appetite
Contusions	bruises
Copious	large amount
Decubitus ulcer	pressure sores/ulcer
Diaphoretic	perspiring
Dyspnea	difficulty in breathing
Edema	swelling
Flatus	rectal gas
Gait	walking style
Geriatric	dealing with the elderly
Hematuria	blood in urine
Hemiplegia	paralysis of one side of the body
Paraplegia	paralysis from the waist down
Productive	coughing up material
Purulent	pus-like drainage
Quadriplegia	paralysis from the neck down
Rales	moist respirations
Sign	change in a client that can be seen or measured
Sputum	phlegm–spit
Symptoms	those changes reported by the clients, which are not visible

FIGURE 3-6 Common vocabulary words seen and used in reports.

Receiving Messages

Many factors can affect how a message is received. Hearing loss, medications, disabilities, and depression can have major effects on how a client receives a communication. Clients with hearing, speech, or visual impairments need special attention.

The following list of techniques can be used to improve communication with these clients:

- Be sure you have the person's attention before beginning to speak.
- Face the person and make eye contact.
- Lower the pitch of your voice; do not mumble.
- Speak clearly and slowly.
- Use short sentences.
- Avoid background noise; turn off the TV or radio.
- Encourage the use of nonverbal communication, such as touch, or hold the client's hand.
- Use written communication or other visual aids if you are unable to communicate verbally.

- Do not shout; use a normal tone, as shouting makes words less clear.
- Do not speak with something in your mouth or with your hands over your lips.
- Restate your sentence when you are not understood.
- If you do not understand a part of your client's message, restate the part that you do understand and ask for clarification.
- Talk toward the "better" ear because many people hear better out of one ear.
- Recognize that illness or fatigue reduces the ability of a person with a hearing or speech impairment.
- Do not exhaust the person with irrelevant noise or chatter.
- Visual cues may assist the client; use hand gestures when appropriate; provide the opportunity for lip-reading.

Touch is an important form of nonverbal communication. In some cultures touching is not appropriate, so talk with your case manager if you are unsure.

Barriers to the Communication Process

The following techniques hinder good communication rather than improve the process.

Not Listening

One reason that a message may not be received correctly is because of poor listening skills. It is interesting how little we are taught about how to listen. Yet listening is one of the most important factors in communication.

A poor listener shows inattention by various means. Some of the behaviors demonstrated by a poor listener are not paying attention to the speaker, listening passively, preparing an answer before the speaker is through talking, rushing the speaker, interrupting the speaker or changing the subject, and becoming emotional.

Changing the Subject

It is often tempting to change the subject because the subject is uncomfortable. The client may be depressed and speaking about things that are discouraging to hear. Stay with the client, who may need to talk about something that is deeply troubling. Changing the subject will not take the problem away, but listening may very well ease the load.

Using Clichés

A cliché is a word or a phrase that people use very often for a lot of different situations, such as the following:

- "Oh, you'll get over it."
- "Just make the most of it."
- "Tomorrow's another day."
- "It's God's will."

You will offer these words of encouragement from time to time, and, at some point in the conversation, these reassurances may be much appreciated. However, when someone comes to you with a problem, clichés may completely invalidate that person's feelings, making her feel that her problems are not important. Clichés may be useful at a later point in the conversation, after the individual has had the opportunity to express feelings.

Giving Advice

Do not give your client advice or make recommendations. Just listening to your client will usually help the person to arrive at his or her own decision.

Talking About Yourself

Caregiver–client discussion is not restricted, but the caregiver's role is to listen to the clients, not to air her own problems.

Showing Disapproval and Passing Judgment on the Client

It is extremely important to remain nonjudgmental of clients. For example, an elderly client is telling you that her children are so wonderful, but very busy. They really do not have the time to see her. You know the client's son and his wife live only a mile away, yet they visit only once a month, if that often. Even though you may think they are ungrateful children, you would be judgmental if you said what you thought to the client. Your negative comment is based on what you are seeing right now in the client's life. You cannot know all of the details of the relationship of the client with her children. In this case, it would be better to just agree with the client that they are busy or to say that she must miss seeing them more often.

Asking "Why" Questions

Often more information is needed before you can understand what someone means. In that case, a "why" question is often used. Care must be taken when asking "why" questions because they can also send the message that you are judging the other person. Such questions include:

- "Why did you do that?"
- "Why are you thinking that?"

These short, direct questions may suggest that you are disapproving of or judging the other person. "Mrs. Jones, I'm not sure why you did that—help me understand so I can do it better next time." Or, "Mr. Smith, why would you think I would do that?" These are softer messages that include the fact that you are inquiring to understand the situation better.

Effective Listening Skills

A person who is an effective listener shows positive behaviors. Paying attention to the speaker; adopting an accepting attitude with a calm, open facial expression and a relaxed nonthreatening body position; and allowing the speaker plenty of time are just a few ways to be an effective listener. We are all very susceptible to distraction when asked to be a listener. Our own needs, fears, values, and beliefs can influence our ability to listen and communicate objectively.

The final factor in good communication is one that is often underestimated. That is when we "interpret the message" that has been sent. At this point, we develop our own understanding of what has been said. Active listening is a tool that will allow the home health aide to become more involved in the communication process. The home health aide can make sure that he or she understands not only what the speaker has said, but also how the person feels. We do this by giving the speaker feedback about what we have heard. The speaker may then confirm or correct our understanding.

We often assume that we know what a person is saying without checking to make sure that we are correct in those assumptions. When we carefully listen, then check to see if we heard correctly, we are participating in active listening. In passive listening, listeners simply sit and hope that they understand what is being said. However, there are many points along the way during which the message may go wrong, so we should work to become active rather than passive listeners. Active listeners become involved in the process, constantly checking to see if they are on target in what they understand.

Active Listening Behaviors

The following four active listening behaviors should be practiced:

- Paraphrasing
- Reflecting the speaker's feelings
- Asking for more information
- Using nonverbal communication

Paraphrasing

Paraphrase what has been said. Paraphrasing involves restating, in your own words, what the other person has said; this gives you a chance to check whether your understanding of what has been said is correct. It also gives the speaker a chance to correct you if you have misunderstood. You might say such things as "Do you mean that . . . ?" or "I understand you are saying. . . ."

Reflecting the Speaker's Feelings

The feelings behind what is being said are often as important as the words, if not more so. Therefore, it is important to try to understand the underlying feelings, attitudes, beliefs, or values. You might make such statements as "That must have made you upset," "I imagine you were thrilled about that," or "Does that worry you?"

Asking for More Information

We often need more information to understand what has been said. In most cases, we simply need to ask for clarification. Responses may include: "I'm interested; tell me more about that," "What happened after that?," or "How did you feel when that happened?"

Aspects of Communication

The average person spends only approximately 5% of the day listening and 30% of the day speaking. These factors can cause us to make assumptions, which may not always be true. As a listener, realize that everyone naturally makes assumptions, but it is important to remain skeptical about these assumptions until they are proven true. Consider the following aspects of communication:

- Certain behaviors on the part of the listener and the speaker communicate that messages are being received. It is important to both listen and observe, as some messages are communicated in ways other than speaking.

- Nonverbal communication reinforces what a client or family member is feeling. It is important to pay attention to facial expressions, posture, and body language. At all times, health care workers need to be aware of their own facial and body expressions, gestures, and posture.

- Eye contact is another important nonverbal form of communication. It is very important to make and maintain eye contact. This shows the client or family member that you are paying direct attention to him or her.

- Posture, the way you sit or position the body, also conveys information. Always try to sit comfortably.

Be sensitive to the client's spatial (space) territory. Sitting too close can be an invasion of personal space, whereas sitting too far away can suggest fear or distrust.

- Verbal input indicates that you are listening and observing. Your response must show that you have listened and can accurately reflect what has been heard and observed.

- Questioning is an excellent way to learn about the client and family. Open questions allow room for response and expression of feelings. Open questions lead to further discussion of a subject or feeling. Examples of open questions include: "Could you describe . . . ?," "Now do you understand that . . . ?," and "Tell me about. . . ." Closed questions generally can be answered with specific information or "yes" or "no." These questions are useful to begin conversations, especially when a client or family member is not very talkative. It is most important to avoid asking leading questions that put words into the client's or family member's mouth.

Observation Skills

In most cases, the client is with the home health aide more than any other person. If there is a problem, the aide may be the only, or at least the most likely, person to notice it. The client may be developing a rash, losing weight, or becoming more disoriented—all indications that there may be a problem. If the problem is noticed and professional assistance is obtained, it may be resolved quickly. If not, the situation may become life-threatening. That it why the home health aide's skills of **observation** are so important.

All five senses—seeing, hearing, touching, smelling, and tasting—should be used in the day-to-day work of the home health aide. Let's consider each sense as follows:

1. **Seeing**
   Look at the client carefully, watching for any change since your last visit. Things you might note are facial expression, posture, skin color, rashes, color of drainage, swelling, way of walking (gait), and steadiness when walking.

   Look at the home for safety hazards (overloaded electrical outlet, throw rugs, loose steps or locks), cleanliness, medications sitting out with covers off, and spots and stains on furniture or floors.

2. **Hearing**
   Listen to the client. What is being said? How is it being said? Is the client's speech clear or slurred? Is

it logical or nonsensical? Are the words sad, angry, friendly, or hostile? Does the client use profane language? Do you hear wheezing, coughing, or gasping for breath?

   Listen to the home. Does the faucet drip? Does the furnace or hot water heater make noises? Are the phone and doorbell loud enough for the client to hear?

3. **Touching**
   Touch the client's hand. Does the skin feel hot, cold, or moist? Is it rough or swollen? What is the pulse rate?

   Feel items in the house: Are the sheets dry? Is the bread stale? Is the water too hot?

4. **Smelling**
   Does the client have bad breath or body odor? Does the odor smell like sweat, urine, feces, alcohol, or fruit? Is there an odor from an open sore or dressing?

5. **Tasting**
   Is the food too salty or too spicy? Is the coffee too strong?

Reporting

Some important instructions that you need during your orientation to an agency are how to **report** information, whom to report it to, and when to report it. The person whom you will most likely report to is your case manager.

If you work for an agency, the agency may provide you with some type of computer to document your visit and the care you completed. Before you start the visit, if there has been any change in the care or condition of your client, the computer will alert you. Some things need to be reported immediately, such as a fall. Currently, because of computers or smartphones, you can communicate a client's fall immediately to your agency. The agency will give you directions on what action you should take. Home health aides can participate in case reviews, consulting with the team members caring for the client—registered nurses, therapists, and other health professionals. Examples of abnormal signs and symptoms that need to be reported and documented are shortness of breath, rapid respirations, chills, fever, pain in the chest, bluish color to the lips, pain in the abdomen, nausea and vomiting, drowsiness, excessive thirst, excessive perspiration, purulent drainage, blood in the urine, pain on urinating, and dark urine with a strong odor. Pain of any kind must be reported.

Throughout your career as a home health aide, and especially as a beginner, you should remember that it is always better to report something than to risk endangering the client, the agency, and yourself by not reporting it. Your case manager will help you learn how to sort out the "crisis" from the "unusual," and develop good judgment in reporting. When you talk over your observations and your feelings with the case manager, you can speak freely and voice your opinions and small details. All of these help your case manager to make decisions; he or she can help you learn to be more concise and accurate in your oral reports as time goes on.

Documenting

The **Health Insurance Portability and Accountability Act**, or **HIPAA**, is federal legislation that protects client records. This act called for the establishment of electronic record systems and privacy rules to legally protect personal health information (PHI). PHI is any information contained in automated records that is transmitted or maintained in any form or medium, including verbal discussions, electronic communications regarding clients, and written communication.

Writing down your observations and actions, or **documentation**, is an important part of your job. Each agency has its own forms that should be used, and the agency will tell you how often you need to document something in writing or on the computer, where to do it, and when to turn it in. Figures 3-7 and 3-8 are examples of forms that are completed by the home health aide.

There is a saying that "The job is not over till the reporting is done." This certainly holds true in home health care. The information you write or transfer over the computer can be in different forms (e.g., narrative, or story form, observation, notes, or charting). The information contained in client records is of significant importance for the following reasons:

1. It is a lasting record of what was done to, for, and by the client. If it is not charted, it is considered not to have been done.

2. It is a record of what was observed about the client.

3. It is a record of how the client reacted to the care that was given.

4. It contains information that can be used by other health team members in evaluating the care that was given and in deciding if changes in the care plan should be made.

5. If the client or family is unsatisfied with services and decide to complain, the client record can be used to show that certain things were done on certain dates and times. It can also show if the client refused to have some treatments done.

6. Always remember that the client record, either on paper or on the computer, is a legal document. It could be introduced as evidence in a court of law in the event that the client or family sues the home health aide or the agency. A well-documented client record can be the home health aide's best protection against false claims.

When you are recording on your report, it is important that you do the following:

1. *Be factual.* Write only those things that you know to be true.

2. *Chart in ink.* Writing or printing in pencil is not allowed in charting if documentation is written by hand.

3. *Use a secure password.* You will be given a password to enter the information into the computer. Do not share this password with anyone. It is your electronic signature.

4. *Be objective.* Record what you actually did, saw, smelled, felt, or tasted. Do not try to interpret the cause or the feelings that went along with the observation. If you feel that you really must put something in the record that is your own interpretation, identify it as such.

   Do not diagnose. If the client complains of pains in his chest and arm, do not write, "Client had a heart attack." Instead write, "Client complains of severe pains in his chest and upper arm. Face is pale and moist."

   If you observed a large discolored area on the client's arm, write a description of it. Do not write, "Mrs. Jones has a big bruise on her arm where I think her husband grabbed her when he got angry with her when she wet the bed." State, "Client has three bruises on her upper right arm. Each bruise is the size of a 50-cent piece." Be specific about the place on the body and the size of each bruise.

5. *Include subjective data.* Subjective data include things that you cannot see or know unless the client tells you (e.g., pain in legs, headache, depression), or remarks that family members might make to you.

Home Health

HOME HEALTH AIDE INSTRUCTION SHEET
Client Information is Confidential / Call RN if change in condition.

CLIENT: *Bill Kane*

✔	**Safety Precautions**	*Clear pathways, lifeline on, w/c locked for transfer*
✔	Bath	*Partial or full sponge as client directs*
	Grooming	*Brush dentures - place in denture cup after supper*
✔	Dressing	*Assist c̄ Teds off and client into pajamas (as he directs)*
✔	Mobility	*Walk c̄ hands on assist as directed - Stop if DOE noted*
	Transfer	
	ROM	
	Splints / Braces	
	Toileted	
	Catheter	
	TPR	
✔	BP	*q̄ M, W, F - list B.P., call R.N. if ↓90/50 or ↑170/98*
	Weight	

	Other as per Instruction Sheet (list)
✔	*Skin care - Client directs the following Topical application (note only if applied)*
	a. DesOwen cream - thin layer on back of ears
	b. Cetaphel cream to hands for dryness/cracking.
	c. Triple Antibiotic ointment to scrapes/skintears on extremities and cover dry dressing (no tape to LE)
✔	*Medications: Set out PM meds as set-up by R.N.*
✔	Housekeeping *"Turn down" bed for sleep, water at bedside, clean-up from supper*
	Meals *Heat supper as client directs*

Additional Instructions:
1. Document any DOE/ need for rest from activities
2. Call R.N. if any S/S infection are noted (i.e. elevated temp, redness @ site, greenish drainage, malaise)
3. Prepare clothes for next A.M. (set-out, put folded tissues in pocket, etc. ask him)

RN Signature:	Date:

FIGURE 3-7   Home Health Aide Instruction Sheet. (Courtesy of Caregivers Home Health)

ABC Home Health Agency
Home Health Aide Documentation
Client Information Is Confidential / Call RN if change in condition.

Home Health

CLIENT: DOB: Sex   :☐

Case Manager: Age :   Allergies:

Date:

| Personal Cares |
| Bath |
| Oral Care |
| Perineal Care |
| Mobility |
| Ambulated 40 ft |
| Cane/Walker |
| —Positioning aides used in recliner |
| Pain Level Scale 0–10 |
| Pain medication is managing pain |
| Medications |
| Did take all as ordered |
| Nutrition |
| % of meals eaten |
| —in-between snack |
| Urinary |
| Incontinent/continent |
| Bowel Movement |
| Lg, med, sm |
| TPR & BP on Friday |
| Initial of HHA |

FIGURE 3-8   Home Health Aide Record.

6. *Be concise.* Plan your words before you write them. Use enough words to give clear information, but do not write a book. You need not write a complete sentence each time; if using a computer, abbreviations are acceptable.

7. *Be neat.* You may either print or handwrite your data, whichever method is most legible. If you make a mistake on the chart, do not erase it, but cross it out with a single line and initial the mistake; this shows you made and corrected the error.

8. *Be accurate.* Be sure the record shows exactly what you did, and if it is appropriate, what the client's reaction was. If you were not able to carry out some treatment that was ordered, give the reason (e.g., "I was unable to apply special lotion to the client's legs as there was no lotion available"). Record vital signs on the designated area in the client's chart.

9. *Sign and date every entry in the record.* You will need to sign or initial at the end of each entry (e.g., John Kane HHA or JK). It is important to

put the date (month, day, and year) and the time the visit began and ended. If you are using a computer, your electronic documentation will record the date and time and your name.

10. *Be descriptive.* "The client was confused" does not give as much information as "The client did not know his name or what time of day it was. He placed his glasses in the wastebasket and his dentures in the toilet bowl."

11. *Be sure what you write relates to the goals set for and by the client.* Do not let yourself fall in the bad habit of continually writing "No change," "Client was okay today," or other meaningless phrases. If the goal is to increase the client's walking ability, you might write, "Walked three times without assistance from bedroom to kitchen."

12. *Use the correct words and abbreviations.* Lists of the correct words and approved abbreviations to use in describing your observations are given earlier in this unit. Try to use these words correctly instead of using slang, and learn their correct spelling. Your reports will be easier to understand and more respected if you learn to use the right words and correct abbreviations.

A twenty-four-hour clock is often used in charting. Instead of charting 1:00 P.M., the time is recorded as 1300 hours (Figure 3-9). This might also be referred to as military time. If using a computer, the time is automatically entered.

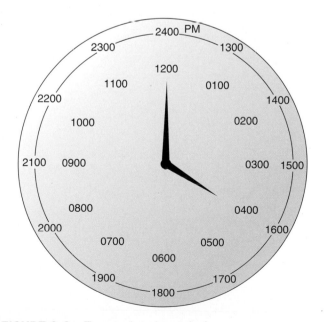

FIGURE 3-9 Twenty-four-hour clock.

Answering the Phone

If the phone rings when you are there and your client asks you to answer it, state "Keane's [client's name] residence." If need be, take the message and relay it to your client, and write the message down. If it is the health care provider and he or she wants to change the client's medication, just state, "I am not allowed to take a health care provider's orders; please call the case manager assigned to this client." Don't give out any information about your client over the phone without the client's permission.

Assessment and Admission

After a client is referred to the home health agency, the case manager will make the initial assessment and admission visit. This visit must include a thorough assessment of the client, family, and home environment, as well as the client's physical, emotional, and social needs. The client's living environment is assessed for adaptations that are necessary. Family members are assessed not only for their understanding of the client's illness, but also for their cultural and social needs as they impact the recovery of the client.

Plan of Care

The plan of care is a legal document that is constructed by the case manager, in conjunction with the client's health care provider, and implemented by the home health aide and other direct care staff. Based on the case manager's admission findings, a plan of care is established. All agencies certified to provide home health care are required to use designated forms, either written or electronic. These forms must be completed upon admission and signed by a health care provider. Unless a client's condition changes radically, this plan of treatment is effective for 90 days for the first two benefit periods. Health care documentation must include the admission sheet, OASIS and comprehensive assessment, nursing plan of care, medication assessment record, and progress notes. Interventions are to be implemented by the client, family, or caregivers, and thus all are involved in the treatment plan (Figure 3-10). The case manager is responsible for coordinating, implementing, and evaluating the care.

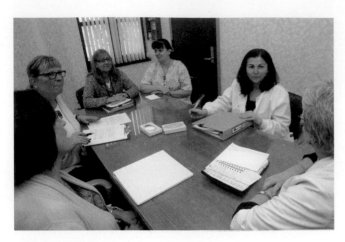

FIGURE 3-10 Case manager having a meeting with the home care team.

- Skin—abrasions, contusions, redness, pressure sores, surgical incisions, color, temperature, elasticity
- Musculoskeletal—activity level, general mobility, gait, range of motion
- Neurological—size of pupils, hand grips, ability to follow commands, level of consciousness
- Respiratory—breath sounds, sputum color, cough
- Cardiovascular—heart sounds, edema, color and temperature of extremities
- Gastrointestinal—bowel sounds, nausea or vomiting, appetite, elimination pattern
- Genitourinary—voiding, color, consistency, and odor of urine, difficulty in urination, penile discharge or vaginal discharge

Although each case manager develops his or her own routine for completing a basic assessment, it should be consistent and complete. The case manager will concentrate on the specific system that correlates with the client's diagnosis:

- Vital signs—temperature, pulse, respirations, blood pressure
- State of comfort—location and intensity of pain, response to medication
- Emotional responses—client behavior and reactions, general mood

WORKBOOK REVIEW

Go to the workbook and complete the review exercises and activities for Unit 3.

REVIEW

For questions 1 through 4, choose the response that illustrates good listening habits.

1. "My daughter wants me to go into the nursing home."
   a. "Well, maybe you should consider it. Things are hard for you here."
   b. "How could she say that! After all you've done for her!"
   c. "How do you feel about that?"
   d. None of the above

2. "I haven't been sleeping well lately."
   a. "Try some of these pills. They work great for me."
   b. "What's keeping you awake?"
   c. "Don't worry; you'll catch up on your sleep later."
   d. "Would a glass of beer before you go to bed help?"

3. "I just can't handle this job anymore."
   a. "Is something at work bothering you today?"
   b. "I know what you mean. I have this client who's driving me crazy!"
   c. "The pay is terrible, and the hours are long; you should just quit."
   d. All of the above

4. "My husband and I had a big fight last night."
   a. "Again? I don't know why you ever married him."
   b. "You're upset about the fight."
   c. "Who started the fight?"
   d. "Why don't you move out?"

5. Mrs. Lindsay is blind. You should
   a. touch her to get her attention.
   b. move furniture and household items around to provide for variety.
   c. provide step-by-step explanations of what you are doing.
   d. have her walk in front of you as you guide her from behind.

6. You are talking to a client with a hearing loss. You should do all of the following *except*
   a. speak clearly and slowly.
   b. speak in front of the client so the client can read your lips.
   c. shout at the client.
   d. use short sentences and simple words.

7. Body language is
   a. use of gestures instead of words.
   b. a form of verbal communication.
   c. of no concern to the home health aide.
   d. used only when a client is unable to hear.

8. Match the abbreviations of diseases in Column I with the correct diseases in Column II.

Column I	Column II
_____ 1. AIDS	a. Alzheimer
_____ 2. CHF	b. acquired immunodeficiency syndrome
_____ 3. DM	c. congestive heart failure
_____ 4. DJD	d. diabetes mellitus
_____ 5. Fx	e. transient ischemic attack
_____ 6. Alz	f. fracture
_____ 7. TIA	g. degenerative joint disease

9. Match the abbreviations in Column I with the correct meanings in Column II.

Column I	Column II
_____ 1. ADLs	a. complains of
_____ 2. TLC	b. activities of daily living
_____ 3. qod	c. four times a day
_____ 4. stat	d. tender loving care
_____ 5. HOH	e. immediately
_____ 6. c/o	f. every other day
_____ 7. qid	g. hard of hearing

10. Match the terms in Column I with the correct colors in Column II.

    Column I   **Column II**
    _____ 1. cyanotic   a. yellow
    _____ 2. necrotic   b. white
    _____ 3. ashen   c. black
    _____ 4. pale   d. gray
    _____ 5. jaundice   e. bluish

11. T   F   If a home health aide shows distaste while changing an adult brief by wrinkling his or her nose, this is sending a nonverbal message through body language.

12. T   F   An example of a subjective observation is a pulse rate of 100.

13. T   F   Home health aides are not responsible for implementation of the care plan for their clients.

14. T   F   An example of effective communication is a home health aide telling a dying client, "Everything will be all right."

15. T   F   Families react differently to the stress of 24-hour caregiving plus the financial cost of care.

16. T   F   If one states it is 1300 hours, that is the same as saying it is 1:00 P.M.

17. Communication is
    a. a written account of the client's illness and response to treatment.
    b. a verbal account of client care and observation.
    c. using the senses of sight, hearing, touch, and smell to collect information about the client.
    d. the exchange of information.

18. Basic components for oral communication are
    a. S.
    b. M.
    c. R.

19. Which of the following gives the most information?
    a. The client has a reddened area on her leg.
    b. The client has a reddened area about the size of a dime right below the kneecap.
    c. The client has a small sore on the front of her left leg.
    d. The client needs to have a nurse look at the area on her left leg below the knee.

Case Studies

20. Your client is a 35-year-old woman whose left leg was amputated. She is usually quite sad and lethargic. Today you arrive and she is cheerful. Her hair has been combed and she has cleaned up and gotten dressed. This is much different from the woman you saw just the day before. This change in mood bothers you. Part of you thinks "Oh, well this is good. It makes *my* work more pleasant." But part of you is uneasy. You know that when someone has a drastic mood change, something serious can be going on psychologically. What would you do first? What questions would you ask to find out more about her emotional state? Who else needs to know about this sudden mood change? What procedures do you follow to communicate your uneasiness?

21. Your older client is a very religious man who uses a wheelchair. He lives with one of his daughters. The other daughter visits regularly. Today you arrive to see that the daughter is visiting and has begun what looks like very heavy cleaning. The client is waiting for his bath and breakfast. You understand from something the daughter says that she thinks the house is dirty and that you have not been doing your job. What would you do first? What is the best attitude to have when approaching the daughter? How do you feel? Can you find out how she feels? Why will it help to know how she feels? What is the main message that you want to get across?

UNIT 4
Safety

KEY TERMS

emergency medical
   technician (EMT)
evacuate

fire extinguisher
hazard
P-A-S-S

peripheral vision
RACE

LEARNING OBJECTIVES

After studying this unit, you should be able to:

- Identify the conditions in aging that contribute to the incidence of accidents

- Identify five causes of accidents around the home

- List five precautions to use when a client is receiving oxygen

- List four ways to make the home safer for a client with dementia

- Discuss the various types of fire extinguishers

- Discuss home health aide safety outside the client's home

- State the basic rules to follow in the event of a home fire

- List five safety tips for the home

Common Hazards

According to the National Safety Council, at least 4 million people are injured each year in home accidents. This means that about 1 person in 50 suffers some kind of injury as a result of an accident that occurs in the person's home.

In addition to actual physical hazards (dangerous), human factors are directly related to many home accidents. Statistics show that certain kinds of accidents happen most often in specific age groups (Figure 4-1). Most of these accidents can be prevented.

Young children must be carefully watched at all times. Parents should be aware of the actions of teenagers. Adults should use good judgment and not attempt to do too many things at one time. Carelessness and accidents go hand-in-hand. Because home health aides care for clients in the home, they should be aware of potential hazards in this environment (Figure 4-2).

An aide should be aware of the effects of medication on the client. Painkillers or tranquilizers can cause clients to become so unsteady that they may fall if they get up from a chair or bed without assistance. If an aide observes that a client becomes disoriented and loses balance easily after taking medication, the aide should inform the case manager. Sometimes clients have such reactions because of the interactions between several medications or too high a dose of a single medication. It is important that the aide is observant for any abnormal behavior the client may exhibit.

Falls and Risks

As the human body ages, the bones become brittle and break easily. Broken hips are a common injury among the elderly.

Many clients may need canes, walkers, or wheelchairs. Before a client uses a cane, walker, crutches, or other device, make certain that each rubber tip is firmly in place and has not worn through.

Some hazards may be avoided by providing a safer environment. Stairways and landings should be kept uncluttered (Figure 4-3). Children's toys, such as skateboards, balls, blocks, and roller skates, must be put away after use. Waxed and polished floors and stairways can be very dangerous. Scatter rugs in hallways should have a skid-proof backing or be removed completely because they pose a safety hazard in the home. Spills on kitchen and bathroom floors should be wiped up at once so that falls may be avoided.

Do not permit the client to walk about with untied shoelaces. Tripping over the laces can result in serious injury. If the client cannot reach the laces to tie them, the home health aide should tie the laces so they do not present a hazard.

The bathroom is one of the most dangerous rooms in the house for accidents. Bath mats should have a rubber backing so they will not skid. Bathtubs should be equipped with nonskid rubber strips to decrease the danger of slipping when getting in and out of the tub. For older adults, special handrails should be installed to assist them as they use the tub or shower (Figure 4-4). A bath chair should be provided for some elderly clients (Figure 4-5). Faucets for hot water should be clearly marked so that accidental scalding will not occur. Special elevated toilet seats and handrails make it easier for clients to use the toilet safely, especially after knee or hip replacement surgery (Figure 4-6). An unused walker can be placed around the toilet backwards, so that a client has something to hang onto when sitting down on or getting up from the toilet.

Another reason clients may fall is due to poor lighting. When elderly clients get up in the middle of the night, it takes their eyes a few more seconds to adjust from the dark to the lightness of the room. Check to make sure the walker and glasses are by the bedside. The path to the bathroom should have good lighting. Many older adults get up in the middle of the night to use the bathroom; they may not wait a few seconds for their eyes to adjust to the light. It is advisable to keep a night-light on in the bedroom so the adjustment from dark to light is minimal. Another reason for falls by the elderly is due to the loss of peripheral vision (side vision), which means they can see only things straight ahead and not on the sides.

If you recognize any unsafe conditions such as loose handrails on outside steps, or if you have suggestions to make the client's home safer, inform the case manager.

Risks for Burns

The older adult client may have an altered sensation due to the natural process of aging. This may be due to decreased nerve impulse transmission or altered circulation, which puts the elderly at risk for burn injury. In the older adult, pain sensation is often lessened, their reaction time is slower, their ability to smell diminishes, and their ability to adjust their sight from darkness to light is slower, which makes them very vulnerable to accidents. Burns may be fatal to both the young and the elderly client. Therefore, it is important for the home health aide to check the temperature of the water prior to the client

Age	Accidents
Infants up to 1 year are physically active and willing to touch or taste most anything.	Falls from a bed or table Burns from stoves or heaters Swallowing small objects Small objects stuffed in ears Smothering in bedding/pillows Cuts from sharp, pointed toys Choking on candies or food, toys, or coins
Preschool children are curious and extremely active. They explore most everything by looking, tasting, and touching. They have few fears and no judgment.	Scalding from pulling pot handles on stove Electrocution from playing with electrical cords and outlets Burns from stove or radiators or playing with matches Poisoning from pesticides or cleaning supplies, lead-based paint chips, medicines Falls from chairs, tables, countertops, open windows, or falls into deep holes in ground Drowning in unattended pools Smothering in discarded refrigerators, freezers, and plastic bags Cuts from kitchen knives
Preteen children are adventurous and not aware of dangers. They become involved in play and do not watch for hazards.	Injuries from bicycle and auto accidents. Hit by car when darting into street or between parked cars Poisoning Drowning
Teenagers like to experiment and are influenced by their peers (others in their age groups). They like to show off and are careless.	Injuries from auto, motorbike, or bicycle accidents because of carelessness, drunkenness, or drug abuse Wounds from accidents with guns Burns from careless smoking habits Injuries from carelessness with tools and machinery Drug overdose
Adults have fewer accidents because learning is based on experiences. Self-control and judgment are better developed, but overconfidence, negligence, and carelessness may cause accidents.	Burns from careless use of outside fire, and inside fireplace; from overloading electrical circuits; from smoking in bed Electrical shock from attempting to repair home electrical problems Using table or chair for climbing instead of sturdy ladder Automobile accidents from carelessness, cell phones, texting, or not wearing a seat belt Overdose of medications from failure to read labels
Old age causes many changes within the body; bones are brittle, eyesight and hearing are impaired. Minor accidents may cause great bodily harm.	Falls Burns Cuts and bruises Overdosing because labels cannot be read due to poor eyesight

FIGURE 4-1   Age-related accidents.

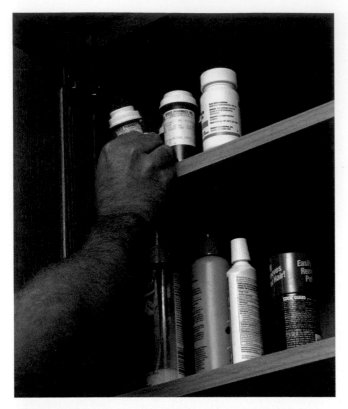

FIGURE 4-2 Keep medication and cleaning supplies in cabinets on a high shelf.

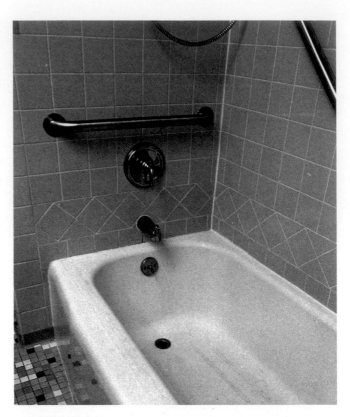

FIGURE 4-4 Grab bars and nonskid strips in the tub prevent falls.

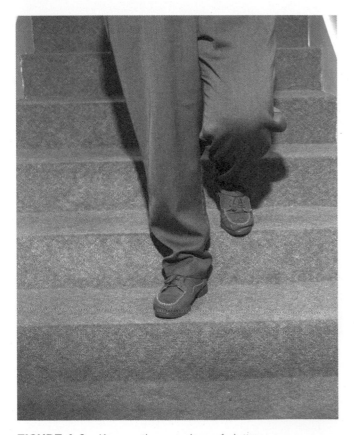

FIGURE 4-3 Keep pathways clear of clutter.

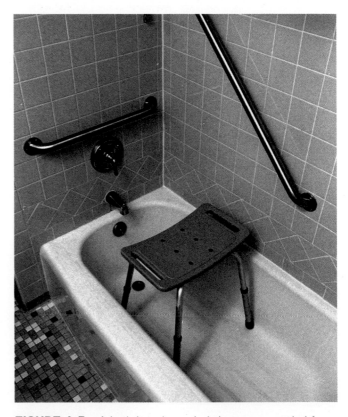

FIGURE 4-5 A bath bench or chair is recommended for the unsteady client.

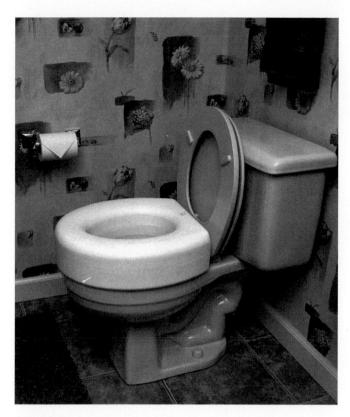

FIGURE 4-6 Raised portable toilet seats are used for clients with hip and knee problems.

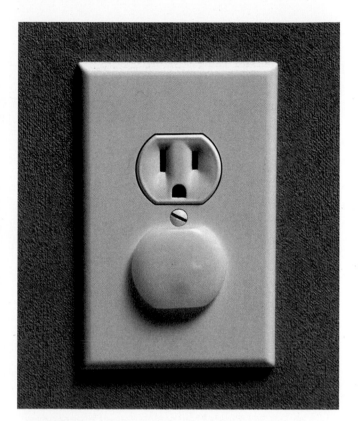

FIGURE 4-7 Electrical outlets should be covered to prevent potential injury to toddlers.

entering the tub or shower, whether the client is young or old. A helpful hint is to run the hot water first and then the cold when preparing for a bath. When cooking in the kitchen, if feasible have the client use the front burners, so there is no reaching over the burners. Oven mitts need to be worn to prevent burn injury when removing food items from the oven. When cooking over the stove, be sure that the client has clothing with short sleeves or closed sleeves. If the client is a little unsteady, fill the coffee cup two-thirds full to prevent the hot coffee from scalding the client's hand.

Matches and lit candles need to be out of children's reach. No youngster should be left unattended while in the kitchen to ensure that no injury can occur from the stove. If the client smokes, make sure there are large ashtrays close by.

Fire

Few words are more frightening to hear than "Fire, fire!" The smell of smoke or the flash of flames from the kitchen stove can cause panic. Some people are stunned and unable to function. Others rush around wildly trying to save their belongings. The home health aide should advise the client and the client's family whenever a fire

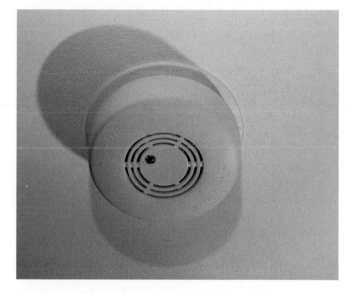

FIGURE 4-8 Smoke alarms should be standard equipment in the client's home.

safety problem is noticed. If there are toddlers in the home, electrical outlets should be covered with plugs, as 2- to 3-year-olds like to touch and feel everything in sight (Figure 4-7). Smoke alarms should be standard equipment in the client's home (Figure 4-8).

As a home health aide, there are basic rules to follow in case a client's home, or something in it, catches on fire. Remaining calm is the first and most important rule. Lives can be saved if an emergency plan has been made beforehand. A home health aide, on entering a client's home, should make note of the nearest exit from each room. In addition to the phone numbers listed in Figure 4-9, there should be a complete list of the client's medication handy in case the health care provider or **emergency medical technician (EMT)** has a question about a possible drug reaction. The emergency numbers posted in the client's home should be in large, easy-to-read print.

The aide must consider the client's condition and decide the best way to move the client in case of a fire. At the time of the fire, other decisions also must be made:

1. Determine if the fire is major. If it is minor, put it out at once, following the directions given in Figures 4-10A, 4-10B, and 4-11.

2. Decide if there is time to call the fire department before you **evacuate** the client. If there is no time, move the client and call the fire department from a phone outside the house or your cell phone.

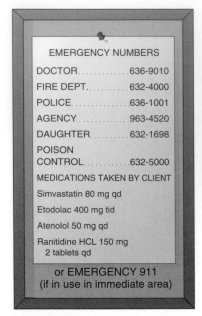
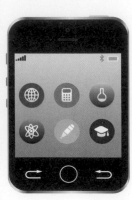

EMERGENCY NUMBERS

DOCTOR	636-9010
FIRE DEPT	632-4000
POLICE	636-1001
AGENCY	963-4520
DAUGHTER	632-1698
POISON CONTROL	632-5000

MEDICATIONS TAKEN BY CLIENT

Simvastatin 80 mg qd

Etodolac 400 mg tid

Atenolol 50 mg qd

Ranitidine HCL 150 mg
  2 tablets qd

or EMERGENCY 911
(if in use in immediate area)

FIGURE 4-9 Important phone numbers and medications taken by the client should be in large print and posted next to the phone, which may save precious moments at the time of an emergency.

Basic Rules in Case of Fire

1. Know the location of the nearest fire alarm box in the area.
2. Know how to phone for the fire department.
3. Remember the location of the nearest exits.
4. Close any door that will tend to confine the fire.
5. See that everyone is out of danger.
6. Know where a fire extinguisher is located and how to operate it. Check batteries of smoke alarms regularly.
7. Never try to fight a fire in a room filled with smoke; the fumes and lack of air are dangerous.
8. Never try to enter a room where much fire is in evidence.
9. Remember that a woolen blanket or other heavy covering will help to smother a small fire.
10. Keep boxes of baking soda handy to extinguish kitchen fires. The boxes can be kept in the refrigerator so you will always be able to find them.
11. Use baking soda instead of water to extinguish small grease, oil, paint, varnish, and similar fires, because water spreads such a fire. Dust the flames with baking soda; this smothers the flames physically and chemically with carbon dioxide gas.
12. Smother small grease fires in cooking utensils by covering them with a lid or long-handled pan, or by throwing baking soda on the blaze.
13. Extinguish small broiling pan fires by first turning off oven and then throwing handfuls of baking soda on the blaze.
14. Throw baking soda on small fires in ashtrays, wastebaskets, or upholstered furniture.
15. Do not try to be a hero. If the small fire does not respond to your efforts to extinguish it immediately, remove the client and yourself from the house as quickly as possible. Call the fire department from a neighbor's house, or flag down passing motorists and ask them to call.

FIGURE 4-10A Basic rules for the home health aide to follow in case of fire in the client's home.

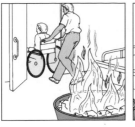
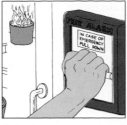
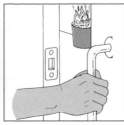
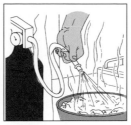
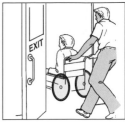

Remove   **A**ctivate   **C**ontain   **E**xtinguish or   Evacuate

FIGURE 4-10B   Remember the sequence of critical actions in case of fire in an assisted-living facility.

First aid—what to do	Home Fire Escape Plan

If you catch on fire:
DON'T PANIC. DON'T RUN–RUNNING WILL INCREASE THE FLAMES. Instead:
 	
1. **Stop.**
2. **Drop** to the ground.
3. **Roll.** Continue to roll until you have completely put out the fire.
4. Remove clothing from the affected area. *Do not attempt to remove clothing that sticks.*
5. Flush area with cool water.
6. Cover with a sterile pad or clean sheet.
7. *Seek immediate medical attention.*
 	
If the burn is from a chemical:
 	
1. Follow steps 4–7 and be sure to flush with cool water for 20–30 minutes.
2. If the eyes are involved, flush the eyes for at least 20 minutes or until medical attention arrives.
3. Remove contact lenses.
 	
If the burn is electrical:
 	
1. Turn off electrical source before touching victim.
2. Check for breathing and pulse. If absent, start cardiopulmonary resuscitation (CPR), if qualified.
3. Follow steps 4–7.
	• Develop a Family Escape Plan.
	• Include two exits from each room.
	• Plan a meeting place outside the home.
	• Practice the plan.
	
	Plan of Escape:
	Evacuate!
	Do not attempt to fight the fire.
	
	1. If in bed, roll off onto the floor.
	2. Stay low! Crawl if necessary. Smoke rises, and oxygen will remain near the floor.
	3. Cover your mouth and nose with some clothing or material to aid in breathing.
	4. Place your hands on any closed door before opening it. If it is hot, *do not open!* Find another exit. If it is not hot, open it slowly, standing to the side. *Do not use elevators.*
	5. *If you are trapped in a room:*
	  a. Roll a rug or other materials and place across the bottom of the door.
	  b. Open a window, both top and bottom, to allow air to enter and smoke to escape.
	  c. Call on cell phone for help, if possible.
	  d. Attract attention and call for help.
	
	(For further information, call The Burn Center at New York Hospital-Cornell Medical Center, 535 East 68th Street, New York, NY at 212-472-6890.)

FIGURE 4-11   First aid—what to do.

3. If the client or family members are in immediate danger, evacuate them at once.

4. If the client cannot be moved safely, and you are trapped in the client's home, go into a room with a door and window. Close the door and place a rolled blanket, towel, or sheets (wet, if possible) at the bottom of the door to keep the smoke out. Place some signal in any available window that will attract the attention of firefighters.

5. An aide needs to be aware of any fire danger prior to it happening. A good way to approach a fire situation is to remember the word **RACE**. As an aide, you might want to post this information on the refrigerator door.

R—**remove** the client from harm

A—**activate** the alarm or call 911

C—**contain** the fire

E—**extinguish** the fire

Waiting for the fire department to arrive is difficult for the home health aide and family members. Under no circumstances should the aide return to the burning building. Family members and neighbors also should be stopped from returning to the building. No personal possession is valuable enough to risk a human life.

Fire Extinguishers. Small fires may be extinguished by using a fire extinguisher. There are four main types of fire extinguishers, each of which is used for a specific type of fire.

1. *Class A extinguishers* contain water that is under pressure. They are used to douse fires involving paper, wood, or cloth.

2. *Class B extinguishers* contain carbon dioxide. They are used to put out fires caused by igniting gasoline, oil, paints or other liquids, and cooking fats. These types of fires would spread if water were used to extinguish them. The carbon dioxide smothers the fire, leaving a white powder residue. These extinguishers should be used with caution because the residue they leave may irritate the skin and eyes. Fumes also may be dangerous to inhale.

3. *Class C extinguishers* contain dry chemicals and are used on electrical fires.

4. *Class ABC* or *combination extinguishers* contain a graphite-like chemical. They can be used on any type of fire. The residue that results from their use can cause irritation of the skin and eyes.

If an aide uses a fire extinguisher on a minor fire, the manufacturer's operating instructions must be followed carefully. Most extinguishers have a lock on the handle that must be unlocked before use (Figures 4-12A and B). The extinguisher should be held firmly and the nozzle aimed at the base of fire. **CAUTION:** Do not aim toward the center of the fire. Discharge the extinguisher, using a slow side-to-side motion, until the fire has been extinguished. Avoid contact with the chemical residues from the extinguisher. To prevent personal injury, the aide always should stay a safe distance from the fire.

An easy-to-remember method for operating a fire extinguisher is to follow the letters P-A-S-S.

P   **Pull** the pin at the top of the extinguisher that keeps the handle from being pressed. Break the plastic or thin wire inspection band as the pin is pulled.

A   **Aim** the nozzle or outlet toward the fire. Some hose assemblies are clipped to the extinguisher body. Release the hose and point.

S   **Squeeze** the handle above the carrying handle to discharge the contents of the container. The handle can be released to stop the discharge at any time. Before approaching the fire, try a very short test burst to ensure proper operation.

S   **Sweep** the nozzle back and forth at the base of the flames to disperse the extinguishing agent. After the fire is out, watch for remaining smoldering hot spots or possible reflash of flammable liquids. Make sure that the fire is completely out.

Once an extinguisher has been used in a fire, it must be replaced or recharged.

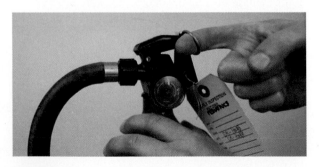
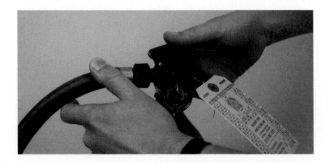

FIGURE 4-12   Use of the fire extinguisher. A. Remove pin. B. Push top handle down.

Safety Checklist

Just by checking one of the following, you may save a life:

- Are all medications in the containers they came in and clearly marked?
- If your client smokes, are there adequate large ashtrays in rooms the client smokes in?
- Are there smoke alarms on every level of the house? If the client is hard-of-hearing, is there a smoke alarm with a louder alarm?
- Are space heaters placed away from furniture and curtains?
- Are oily rags disposed of correctly?
- Does the home have a carbon monoxide alarm?
- Are cleaning supplies stored in a safe place and clearly marked?
- Are flammable items—gasoline, paint remover—stored in proper containers in a safe place?
- Are the outside steps and sidewalks free of ice and snow?
- Do light fixtures have the correct wattage bulb? (As clients age, they require more light.)
- Do the door locks work?
- Is the furnace in good working order? Have the filters been changed? Does the thermostat work and is it set at the proper temperature?
- Is the water temperature set at 120° or less?
- Is it easy for the client to get mail?
- Would a night-light be useful?
- Are doorways, hallways, and steps unobstructed?
- Do frequently used steps have nonskid strips?
- Are electrical outlets covered, if there are toddlers in the house?
- Are electrical outlets overloaded? Are electrical extension cords placed in safe areas?
- Are grab bars needed and in place in the bathroom?
- Would a sturdy shower or tub bench be beneficial in transferring?
- Would your client benefit from a lifeline or a cell phone?
- Is the client's furniture functional? Can he or she easily sit down and get back up?
- Are guns stored in a locked cabinet with shells removed?
- Do scatter rugs have nonskid backing if client insists on using scatter rugs?

Tips for Handling Oxygen Equipment

The following do's and don'ts apply to oxygen equipment in the client's home:

- Do not allow smoking around oxygen equipment; this includes friends and relatives of client.
- Do treat all oxygen-handling equipment with care. Store the equipment in a clean, dry location. Remember, oxygen is combustible.
- Do maintain the oxygen-handling equipment exactly as instructed.
- Don't allow the oxygen equipment near grease or oil.
- Turn off the oxygen tank if not in use, as it is quite expensive.
- Don't use equipment that is visibly dirty, in poor repair, or damaged.

Tips for Home Safety with Client with Dementia

Here are a few tips to make a home safer for a client with dementia:

- Place additional locks on inside doors, preferably high up, so that the client cannot easily locate them (if the client is living with someone).
- Lower the temperature of the hot water to less than 120 degrees to prevent the client from being burned.
- Decorate with solid colors, as patterns make the home more confusing.
- Put safety knobs on top of the stove, so the client cannot turn it on when someone is not there.
- Put safety locks on cabinets or drawers that contain potentially dangerous items such as knives and cleaning supplies.

- Keep a night-light on at night, as this will reduce confusion if the client with dementia wakes up.
- Make sure client has an ID bracelet.
- Remove locks on bathroom doors, as the client might lock the door and forget to know how to unlock it.
- Keep furniture in the same place and try to create a clear path for the client to walk.
- Do not overly decorate for holidays, as the decorations can cause further confusion for the client.
- Replace live indoor plants with artificial plants, as the client may like to pick and chew on leaves.

Safety Outside the Client's Home

The home health aide must be aware of safety issues outside the client's home as well as within. The aide must be "streetwise" and safe. To be streetwise, each aide must:

1. Be alert.
2. Be observant.
3. Trust his or her own instincts.
4. Know how and when to call 911.

Do's and Don'ts

- Do have identification on.
- Do not bring money or credit cards into the client's home.
- Have a cell phone to easily access your case manager or client.
- Do not wear flashy jewelry.
- Do leave the client with access to a phone.
- Do track your visit to the client's home with your home care agency with the use of your computer or cell phone.

Safety When Walking

- Plan the safest route.
- Choose well-lighted streets, not alleys.
- Take the long way if it is the safest.
- Cross the street and head for a busy, well-lighted area if you are followed.
- Do not hitchhike.
- If you feel at all threatened, leave the area immediately and call your case manager.

Safety When Driving

- Keep your car in good running condition.
- Plan the safest route and have an alternative route in case of highway closure, and use your global positioning system (GPS) if you have one.
- Have your keys ready when approaching your car.
- Drive with your doors locked. Pull over if you need to use your cell phone.
- Park in well-lighted areas.
- Stay in your car when you see a street or motorist problem; use your cell phone to call for help.
- If you leave valuables in your car, be sure to lock it.
- Keep a flashlight, map, and water in your car. Many times home health aides are making visits after dark and in rural areas. Directions to clients' homes may not be clear.

WORKBOOK REVIEW

Go to the workbook and complete the review exercises and activities for Unit 4.

REVIEW

1.   T   F   Hazards may be avoided by providing a safer environment.

2.   T   F   The most common accidents for older adults are falls, burns, cuts and bruises, and poisoning because labels cannot be read due to poor eyesight.

3.   T   F   The bathroom is the most dangerous room in a home.

4.   T   F   Grab bars, nonskid strips, and bath chairs are assistive devices that can increase the safety and security of the elderly client.

5.   T   F   Painkillers or tranquilizers can cause a client to become unsteady and fall.

6.   T   F   A common cause of accidents with preschool children is scalding from pulling pot handles on the stove.

7.   T   F   Clutter on stairways can cause an older adult to fall and fracture a hip.

8.   T   F   In case of fire the aide should remember the following:
Remove the client from harm
Activate the alarm or call 911
Contain the fire
Extinguish the fire

9.   T   F   If a client is receiving oxygen, the client is not allowed to smoke, but it is okay for relatives and friends to smoke while visiting with the client.

10.   The types of fire extinguishers available for home use are
   a.   Class A extinguishers that contain pressurized water and are used for paper, wood, and cloth fires.
   b.   Class B extinguishers that contain carbon dioxide and are used for gasoline, oil paint, and cooking fat fires.
   c.   Class C extinguishers that contain dry chemicals and are used for electrical fires.
   d.   all of the above.

11.   List six items to check in order to make the home safer for an elderly client.

_____

_____

_____

_____

_____

_____

12. List four ways to make the home safer for a client with dementia.

_____

_____

_____

_____

13. Explain what the following initials stand for in P-A-S-S.

P _____

A _____

S _____

S _____

Case Studies

14. You are scheduled to service a client who lives alone in a small house. The client has just had eye surgery and should not bend over. The bedrooms and bathroom are on the upper level; the living room, dining room, and kitchen are on the lower level. Some of the flooring is linoleum, and some is wood. There are rugs in some of the rooms. The client often leaves things on the stairs so that she will remember to transfer them. There is an overhead light in the bedroom and bathroom and a smoke detector in the hallway near the bedroom. Next to the rear exit the client saves newspapers, glass, plastic, aluminum, and tin containers for recycling. How would you make her environment safer?

15. What actions can you as a home health aide take to remain safer when you are traveling to and from your client's home?

UNIT 5
Homemaking Service

KEY TERMS

chronic obstructive
  pulmonary disease
  (COPD)

closed bed
dyspnea
fanfold

incontinent
mitered corner
occupied bed

open bed
unoccupied bed
vomitus

LEARNING OBJECTIVES

After studying this unit, you should be able to:

- List at least four tips used to plan and organize tasks

- Explain how to care for major home appliances

- Name three factors that determine the home health aide's cleaning plan

- List five cleaning tasks done daily

- List five cleaning tasks done weekly

- Describe the correct method for separating and disposing of garbage

- Identify at least four steps used in cleaning a kitchen

- Identify at least four steps used in cleaning the bathroom

- Explain how you would clean up a blood spill

- Discuss extra tasks that need to be done if there are pets in the home

- List in order the linens used to make a regular bed using a lift sheet

- List five guidelines for bed making

- Describe the differences between a closed, open, occupied, and unoccupied bed

- Demonstrate the following:

  PROCEDURE 1 Changing an Unoccupied Bed

  PROCEDURE 2 Changing an Occupied Bed

Household Management

Managing a household is like operating a daily 24-hour business. Homemakers raise children, manage a budget, provide a clean and livable house, prepare and serve meals, and handle home accidents. This requires intelligence, understanding, and physical labor. Homemakers are good at multitasking.

Many home health aides have a basic knowledge for keeping up a house. However, the habits developed in their own homes may not be suitable in all work situations.

The units covering homemaking skills are presented to introduce homemaking techniques to the beginner. However, even the experienced homemaker may learn some helpful new tips.

The home health aide should realize that each home situation may offer different challenges. A professional home health aide must adapt to the physical surroundings of each job. This adjustment requires the use of whatever environment and supplies the client has available. The home health aide must remember to show as much care for the property of others as is shown for his or her own personal property. The equipment and furnishings used by the home health aide belong to the client. Considerate and cautious care must be used. If equipment has frayed cords or if appliances do not work, they should be repaired.

When performing regular household duties, the aide should make a list of any items in short supply. Toilet paper, laundry products, food, or other necessities should be purchased before the house supply runs out.

Sometimes a home health aide handles the client's money. Always get a receipt for any purchases you make and place the receipts in a special place. If there is any doubt about what an item costs, or if the client has any questions as to where the money was spent, you can quickly verify your expenditures. Honesty in money matters is an absolute necessity.

When you are in a client's home and the client requests a cleaning job done a certain way even though you know a better way, you should follow the client's directions.

A few of the homes you will be going to might be very dirty and unkempt; if you are assigned to work at such a home for 3 hours, for example, you will not be able to clean it in that short time and get everything spotless. Your client might think differently and expect you to complete all cleaning tasks. If this situation exists, you need to discuss it with your case manager.

Planning and Organization

An important duty of the aide is to plan, organize, and carry out tasks completely. The aide who plans the work,

organizes the tasks, and starts doing them will find the workload lightened. A home health aide will be given instructions for each assignment. The care of the client is of primary importance, but the household tasks cannot be ignored. The aide should take a few minutes each morning to plan the tasks that should be completed by the day's end (Figure 5-1). This can save time and energy.

- Carry a pad and pencil. Make a note of household supplies that may be needed in each room.

- Before starting to clean a room, the home health aide should stop to think which cleaning supplies may be needed. All the supplies needed to complete the work in a particular room should be taken to the room at one time. Carry cleaning supplies from room to room in a plastic container or basket.

- Prevent buildup of dirt by tidying rooms, dusting, wiping surfaces, and sponging up spots as soon as possible.

- Keep a sponge in the kitchen and bathroom for quick wipe-ups.

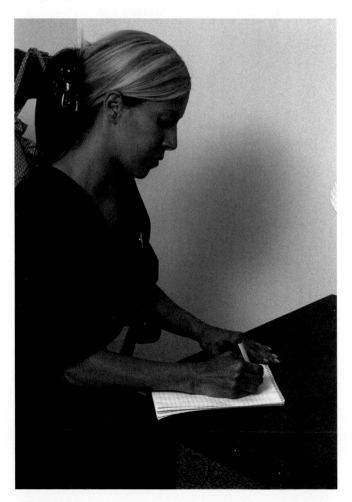

FIGURE 5-1 An aide planning her work and listing the supplies she will need.

- Schedule major jobs for a certain day of the week. For example, vacuum and wash floors on Friday so the house will be ready for weekend use; launder and iron one day; plan weekly shopping trips for Mondays or Wednesdays.
- Learn how to use and care for the equipment in the home (Figure 5-2). Most appliances have an instruction manual; read the manual before using an appliance. After using equipment, clean it so it will be ready for the next use.

Basic Cleaning Supplies

The following is a list of supplies needed to maintain a clean home and do laundry. There are many brands of each available on the market—whatever is available in the client's home is what you will use. Always read the labels.

- all-purpose cleaner
- baking soda
- bleach—liquid or powder
- broom and dustpan
- cleaning cloths
- stain remover for carpets
- stain remover for clothing (e.g., Spray 'n Wash)

- dishwashing soap
- dishwasher soap (automatic)
- disposable gloves
- fabric softener for clothes
- furniture polish—spray or liquid
- glass cleaner
- laundry detergent
- paper towels
- scrub pail
- steel wool or small scrubber
- toilet cleaner and brush
- vacuum cleaner
- vinegar

Combining Client Care and Household Tasks

The order in which tasks are done is not always important. If you know what should be completed by the end of the day, the work can be arranged around the client's needs. For example, after the client's bath and after the

Dishwasher	Clean exterior with mild cleaner and wipe dry. Clean interior with wet cloth. Use only recommended amount of soap when running a load.
Dryer	A full load of wet clothes placed in a dryer contains about one-half gallon of water. As water is removed from the clothes, lint is created. A clothes dryer is one of the most expensive appliances in the home to operate. The longer it runs, the more money it costs. Clean the lint filter after each load to increase dryer efficiency.
Freezer	Defrost at least once a year. If frost-free model, remove foods and wipe inner surface with damp cloth and baking soda. Look at the dates on food items and if outdated items are found, with the client's permission, place them in the garbage.
Garbage disposal	Run cold water during disposal and for a minute after. Never put glass, metal, or rubber into the disposal unit. If odors should occur, they can be removed by running orange or lemon peel through the unit.
Microwave oven	Wipe clean with wet cloth and soap. Rinse and wipe dry.
Refrigerator	Clean outside and inside with soft wet cloth and mild soap or baking soda. Open the refrigerator door and scan the inside for rotten or spoiled food. Dispose of any rotten or spoiled food.
Stove/oven	Wipe up spills and grease at once especially around the burners.
Washing machine	Wipe the exterior with a soft wet cloth. Remove the lint filter, turn it inside out, and wash the lint off.

FIGURE 5-2 Guide for cleaning and maintenance of household appliances.

bed linens are changed, the home health aide may decide to clean the client's room. The kitchen could be cleaned after the breakfast meal. The client's bathroom cleaning could be done after the bedpan has been used and emptied into the toilet bowl. These examples show how to pair client care procedures with homemaking duties. This technique saves time and energy by eliminating many extra steps each day.

Maintaining a Clean Home Environment

The home health aide is not normally expected to do general cleaning in the client's whole home; these tasks are often done by a cleaning service. However, if you are assigned to do the cleaning, here are a few factors to consider:

- Needs of the client
- Size of the home
- Ages of people living in the home
- Number of people living in the home
- Time allowed for you to complete the assigned tasks
- Cleaning supplies available

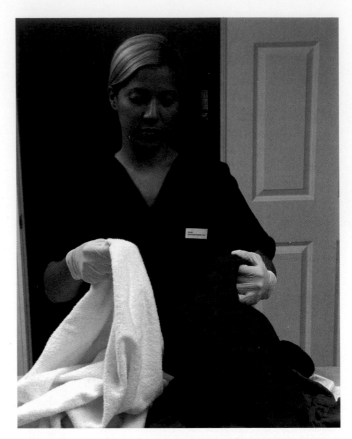

FIGURE 5-3   Sorting laundry.

The Client's Laundry

First check the clothes for stains and sort out the clothes that need to be presoaked (those with stains) or sprayed with a stain remover (Figure 5-3). Separate the whites from the colors; then separate light colors from dark colors. Then separate the lint generators—towels and sweatshirts—from lint magnets, such as corduroy or permanent-press clothes. If you have delicates like bras, silk shirts, or silk pajamas, wash them separately. As you sort, remember to close zippers to prevent snagging and to empty all pockets. For dark clothes like black jeans, turn the jeans inside out when washing, as this will prevent the jeans from picking up lint. As each item is sorted, check it for spots that may need special care. Collars of shirts and dresses and spots from food or other stains may need special care. Take special precautions if washing red clothes. Liquid bleaches should only be used on white cotton; use only the amount stated on the container.

Wear gloves if handling contaminated linens. Don't shake the linens. When loading the washing machine, don't just dump the clothes into the machine. It's important to distribute the clothes evenly. The weight of the

clothes should be evenly balanced around the inside cylinder in order to prevent the cylinder from spinning off its track during the wash, and to ensure that the clothes are washed evenly. Be careful not to overload the washer. It is better to do two loads, as in the long run it will save wear and tear on the machine. Read the directions on the label to determine how much detergent to use. Most manufacturers include a scoop for powdered detergent and a measured cap for liquid detergent. However, keep in mind that each detergent is different, and hence should be used according to the manufacturer's instructions or the machine's user's manual. Too much detergent can cause overflow problems or form clumps in the folds of the clothes, which may not wash out. Add a sufficient amount of fabric softener; this will depend on the make and style of the washing machine. Close the machine and turn the dial to the correct setting. Use the proper water temperature: hot for white, warm for colors, cold for bright colors.

Drying Clothes

Place the clothing into the dryer. Do not put items such as bras, silk pajamas, and other delicates into the dryer, unless your client directs you to do so. Most dryers have a range of minutes you can set, depending upon what types of material are in the dryer.

Once the clothing is dry, remove and fold the laundry and place it in a designated location. If you remove the items right away, there is less chance of wrinkles setting in. Permanent-press clothing needs to be removed right away or it will become quite wrinkled.

Ironing

Today there are very few items that need to be ironed. If you need to iron a dress shirt or a dress, turn on the iron to the correct setting according to the fabric you are ironing. Once the iron has reached the desired temperature, start ironing. If it is a shirt, iron the collar first, then the sleeves, and then the body of the shirt. Spray starch may be used to give the shirt a smoother, nonwrinkled appearance. Finally, place the item on a hanger until thoroughly dried and return it to the closet.

Laundry tasks are rather easy if you have good working equipment and the equipment is located conveniently in the client's home. Timing is important, as it will take at least 30 minutes to wash one load and at least 30 to 45 minutes to dry the load. Potential problems arise when the dryer no longer dries clothes or the washing machine does not drain the water out as it should—in such cases you will not be able to complete your tasks in the time allocated. Another problem that could occur is if the client lives in a multiunit apartment building and you must use the commercial machines in the basement or common area of the building. You will need to run back and forth from the laundry room to the client's apartment, which can be a time-consuming task. Also, you need to arrange a time to do the laundry when other individuals are not using the machines. On some occasions you will need to leave the client's home and do the laundry at a laundromat.

Cleaning the Bathroom

You may clean the toilet first or last. When cleaning the toilet, place the toilet cleaner etc. Starting with the toilet first, place toilet cleaner, bleach, or vinegar in the bowl and swish the solution around with a toilet brush, paying special attention to the area under the rim of the bowl (Figure 5-4). If time allows, leave the solution to set a while and then flush the toilet. Clean the sink, countertops, and shower or tub with a disinfectant solution. This will help kill the germs. Everything in the bathroom except the mirror can be cleaned this way in just 3 to 4 minutes

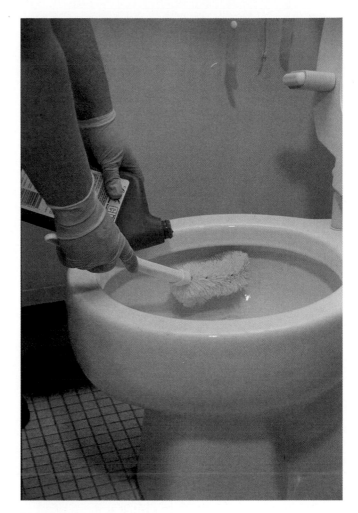

FIGURE 5-4 Cleaning the toilet bowl.

a day. Use a large sponge and clean the floor with an all-purpose cleaner or spray, unless the floor is carpeted. Also, a squeegee can be kept in the shower so that everyone can wipe it down when they are done. If the bathroom has an unpleasant odor, place a fabric softener sheet in the wastebasket or add a dab of fragrance on a light bulb. When the light is on, the heat releases the aroma.

Cleaning the Kitchen

The best advice is to clean as you go; work from the cleanest to the dirtiest areas.

Dishes

Separate dishes and wash them in the following order—glasses, silverware, plates and cups, and, last, do the pans. Rinse the dishes under hot water and let them air-dry, if possible. Air-drying is more sanitary than drying with a dish towel. If you are unable to wash the dishes right after a meal, rinse the dishes and soak the pans in warm, soapy water.

Many homes are equipped with dishwashers. Before placing dishes in the dishwasher, scrape and rinse them well. Place the correct amount of automated dishwasher soap into the correct location. Close the door tightly and push the correct button to start the machine. Run the dishwasher only if it is full to conserve energy. It is better to wash sharp knives and plastic glasses by hand.

Cleaning Kitchen Countertops

Use a mild dishwashing liquid on countertops and rinse well afterward to prevent residue from getting on food. After cutting fresh meat or vegetables directly on a countertop, be sure to wipe it off with hot water and soap immediately to prevent the spread of germs.

Cleaning Kitchen and Bathroom Floors

If time and space allow, move chairs and other items on floor before mopping. Sweep first, then mop with a mild soap and rinse with clean warm water or plain diluted vinegar. An old toothbrush works well for cleaning off dirt that may have accumulated in certain areas of the floor.

Cleaning Cabinet Exteriors

The cleaning product used for cabinets will depend on the type of material the cabinets are made of. If wood, clean with a solution of warm water and a small amount of mild soap (like Ivory) on a soft cloth. Dry with another soft cloth. If painted or other artificial finish such as Formica, use a mild cleaning solution or spray on the cabinets and dry with a clean cloth. If in doubt, ask your client what you should use to clean the exterior. Remember that kitchen work never ends, but it still can be challenging and satisfying when done well.

Cleaning Safety Tips

Don't mix cleaning products such ammonia and bleach. Such mixtures can be toxic. If you need to clean up blood on a kitchen or bathroom floor, use a solution of 1 part bleach to 10 parts water and wipe up the blood spill while wearing disposable gloves (Figure 5-5). Cleaning supplies should be stored in a place that children and disoriented adults cannot reach.

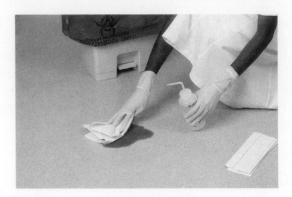

FIGURE 5-5 To clean up blood and body fluid spills, use a solution of bleach and water.

Cleaning Tasks If There Are Pets in the House

As much as your clients love their pets, they can create cleaning headaches. Due to mud-spattered paws, hair on the furniture, pet odor, and occasional accidents, the home health aide could spend quite a bit of time cleaning up after the pet.

Bathe and brush the pet regularly to minimize the amount of pet hair and pet dander, and to help with odors. Keep a wet sponge handy to quickly pick up loose pet hairs. A vacuum cleaner with a beater brush is necessary to pick up the hair in the carpet; a vacuum cleaner without a beater brush will not do the trick. Use a pet rake, a brush with crimped nylon brushes, to remove pet hair from fabrics and upholstery. To remove pet urine stains from carpeting, dilute the spot using a cloth dampened with water. Then clean the area with a solution of vinegar and water—1 teaspoon of vinegar to 1 quart of water.

Daily Cleaning Tasks

The following are duties that should be done every day. Daily cleaning should not require longer than an hour a day.

- Pick up toys, magazines, newspapers, wet towels, and clothing. Do not discard any of these items without the permission of the client.
- Make the beds.
- Empty ashtrays and wastebaskets. Separate cans, glass containers, and other recyclables from the garbage.

- Do the dishes and wipe off the countertops.
- Clean the top of the stove.
- Sweep the kitchen floor.

Weekly Cleaning Tasks

Weekly care can be done in more than one way. A load of laundry can be done every day or done all in one day. How and when the laundry should be done will be clearly stated in the care plan. The following tasks need to be done on a weekly basis:

- Change the bed linens.
- Water the plants.
- Dust the furniture—use a flannel or other soft cloth for dry dusting and another for polishing. Pour polish onto the polishing cloth.
- Vacuum floors and carpets, getting under the furniture; if need be, move furniture to vacuum completely.
- Damp or wet mop the floors in the kitchen and bathroom.
- Clean all mirrors with glass cleaner.
- Wipe the television screen off with soft cloth—be sure the TV is turned off before cleaning.
- Wipe off switch plates and door handles with a soft, wet cloth.
- Using a brush and bowl cleaner, clean the inside and the outside of the toilet. Be sure to scrub the area under the top rim of the bowl and also the toilet seat.
- Wipe out the tub or shower and sink with cleanser and disinfectant.

Periodic Cleaning Tasks

Certain areas in the home do not require frequent cleaning. The following tasks can be done on an occasional basis:

- Remove cobwebs from ceilings, walls, and drapes.
- Clean the window blinds.
- Remove pictures from the walls and dust behind them. Dust the frames and glass.
- Clean the light fixtures.
- Remove books from shelves and dust both the books and the shelves.

- Clean the inside of windows.
- Straighten up drawers and closets.
- Launder small area or throw rugs.

Variables When Changing Bed Linens

If you work in a hospital or long-term care facility, there are usually only one or two different types of beds requiring linen changes, and a supply of clean bed linens will be readily available for your use. In home care, however, this will vary greatly. Every home will have a different type of bed and different size and texture of bed linens to work with (Figure 5-6). In some cultures, individuals do not sleep in beds but rather on mats that they roll up during the day. In a few homes, you may find regular hospital beds that can be either electrically (Figure 5-7) or manually operated. You will need to be flexible and versatile in when and how you change the bed linens.

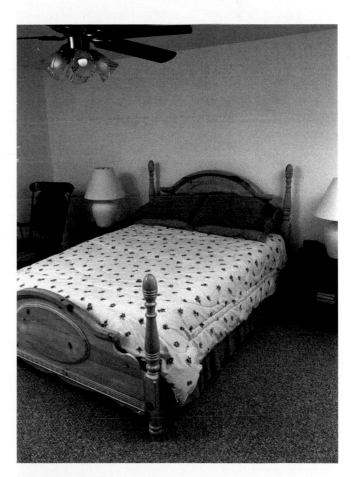

FIGURE 5-6 Closed bed.

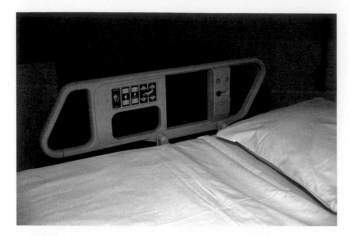

FIGURE 5-7   Hospital bed with electrical controls.

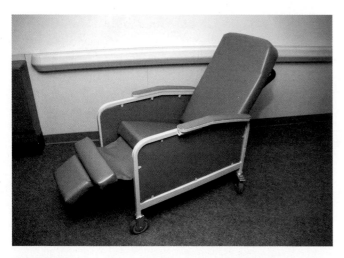

FIGURE 5-8   Clients with respiratory problems often sleep in a lounge chair like this one.

One client may have 10 sets of sheets, whereas the next client will only have one set. As a home health aide, you will never find two homes alike, two clients alike, or two families alike. Every time you start working with a different client, you will encounter a different set of variables to work with. Occasionally, you may have a client with respiratory problems such as **chronic obstructive pulmonary disease (COPD)**. These clients suffer from **dyspnea** (difficulty breathing) and shortness of breath. They are unable to sleep in a regular bed and often spend 24 hours a day in a lounge or recliner chair (Figure 5-8). The chair is their bed, and in this scenario, instead of changing linens on a bed, you will change them right on the chair.

Be sure to ask input from your client on how he or she wants the bed made. If your client is 80 years old and has been making the bed a certain way for all of his or her life, follow the client's directions unless told otherwise. Your case manager will help to work through each different

circumstance, and as you gain more experience, you will be able to problem-solve the situations you are placed in.

Linens

Following is a list of linens generally needed to change a regular bed:

- mattress pad
- fitted sheet
- chux or lift sheet
- flat sheet
- blanket
- bedspread
- two or more pillowcases

Guidelines for Bedmaking

These bedmaking guidelines should be followed:

- Collect the linens in the order you will use them.
- Remember to hold linens away from your uniform.
- When making a bed, do not shake the linens, as this will spread germs.
- A flat sheet may be used in place of a fitted sheet on the bottom of the bed.
- Textures of linens vary greatly—they generally are made from cotton, flannel, or jersey knit.
- Bed linens come in a variety of colors—try to match the colors in a set.
- Blankets can be cotton, wool, down, or handmade quilts.
- If the client has an air mattress or foam egg-crate mattress on the bed, a fitted bottom sheet will stay in place better than a flat sheet.
- If the bed linens are soiled with urine or **vomitus** (material vomited), wash the soiled bed linens as soon as possible to prevent germs from spreading and decrease odor in the home. Always wear gloves if linen is soiled with body fluids.
- Place soiled linens on a chair or in a plastic bag, rather than on the floor.
- To preserve bed linens and decrease unpleasant odor in the home, use adult briefs on clients who are **incontinent** (unable to control urination).
- Plastic protective covers on pillows may be used if the client is incontinent.
- If the pillow has a zippered end, place this end in the pillowcase first.

- A hospital bed can be elevated to the aide's working height when changing bed linens, which will prevent back injuries. When finished changing the unoccupied bed, always check to see if the bed looks neat and wrinkle-free.
- Check the client's care plan for positioning the head and foot of the bed, the number of pillows to use, and the use of pillows in positioning.
- Mattress pads, blankets, and bedspreads generally do not need to be routinely changed unless they are soiled.

Bed Terminology

When changing linens on a bed or making the client's bed, the home health aide needs to be familiar with the following terminology:

occupied—the bed is being made with the client in it.
unoccupied—the bed is being made without the client in it.
closed—the client is out of bed and the linens are pulled up to the top of the bed (see Figure 5-6).
open—the client is out of bed, but the linens are **fanfolded** (folded in pleats; Figure 5-9) to the foot of the bed (Figure 5-10).
mitered corner—special corner made on beds to keep the linens in place and give a neater appearance to the bed; sometimes called a hospital corner.

See Procedure 1: Changing an Unoccupied Bed and Procedure 2: Changing an Occupied Bed.

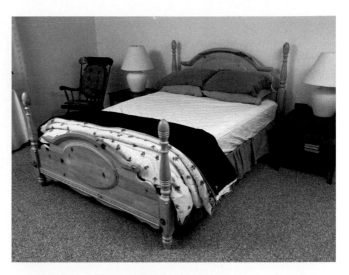

FIGURE 5-9   Open bed.

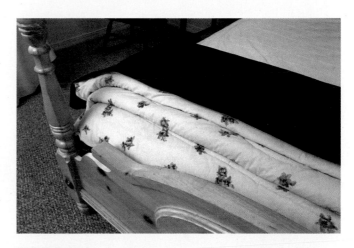

FIGURE 5-10   Fanfold top linens to the foot of the bed.

PROCEDURE 1   CHANGING AN UNOCCUPIED BED

Purpose
- To apply clean and fresh linens to a bed
- To add to the client's comfort by removing wrinkled or soiled sheets

Procedure
1. Wash your hands and assemble supplies:
   - 2 pillowcases
   - bedspread (optional)
   - top sheet
   - blanket (optional)
   - lift sheet or Chux
   - fitted sheet
   - mattress pad (optional)
   - disposal gloves (optional)

2. Strip bed of soiled linens and place in laundry. Blanket and bedspread can be reused, if not soiled. Do not allow dirty linens to rub against your uniform. Roll linens in and away from yours body. Wear gloves if there is a chance of contact with blood or body fluids.

(continued)

PROCEDURE 1   CHANGING AN UNOCCUPIED BED (*continued*)

3. Wash your hands.
4. Place mattress pad on bed (if it needed to be changed) and then put a clean fitted sheet or flat sheet on bed. If a flat sheet is being used, unfold the sheet with the long fold at the center of the bed. Place the lower hemline even with the bottom of the mattress (Figure 5-11). If a fitted bottom sheet is used, fit it properly and smoothly around one corner (Figure 5-12).
5. Apply the lift sheet or Chux, if used.
6. Place the top sheet on the bed. Place the hem even with the top edge of the mattress.

Place the center fold at the center of the bed. Tuck in the top sheet at the foot of the bed.
7. Place the blanket back on the bed. Put the top edge 12 inches from the top of the mattress. Place the bedspread on the bed.
8. Tuck the blanket, spread and top sheet under the bottom of the mattress at the foot end of the bed. Miter the corners (Figures 5-13A–I). Fold the top sheet over the top edge of the blanket.
9. Walk over to the opposite side of bed and make the remaining part of the bed.
10. Put pillowcases on the pillows. Do not hold the pillow under your chin while putting it into the case.

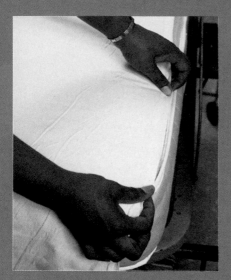

FIGURE 5-11   Place the flat bottom sheet even with the end of the mattress at the foot of the bed.

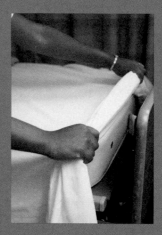

FIGURE 5-13A   Gather about 12 to 18 inches of top sheet at the bottom of the bed.

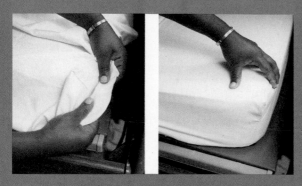

FIGURE 5-12   If a fitted bottom sheet is used, fit it properly and smoothly around the corner.

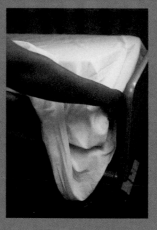

FIGURE 5-13B   Face the foot of the bed and lift the mattress with your nearest hand.

(*continued*)

PROCEDURE 1   CHANGING AN UNOCCUPIED BED (*continued*)

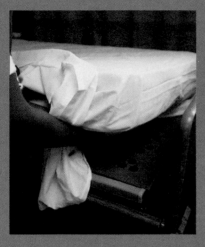

FIGURE 5-13C   With your opposite hand, bring the sheet smoothly over the end of the mattress, continue to the mitered corner.

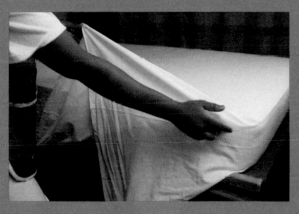

FIGURE 5-13D   To make a mitered corner, pick up the sheet hanging at the side of the bed, about 12 inches, forming a triangle.

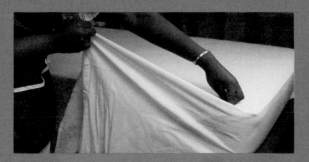

FIGURE 5-13E   Place your finger on the bed to form a sharp corner.

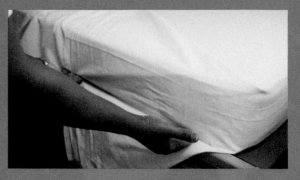

FIGURE 5-13F   Using two hands, tuck the sheet well under the mattress.

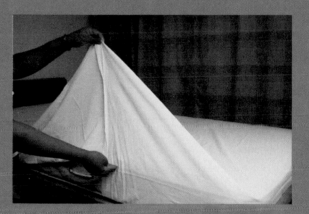

FIGURE 5-13G   Using your fingers as a guide, allow the sheet to drop straight down,

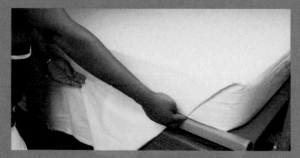

FIGURE 5-13H   The finished corner will look like this for a top sheet.

11. Wash your hands.
12. Document the completed tasks.

(*continued*)

PROCEDURE 1   CHANGING AN UNOCCUPIED BED (*continued*)

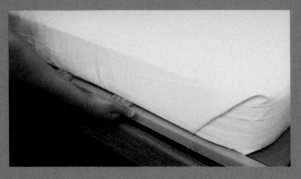

FIGURE 5-13I   The finished corner should look like this for a bottom sheet.

PROCEDURE 2   CHANGING AN OCCUPIED BED

Purpose

- To apply clean linens while the client remains in the bed
- To add to the client's comfort by removing soiled and wrinkled linens.

Procedure

1. Wash your hands and assemble supplies. Wear gloves is there is a chance of contact with blood or body fluids.
2. Assemble clean linens—flat sheet and fitted bottom sheet (if available) and extra flat sheet or Chux if used by the client.
3. Tell the client what you plan to do and provide for the client's privacy by closing the bedroom door.
4. Place clean linens on a clean chair or table in the room in the order in which you plan to use them.
5. Loosen bedding from under the mattress by lifting the mattress with one hand as you pull out the bedding with the other hand.
6. Remove the top covers one at a time, folding each to the foot of the bed.
7. Leave the top sheet covering the client to prevent chilling and to afford privacy.
8. Place two straight chairs against one side of the bed; this helps protect the client from falling out of bed. If the bed has side rails this is not necessary; simply raise the side rail on the opposite side of the bed.
9. Assist the client to turn to the side facing the chairs or side rail. Assist the client to move near the edge of the bed by the chairs. Stand at the other side of the bed.
10. Roll or fanfold (fold in pleats) the soiled bottom sheet to the center of the bed beside the client's back.
11. Fold the clean bottom sheet lengthwise and place the fold at the center of the bed. Fanfold half of the clean sheet next to the soiled sheet. Tuck the other half under the mattress. Make a mitered corner at the top. Tuck the sheet from the top or head of bed and move toward the foot of the bed.

(*continued*)

PROCEDURE 2 CHANGING AN OCCUPIED BED (*continued*)

12. Help the client turn toward you onto the clean sheet. Bring the chairs to the other side of the bed for the client's protection (or raise the side rail).
13. Go to the other side and remove the soiled sheet. Place soiled linens in a large plastic bag.
14. Pull a clean sheet across the bed and tuck it under the mattress. Make a mitered corner at the top and tuck alongside from the head to the foot of the bed. Make certain the sheet is tight and wrinkle-free.
15. Turn the client onto his or her back in the center of the bed. Place a clean top sheet over the soiled top sheet. Slide the soiled sheet out from under the clean sheet. Have the client hold the fresh top sheet in place.
16. Place the soiled sheet in a large plastic bag.
17. Unfold the blanket and bedspread and place them over the top sheet.
18. Tuck in the bottoms of the sheet, blanket, and bedspread at the foot of the bed. Miter the two corners; leave extra room for foot and toe movement.
19. Change the pillowcases and replace the pillows under the client's head. Put soiled cases in a large plastic bag.
20. Be sure the client is comfortable and that the room is neat. Remove the soiled linens from the room.
21. Wash your hands.
22. Document the procedure completed.

WORKBOOK REVIEW

Go to the workbook and complete the review exercises and activities for Unit 5.

REVIEW

1. When deciding on a cleaning plan, you should consider which of the following?
   a. The needs of the client
   b. The size of the home
   c. The ages of the people living in the home
   d. All of the above

2. Which of the following is *not* a tip for loading the automatic washing machine?
   a. Empty shirt pockets and pants pockets.
   b. Distribute laundry equally in the drum.
   c. Unzip all zippers.
   d. Check collars and the fronts of shirts for stains.

3. List five daily cleaning tasks.

   _____

   _____

   _____

   _____

   _____

4. List five weekly cleaning tasks.

   _____

   _____

   _____

   _____

   _____

5. T   F   Always wear gloves when handling wet linens.

6. T   F   It is wise to add twice the amount of laundry soap to the washing machine, as this will make the clothes much cleaner.

7. T   F   Leaving the clothes in the dryer for at least an hour after drying will prevent wrinkles from forming.

8. T   F   Use only a strong all-purpose cleaner with hot water when scrubbing a kitchen floor.

9. T   F   To decrease the amount of germs in the bathroom, use a disinfectant cleaner when cleaning the sink and tub.

10. Name five different types of linens needed to change a client's bed.

    _____

    _____

    _____

    _____

    _____

11. List five guidelines to remember when changing the linens on a client's bed.

    _____

    _____

    _____

    _____

    _____

12. Describe the following different types of beds:

Closed bed _____

Occupied bed _____

Unoccupied bed _____

Case Studies

13. You are scheduled to service an incontinent client. When you arrive you encounter piles of laundry, dirty floors, cluttered rooms, soiled bed linens, dirty dishes in the sink, and no food in the refrigerator. The client needs a bath and is hungry but wants to go for a walk to the park. How would you respond to the client's request? How would you organize the other chores on your care plan?

14. You are assigned to do the following tasks in the home for Mr. Tan, a 95-year-old man who is paralyzed on his right side: shower, oral care of dentures, shave, apply topical ointment to both legs, change his bedding, walk outside for at least two blocks, cook two balanced meals, do his laundry for the week. You are allowed 4 hours to do the tasks. How would you plan your work?

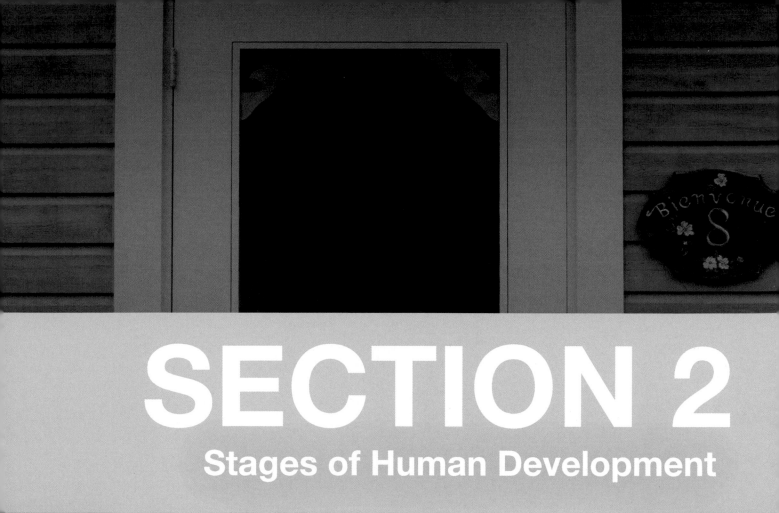

SECTION 2
Stages of Human Development

Unit 6
Infancy to Adolescence

Unit 7
Early and Middle Adulthood

Unit 8
Older Adulthood

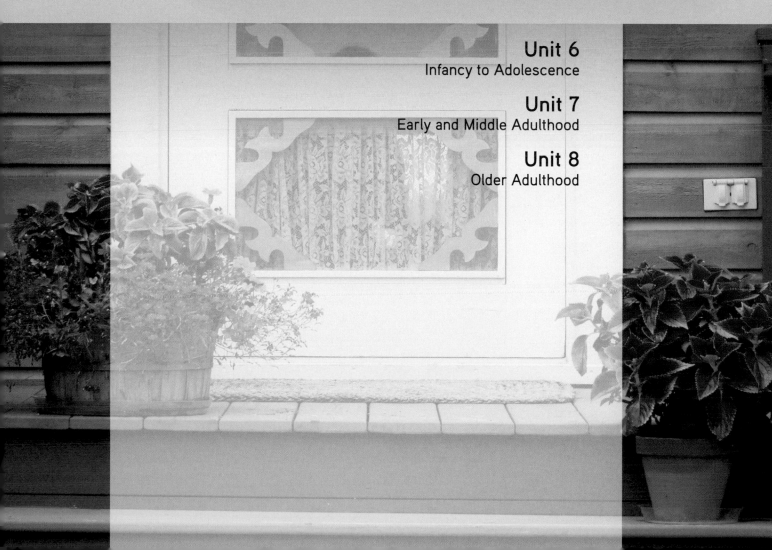

UNIT 6
Infancy to Adolescence

KEY TERMS

adolescence
autism or autism
  spectrum disorder
bonding
cerebral palsy
child abuse
conception
cystic fibrosis

developmental
  disabilities
fetal alcohol syndrome
  (FAS)
fetus
gestation
gestation period
hierarchy

learning disorder
low-birth-weight
obstetrician
physiologic
premature
puberty
self-actualization

sexually transmitted
  disease (STDs)
sibling rivalry
substance abuse
sudden infant death
  syndrome (SIDS)
whooping cough

LEARNING OBJECTIVES

After studying this unit, you should be able to:

- Discuss issues dealing with pregnancy and childbirth

- Explain the bonding of the father, mother, and infant

- Discuss Maslow's five basic needs

- List four abnormal conditions or diseases of infancy and early childhood

- Describe four common childhood illnesses

- List three signs of fetal alcohol syndrome

- List five safety checks for young children

- Describe three characteristics of toddlers

- List three characteristics of preschool-aged children

- Discuss the seat-belt requirements for infants and preschool children

- List three developmental tasks of adolescence

- Discuss smoking, use of illegal drugs, and alcohol abuse in adolescence

- Define child abuse

- List four behavioral patterns associated with abused children

- Discuss when and how to report cases of child abuse

Becoming a Family

An aide who is assigned to care for a newborn infant and the mother is usually going into a happy environment. If it is a first child, both parents may be very attentive toward the baby and watch its every move. Of course, the newness wears off, and suddenly they are faced with a demanding, dependent human being for whom they are entirely responsible. Even so, this is usually a positive assignment.

Pregnancy

Conception is the fertilization of the female egg by male sperm. This union forms the fetus. The time from conception to birth is called the gestation period. When a woman is pregnant, it is essential that she receive prenatal care either from a health care provider or a midwife. Many complications of pregnancy and birth disorders may be prevented by proper prenatal care. It is an important duty as a home health aide to encourage your client to seek prenatal care. If the client is pregnant, the aide should encourage the client to eat a balanced diet, not smoke or drink alcoholic beverages, and only take medication ordered by the health care provider.

Labor and Delivery

Infants are most often delivered by a health care provider in the hospital. However, in some areas, this situation is changing. There has been increasing use of midwives and other birthing options as alternatives to hospital births. Normally, a woman goes into labor and delivers the baby with the assistance of an obstetrician. The baby moves from the uterus into the vagina and passes out of the body. This normal process can be eased, however, by use of medications, health facilities, and trained personnel.

Bonding is a process of attachment of mother, father, and infant that occurs after birth of the child. It is important to remember that each family member bonds differently and at different rates. The newborn infant is placed on the mother's abdomen skin-to-skin so that both parents can make eye contact with the child and feel and cuddle the infant. This initial contact is important because it assists in creating positive emotional ties between the parents and child and the child and the parents. Cuddling and fondling are important in the first few months of the newborn's life. The home health aide needs to encourage a new mother and father to hold, talk, and play with the baby often. The newborn needs to develop a sense of trust and security to develop into a trusting and secure adult (Figure 6-1).

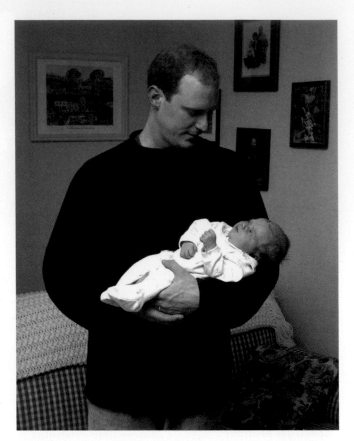

FIGURE 6-1   Father bonding with infant.

Normal Infant Growth and Development

As an infant grows, both physical and mental abilities develop. In the first month, infants are quite helpless. They totally depend on others to meet their basic needs. According to American psychologist Abraham Maslow, all human beings have a hierarchy (ladder) of five basic needs. He suggests that higher types of needs can only be gratified after a person's basic needs have been met. Maslow's hierarchy is best understood by imagining a triangle shape. At the base of the triangle is the first basic human need, which is physiologic in nature, that is, the need for food and shelter. After the physiologic needs are met, the second basic need is for safety. Moving up the hierarchy triangle, the third basic need is the need for love and belonging. The fourth basic need is for esteem, which refers to achievement and recognition. The fifth basic need, at the tip of the triangle, is for self-actualization, the highest human need, which is the desire to reach one's fullest potential (Figure 6-2).

Maslow's hierarchy of needs shows the importance of meeting basic human needs beginning in infancy

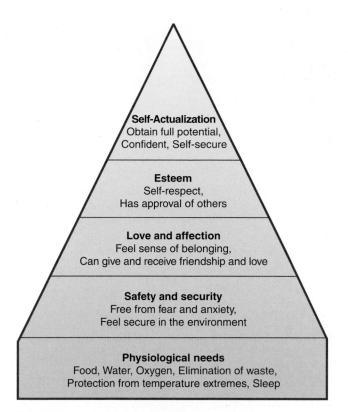

FIGURE 6-2   Maslow's hierarchy of needs.

and moving throughout the life cycle. For instance, the newborn must be fed, changed, cleaned, kept warm and clothed properly, and kept safe and secure. Infants also need to be held and cuddled. Giving love to the infant fulfills a basic need. When these needs are met, the child should have every chance to grow up to be a happy, confident, and fulfilled person.

By age 2 months, babies can raise their heads and may cry when they want to be picked up. Crying is the infant's way of communicating that he or she needs something. Through trial and error, parents gradually come to understand the needs of their infants. As infants develop, they notice lights and sounds and begin to babble. They get used to certain patterns, especially the times to eat and times to sleep. Usually by the fourth month an infant sleeps 8 to 12 hours at night and naps during the day. Regular schedules of meals, activities, and sleep are needed and should continue throughout the first year.

Normal Weight Gain

Normally, infants weigh between 5 and 9 lb (2.3 to 4.1 kg) at birth. During the first 5 days, a weight loss of several ounces is expected. Until birth, all the baby's needs are supplied within the uterus through the umbilical cord.

Birth is a shock to the baby's system, and it takes a few days for the infant's body to adjust. When the body starts to function normally, a weight gain of 6 to 8 oz (0.17 to 0.23 kg) a week is normal. Birth weight is usually tripled by age 1. In the second year, weight increases at a rate of 0.5 lb (0.23 kg) per month.

Health Problems in Infancy and Early Childhood

Some infants are born with diseases, injuries, or malformations. These abnormalities may be inherited through the parents' genes or may result from diseases or drugs present in the mother's body during pregnancy. Common abnormal infant conditions are described in Figure 6-3. Children with these conditions need special medical and emotional care. The aide may need to help the mother and family members adjust to meeting the child's special needs.

One condition that often causes problems is premature birth. An infant born before full term (before 37 weeks of gestation) is considered premature. A newborn weighing less than 5 lb may be premature. However, some babies are full term yet weigh less than 5 lb. A newborn with this condition is called a low-birth-weight baby. The average weight of newborns is between 6 and 9 lbs.

Another condition of infancy that caregivers should be knowledgeable about is sudden infant death syndrome (SIDS), which is when an infant stops breathing for unknown reasons while asleep. This condition usually occurs in infants under 1 year of age. It is now recommended that babies be placed on their backs, rather than their stomachs, when sleeping to help prevent SIDS. If breathing disorders are suspected in an infant, a monitor may be placed on the infant so that an alarm is sounded if the baby stops breathing.

Common Childhood Illnesses

Strep Throat

Strep throat is a bacterial infection that is spread via droplets in the air from the nose or throat. A throat culture is usually done to identify the strep organism. If the culture is positive, the child is placed on a 10-day course of antibiotics. Clinical manifestations may include sore throat, enlarged lymph nodes (swollen glands), headache,

Condition	Description	Treatment
PKU Phenylketonuria	Body is unable to break down a certain amino acid. Mental retardation, convulsions, and eczema are common.	Specific diet begun early in infancy prevents symptoms. Test for PKU at birth.
Cerebral palsy	Defect, injury, or disease of the brain tissue, which causes lack of muscle coordination and possible paralysis; person has shaking and muscle spasms with poor balance.	No cure, but treatment varies and may include muscle relaxants, orthopedic surgery, use of casts or braces, exercises.
Congenital heart disease	Malformation of vessels, valves, or chambers in the heart; results in faulty circulation and usually cyanosis.	Surgery often is successful in restoring normal functioning.
Down syndrome (trisomy 21)	Chromosome abnormality causing various degrees of retardation and typical physical malformations such as slanted eyes, broad hands with short fingers, and a protruding tongue.	No treatment, but many people can be taught to live with some independence.
Hydrocephalus	Defect in the absorption of cerebrospinal fluid; fluid builds up and increases the size of the head.	Common treatment is with surgery. Shunts are commonly used to divert fluid away from brain and into the abdomen.
Sickle cell anemia (thalassemia)	Abnormal sickle-shaped red blood cells break down easily and cannot transport oxygen efficiently; causes fever, blackouts, and pain. (More prevalent in African American populations.)	Blood transfusions. No cure.
Leukemia	Overproduction of immature white blood cells, anemia, internal bleeding; person has increased risk of infection, fever, pain in the joints, and swelling of the lymph nodes, spleen, and liver.	Chemotherapy
Tay-Sachs	Degeneration of the central nervous system; infant does not develop mentally; disease more often affects those of Jewish ancestry.	No cure; infant usually does not live beyond age 1 year.
Cystic fibrosis	Inherited malfunction of the pancreas, intestine, sweat glands, and respiratory system.	No cure; special diet and respiratory care to prolong life.
Cleft lip/cleft palate	Fetal growth is incomplete. Infant may have problems feeding. Cleft palate may alter tooth formation and cause speech problems.	Surgical repair; special feeding nipples and special therapy.
Fetal alcohol syndrome (FAS)	Set of signs, symptoms, and problems that newborn babies have if the mother drinks during pregnancy: (1) smaller baby, (2) small head, (3) weak heart or kidney problems, (4) failure to thrive, (5) peculiar-appearing flat face with narrow eyes and drooping lips.	No cure—supportive care. The child may experience some degree of mental retardation for the rest of his or her life.
Sudden infant death syndrome (SIDS)	Infant stops breathing while asleep.	Place monitor on infants with suspected breathing problems.

FIGURE 6-3 Abnormal conditions in infants that may require medical attention, long-term adjustments, and services of the home health aide for the child and family.

and fever. Treatment is necessary to prevent the spread to other individuals, as well as to prevent rheumatic fever, a serious complication. Rheumatic fever can occur 5 to 6 weeks after an untreated strep infection. Clinical manifestations of this disease include joint pain, and eventually it may affect the valves of the heart. Children can return to day care or regular school after being on the antibiotic for 24 hours with no fever present.

Pinkeye—Bacterial Conjunctivitis

Pinkeye appears as redness of the white part of the eye with development of pus in the eye. There is little or no pain felt by the child. It is treated with antibiotic eye drops. Pinkeye is highly contagious, and children are usually kept out of school or day care until their eyes have had time to heal.

Croup

Croup is caused by several respiratory viruses. Cold symptoms are followed by a "barking" cough, and the child typically wakes at night with cough and some difficulty breathing. Treatment consists of cool humidified air. For persistent coughing at night, take the child outside into the cool night air or open a window in the bedroom (bundle up as needed to prevent chilling). Seek medical help for any labored breathing.

Whooping Cough

Whooping cough is an acute contagious respiratory illness that affects children and older adults. Respiratory symptoms include a runny nose and a repeated cough that ends in a forced intake or breath of air, or "whoop" sound. Treatment is symptomatic and supportive. Whooping cough can be prevented by immunizations.

Influenza

Influenza is a contagious respiratory illness that most often occurs during the winter and early spring. Respiratory symptoms include sudden onset of fever, chills, congestion, cough, sore throat, body aches, and headache. Treatment depends on the degree and severity of symptoms. Medical doctors recommend a yearly flu injection to prevent this contagious disease.

Rotavirus (Diarrhea/Vomiting)

When a small infant or child has mild to severe vomiting, diarrhea, abdominal cramping, and foul-smelling stools, it is often caused by this virus. Treatment depends on the severity of the diarrhea and vomiting.

Otitis Media (Middle Ear Infection)

Otitis media is caused by an increased amount of fluid and inflammation in the ear, causing the eardrum to bulge. It can be quite painful. A small child may tug his or her ear and be fussy due to the discomfort. Other signs include drainage from the ear and fever. A mild analgesic such as Tylenol® may be given for pain. A culture is taken from the ear and the child is usually placed on a regimen of antibiotics. If untreated, otitis media can lead to hearing loss or other serious complications of the ear canal and brain.

Developmental Disabilities and Learning Disorders

Developmental disabilities are mental or physical impairments, usually apparent at birth or before the age of 7, that are likely to continue indefinitely and may result in substantial functional limitations that require lifelong or extended care. Examples of these disabilities are cerebral palsy, mental retardation, and autism.

A learning disorder is a condition that affects an individual's ability to either interpret what is seen and heard or to link information from different parts of the brain. These disorders can cause difficulties with speaking and writing, coordination, self-control, and attention. Such difficulties extend to schoolwork and can impede abilities in learning to read, write, and/or do math.

Attention-Deficit/Hyperactivity Disorder (ADHD)

ADHD is a childhood mental disorder that is marked by inattention, hyperactivity, and impulsivity. Children who are inattentive have a hard time focusing their attention and may be bored with a task after only a few minutes. Children who are hyperactive always seem to be in motion; they cannot sit still and may display restlessness. Children who are overly impulsive seem unable to curb their immediate reactions or to think before they act. This disorder is more common in boys than girls.

Autism

Autism or autism spectrum disorder (ASD) is a disorder with a wide range of symptoms and severity seen in children. The child has difficulty in social communication and social interaction. *Example* would be failure of normal back-and-forth conversation; failure to initiate or respond to social interactions. The child's speech is often repetitive and stereotyped. The child displays repetitive behaviors, interests, or activities. *Example* would be lining up or flipping objects continuously. The child may insist on sameness and wants the routine the same. The child maybe hyper-aware of a jumble of details, yet they are often clueless about the big picture, missing social cues other kids perceive automatically. The child requires close adherence to specific routines and rituals. Treatment and care is individualized depending upon the communication and behavior deficits seen in the child.

Responsibilities of the Home Health Aide

Often a mother must leave one or more children at home while she is at the hospital. The aide may be assigned to attend to the children during this time period or after the mother has returned home with the newborn. The children are likely to want to be near the mother and may want to play with the baby. Sometimes older children are too rough with the baby even though they do not intend to be. The children also may be jealous of the new member of the family. This jealousy is called **sibling rivalry**. If such jealousy is noted, the home health aide should give the children extra attention. The aide can make the children feel important by giving them chores to do for the baby or mother. They should be praised for being helpful. Children may need help adjusting to the role of being a big brother or sister. The aide should be sure that the older children wash their hands before touching the baby to prevent the spread of germs and infections. If they have colds, they should be kept away from the baby until they are no longer contagious.

In addition to the older children, the aide cares for the mother and the newborn. These duties include:

- Bathing the infant
- Diapering
- Feeding the infant
- Preparing the formula
- Doing added laundry
- Caring for the mother
- Assisting the mother if she is breastfeeding
- Preventing accidents

Toddlers and Preschoolers

Ages 1 and 2 are known as the toddler stage. The toddler approaches life with a great deal of interest (Figures 6-4A and B). A favorite activity is exploring the immediate environment, which makes safety precautions a necessity. Toddlers want to be more independent and experiment with control—testing their parents' limits and discovering their own. This is a time when children start to show possessiveness with belongings and people close to them. At about age 18 months, their favorite word will often be "No!" As infants grow into toddlers, muscle coordination increases, and physical skills expand and improve greatly. Toddlers can speak several understandable words and can refer to themselves by name. They can recognize themselves in the mirror, they can walk well, and they feed themselves with a spoon and drink from a cup. By the time the child is 3 years old, he or she should be able to follow simple directions, be toilet trained, and

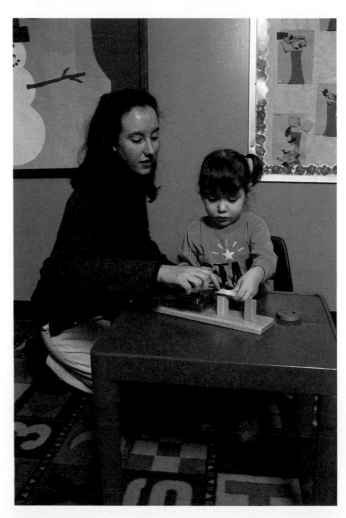

FIGURE 6-4A   The toddler begins to develop manual skills.

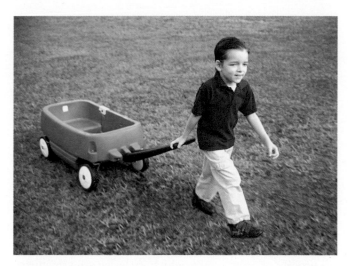

FIGURE 6-4B A child enjoys being outside engaging in active play.

communicate with others in short sentences or phrases. The child's attention span is longer and he or she enjoys playing alone but also likes to play with an adult. Most toddlers like to be outdoors to run and play. Remember that they need constant watching, whether indoors or outdoors, and they love one-on-one attention.

The period of time from 3 until 5 years is known as the preschool years. The child has never-ending energy and is always on the go. Preschoolers start playing with other children their age for a longer period of time and are able to do more complex physical tasks such as riding a tricycle, climbing a jungle gym, and tying their shoes (Figure 6-5). They can print their names and begin to recite the ABCs, and they love to ask questions. By the time the child is 5, he or she should be able to hop and skip on one foot, speak clearly, and be understood by others not in the family. The child can count to 40 and recognize various shapes. The caregiver needs to continue to monitor the child closely; be consistent, firm, and gentle in disciplining the child; and reinforce good social skills. If time allows, the aide may spend time coloring, playing ball, or engaging in other similar activities with the child.

Safety Concerns

Keeping a child physically safe is an ongoing responsibility. Accidents are the primary cause of death in children under 5 years of age, with the main cause being automobile accidents. Each year 1 million children are brought for medical care due to accidents; 40,000 to 50,000 children suffer permanent damage and 4,000 die. We know that most accidents can be prevented and that injuries from all accidents can be minimized.

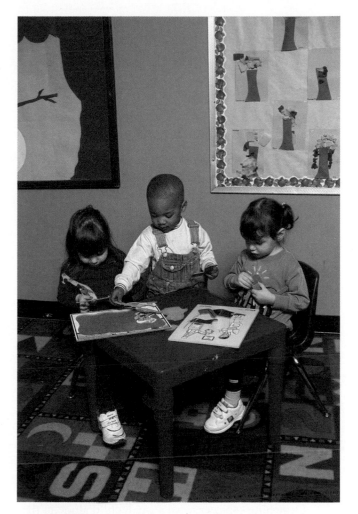

FIGURE 6-5 Learning to play with peers is important for preschoolers.

Childhood injury involves three elements: the child, the object that causes injury, and the environment in which it occurs. Here are several safety checks to ensure a safe environment for young children:

1. Infant car seat—Make sure the child rides in the backseat. The backseat is generally the safest place in a crash. Infants, car seats are positioned facing the rear until they are about age 1 and weigh at least 20 to 22 pounds. Children over the age of 1 who weigh at least 20 pounds may ride facing forward. Put the belt through the correct slot. The safety belt must stay tight when securing the safety seat. Make sure the harness is buckled snugly around your child. The harness should be adjusted so you can slip only one finger underneath the straps at the child's chest. Keep the straps over the child's shoulder. Have toddlers who weigh over 40 pounds use a booster seat. A belt-positioning

booster seat, used with the adult lap and shoulder belt, is preferred for children weighing 40 to 80 pounds. Seat belt rules vary from state to state. Check with your highway patrol office for your state's requirements.

2. Fire prevention—Do not let children play with matches. Check to ensure that the smoke alarm is working.

3. Choking—Do not put a pacifier or any object on a string around the baby's neck. Check toys for sharp edges or small parts. All foods for the baby should be mashed, ground, or soft enough to swallow without chewing.

4. Poisoning—Keep all medications and household cleaning products out of reach. Use safety latches on cupboards or drawers that contain items that might be dangerous.

5. Burns—Always check the water temperature before placing the baby in the bath. Never hold the baby while cooking at the stove or oven, drinking a hot liquid, or smoking.

6. Falls—Use gates at the bottom of stairways. Do not leave the baby on the changing table alone. Never leave a baby unattended on any surface above floor level.

7. Drowning—Never leave a small child alone in the bathtub or around any container with water in it, no matter the level of the water. This includes buckets, wading pools, and the toilet.

8. Strangulation—Keep strings from window blinds up and out of the way of a crawling or toddling baby. Do not place the baby's crib near window blinds, where the baby can reach the cords.

9. Have the child wear a helmet when riding a tricycle or bike.

School-Aged Children

A child beginning school often needs time to adjust to the new situation. The child may one day seem confident and secure and the next day be clingy and dependent. Some children find it difficult to leave the familiarity of home. However, most children enjoy school and being with other children. A school-aged child generally can follow simple instructions and be fairly independent.

It is important that children be given small jobs so that they feel a sense of responsibility. They learn that rules are necessary to make groups (family or school) work. Praise for achievements is better than punishments for mistakes. The school-aged child enjoys activities at home and away from home.

Adolescence

Adolescence refers to the years between the ages of 13 and 19, during which broad developmental changes occur, including intellectual, emotional, social, and physical changes. **Puberty**, on the other hand, is the physical process of growing up, which includes growth spurts, changing body shape, and maturation of the reproductive system. Pubertal changes occur gradually; they may start as early as age 9 or 10 and not be completed until about age 20 or even a little older in some people.

Physical Changes in Puberty

Puberty begins sometime between the ages of 10 and 15 when the endocrine system releases hormones in both boys and girls. At this time, the secondary sexual characteristics begin to emerge. In boys, hair on the face, underarms, and pubic region starts to grow and the voice deepens. There is usually a marked growth in both height and weight. At puberty, the testes, scrotum, and penis enlarge and the youth is able to produce sperm.

In young girls, the breasts develop and pubic and underarm hair grows. About every 28 to 35 days the mature female reproductive system releases one or more eggs (ova), and the menstrual cycle begins.

How easily adolescents deal with these changes will partly reflect how closely their bodies match the well-defined stereotypes of the "perfect" body for young men and young women. Adolescents who do not match the stereotypes may need extra support from adults to improve their feelings of comfort and self-worth. If a teenager is dependent on a home health aide for his or her personal care and other needs, this teenager will definitely need emotional support to accept his or her less-than-perfect physique.

Mental and Emotional Changes

The teenage years are profoundly influenced by both the physical and mental changes of adolescence. In our society, an adolescent reaches adult status when he or she is financially able to support oneself. Today, financial independence is generally not achieved until late adolescence or early adulthood, after the individual has completed some type of education and gained some entry-level work experience. Adolescents start to develop their own set of values and beliefs during this period.

Adolescents face many other challenges. They are trying to establish their sexual identities and feel comfortable with their bodies. Allow them privacy to do their personal care. They are testing independence; yet they are not, and do not want to be, totally independent. This is also the time when a teenager starts to drive, which is quite a hallmark in the teenager's life, along with a major social event, the school prom. Parents need to provide a supportive environment for adolescents to search and explore their identities and their new social roles in the community. Status within the community, beyond that of family, is an important achievement for older adolescents. The adolescent should be given an opportunity to make some decisions and be accountable for the consequences of those decisions. Teenagers are strongly influenced by their peer group (Figure 6-6). Open communication between parents and teenagers is healthy and important. If teenagers have a previous history of good communication with their parents, they will be willing to share their concerns and feelings with them. Parents and adults have an important role to play and can have a positive impact on the lives of adolescents. If you are a home health aide in a home where there is not good rapport between the adolescent and parents

and the teenager wants you to take sides, this may put you in a rather awkward position. The best advice is to stay neutral. Listen to what he or she has to say, which will convey your interest in the teenager's side, and that might be all that is needed.

As a home health aide, you rarely will be assigned to care for an adolescent unless there is a physical problem with the youth's health, such as an accident (body in a cast), childhood cancer, or other severe physical condition or behavior problem.

Common Health Problems

Adolescents are at an age of experimentation. They often express their independence by trying new things. For some adolescents, this experimentation leads to smoking, abuse of drugs or alcohol, gang involvement, or sexual experimentation.

Sex-related health problems are especially common with adolescents. An active sex life may pose health and emotional problems. **Sexually transmitted diseases (STDs)**, including the human immunodeficiency virus (HIV) and chlamydia, may bring about serious health problems. In addition, teenage girls must consider the possibility of becoming pregnant. Sex-related health problems often result from the adolescent having insufficient and inaccurate information.

Teenage Pregnancy.   In addition to an increase in STDs among teenagers, there is also the issue of unplanned teenage pregnancies. Many teenagers have sex without using contraceptives, and when they do seek family planning services, it often is too late.

Few teenagers are ready to handle the emotional and financial responsibilities that accompany pregnancy and parenthood. The decision to raise a child, place the child for adoption, or have an abortion is usually difficult for a teenage girl and her boyfriend.

Teenage girls are still growing themselves, both emotionally and physically. Even a healthy, well-adjusted teenager will feel the stress that pregnancy puts on her body. A teenage father may feel emotional stress.

Pregnancy can be prevented through use of planned birth control methods as well as abstinence from sexual intercourse. Teenagers who are sexually active should be made aware of the options available. Common birth control methods are the oral contraceptive pill, the diaphragm, the condom, and foam spermicidal. The rhythm method, which refers to using a calendar to plan not to have intercourse during a woman's ovulation

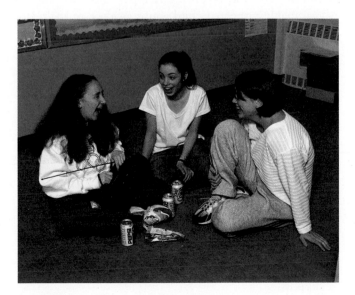

FIGURE 6-6 Peer relationships are important to adolescents.

period, is not very reliable. Condoms are recommended for the male to prevent unwanted pregnancy, and can reduce but not eliminate the risk of the STD transmission.

Religious and cultural practices may determine the type of birth control used. In any case, it is wise for the teenager to consult a health care provider, family planning clinic, or school nurse. The only advice a home health aide should offer is to mention that one of these professionals should be consulted.

Substance Abuse. Substance abuse is the use of alcohol or drugs that results in poor treatment of the body. Drug use among adolescents has been on the increase over the past 20 years. Smoking has increased, particularly among teenage girls, who often use it as a way to lose weight. The use of marijuana can lead to the use of harder drugs such as heroin and ecstasy. It is recognized that "pot" smoking, "pill popping," and the use of hard drugs have increased the crime rate and caused serious physical and mental health problems. Many families have been destroyed because of the aftermath of drug abuse by family members. Drug awareness programs are provided in schools to alert young people to the dangers involved in drug use.

Alcohol abuse has also become a major problem. Children as young as 6 and 7 years of age are abusing alcohol. Parents often are not as concerned about drinking as they are about other drugs. They seem to think that alcohol is less harmful than taking illegal drugs. In fact, youthful drinking is a serious and dangerous problem. Drinking can lead to cirrhosis of the liver in later life. It also can lead to permanent brain damage. Moreover, drinking is a major cause of death due to driving while intoxicated (DWI). Although it is illegal to drink under the age of 21, the consumption of alcohol by minors is still a problem. Alcohol is an accepted part of our adult society, but all too often its negative influence reaches the younger generation. Organizations such as Al-Anon and Alateen are educating drinkers and helping them to stop drinking for at least "one day at a time." DARE, or Drug Awareness Resistance Education, is a program organized to prevent young people from using illegal drugs and alcohol.

Child Abuse, Maltreatment, and Neglect

All states have child abuse and neglect laws that protect children under the age of 18 years. These laws regulate the conduct of the parent, guardian, custodian, or caretaker.

Most states define child abuse by a responsible person (parent, caregiver, friend, or relative) as the commission of any of the following acts:

- Inflicts or allows to be inflicted upon the juvenile a serious physical injury by other than accidental means
- Creates or allows to be created a substantial risk of serious physical injury to the juvenile by other than accidental means
- Uses or allows to be used upon the juvenile cruel or grossly inappropriate techniques to modify behaviors
- Commits, permits, or encourages the commission of crimes against the juvenile, including, but not limited to, the following: rape, any sexual offense, a crime against nature, incest, and preparation of obscene photographs, videos, or motion pictures
- Employs or permits the juvenile to assist in a violation of the obscenity laws or gives obscene material to the juvenile
- Sexually exploits the juvenile, including the promoting of prostitution of the juvenile or the taking of indecent liberties with the juvenile
- Creates or allows to be created serious emotional damage to the juvenile
- Encourages, directs, or approves of delinquent acts of the juvenile

There is always a duty to report child abuse, neglect, or maltreatment. Failure to report is itself a criminal act. Accordingly, you must promptly report any such known or reasonably suspected child abuse, neglect, or maltreatment to your case manager. If you are self-employed, the law requires you to report directly to the Department of Social Services in the county where the juvenile resides. Every state protects the person who makes these reports by giving the person immunity from any civil or criminal liability so long as the reporting person was acting in good faith. Occasionally, if prior abuse or neglect has been found in the home, a home health aide will be asked by the child protective service to verify that the family is meeting the requirements of the case plan developed jointly by the protective service worker and the family.

Examples of maltreatment and neglect of children include cases in which children are:

- Improperly fed, clothed, or deprived of any emotional support
- Allowed to drink alcohol or given illegal drugs

- Chained or locked in a closet
- Kept in an environment where mice, rats, cockroaches, or other pests can harm the child
- Left alone in an apartment or house or locked in a room while the legally responsible adult is away
- Left with unexplained bruises, welts, or other injuries

Abusive parents or caretakers may have been raised in abusive families themselves. The husband or wife may abuse the spouse. Life crises such as loss of job, debt, housing problems, substance abuse, and gambling losses can lead to abusive behavior; physical or mental health problems may cause a parent to become abusive; and parents who are too young themselves may lack the self-discipline to deal with their own children. Many of these parents are not aware of the damage they are doing to their children and may need help to develop better parenting skills. Parents of mentally or developmentally disabled children may be unable to cope with their children's problems. These parents should be encouraged to join support groups for parents with similar problems.

Abuse comes in many forms. It may be categorized as physical, sexual, emotional, or neglect. Figure 6-7 lists typical behavior for abused or mistreated children. Child abuse may take place in the homes of any group of people, regardless of income, ethnic origin, or religion. It is most important to remember that if you suspect it, you must report it.

Avoid contact with parents or other adults
Become upset when other children cry
Are extremely aggressive
Are extremely withdrawn
Suffer mood swings
Fear going into the home—run away from home
Are overly demonstrative and loving to the abusive parent
Blame them for being "clumsy" or "bad"
Wear long sleeves to conceal injuries
Appear to have low self-esteem
Attempt suicide
Grades go down in school

FIGURE 6-7 Observable patterns of abused or mistreated children.

WORKBOOK REVIEW

Go to the workbook and complete the review exercises and activities for Unit 6.

REVIEW

1. What are the five basic needs of humans described by Abraham Maslow?

_____

_____

_____

_____

_____

2. Why is it important for the aide to allow the mother to assume as much of the care of the newborn baby as possible? What would you look for and document relating to the mother's bonding with her infant?

3. What kind of observations would you likely make in caring for an infant? A toddler?

4. List four abnormal conditions in infancy and early childhood.

   _____

   _____

   _____

   _____

5. List two signs or symptoms of the following childhood illnesses:

   Influenza _____

   Otitis media _____

   Conjunctivitis _____

   Croup _____

6. How many pounds should the child weigh before the child can be safely placed in a booster seat?

7. Identify four behavior patterns of abused or mistreated children.

   _____

   _____

   _____

   _____

8. List three types of child abuse.

   _____

   _____

   _____

9. What is a home health aide's responsibility, when employed by an agency, if child abuse is suspected?

10. An infant needs to be
    a. toilet trained immediately.
    b. weaned to a cup by 6 months.
    c. kept awake during the day so he or she will sleep at night.
    d. loved, held, and fed regularly.

11. Typical characteristics of adolescents include which of the following?
    a. Strongly influenced by peers
    b. Growing desire for independence from parents
    c. Possible problems with substance abuse
    d. All of the above

12. Match the childhood illnesses in Column I with the correct descriptions in Column II.

    Column I

    ____ 1. PKU

    ____ 2. Hydrocephalus

    ____ 3. Down syndrome

    ____ 4. cystic fibrosis

    ____ 5. sickle cell anemia

    Column II

    a. an inherited malfunction of the pancreas

    b. caused by a chromosome abnormality

    c. affected individuals are unable to break down a certain amino acid

    d. defect in the absorption of brain fluid and the head is enlarged

    e. caused by abnormal sickle-shaped red blood cells that are very fragile

13. Signs and symptoms of fetal alcohol syndrome include which of the following?
    a. Small head
    b. Weak heart
    c. Flat face with drooping lips
    d. All of the above

Case Studies

14. You are helping a 16-year-old new mom who does not know much about babies. She appears uncomfortable and awkward holding her baby, and does not want to cuddle the baby. Why might she be behaving this way? What would you do? Why?

15. You are making your first visit to a new client, who is a young mother with two children, ages 18 months and 3 years. What observations could you make to assess whether the mother is attending to basic safety issues for her young children? What recommendations would you make to the mother to improve the safety of her home for her children?

UNIT 7
Early and Middle Adulthood

KEY TERMS

bone density test
cholesterol level
colon
Division of Vocational
  Rehabilitation (DVR)
early adulthood

electrocardiogram (ECG)
empty nest
  syndrome
mammogram
menopause
middle adulthood

osteoporosis
Pap smear
preventive health
  measures
prognosis
prostate

psychologist
Special Olympics
testicles
thyroid-stimulating
  hormone (TSH) test

LEARNING OBJECTIVES

After studying this unit, you should be able to:

- Discuss three major decisions that a young adult will need to make during early adulthood

- List five preventive health checks that are recommended to be done before the age of 50 for women

- List five preventive health checks that are recommended to be done before the age of 50 for men

- Discuss three life changes that occur with middle adulthood

- List two reasons why a middle-aged adult should be involved in an exercise program or other social activities

- Discuss emotional needs of disabled adults

- Discuss recent changes in society and technology that have helped enhance the lives of clients with special needs or disabilities

Early Adulthood

Early adulthood generally refers to the ages of 20 to 39 years. This is the time when an individual starts planning his or her life and making major decisions that will affect the years to come. The person assumes more responsibility for his or her future. Young adults are no longer required to further their education and must decide whether to attend a 4-year or technical college, or enter the workforce without any additional training. This is the time when some couples, including lesbian and homosexual couples, may marry or may live together without a formal marriage contract. Individuals, are now delaying marriage and having children later in life. The average age of individuals getting married today is in the middle 20s. The average age of first-time mothers is now 25. The size of families has been gradually decreasing, with the average family having only two children (Figure 7-1). Another recent change in society is the increase of single mothers caring for their children. It is quite difficult for a single mother of a child with a disability to care for the child 24 hours a day, 7 days a week. Thus, single mothers of children with disabilities often rely on a home health care agency to assist them part-time.

During early adulthood, many individuals are interested in establishing a career, joining various social groups, and serving their community or country in various roles. Some might join a golf group or a church group; parents might become active in the parent–teacher association (PTA) or assist with the Boy Scout or Girl Scout programs in their area. A few young adults might join the armed forces and elect to see the world before settling down. It is a time in life when many choices are available.

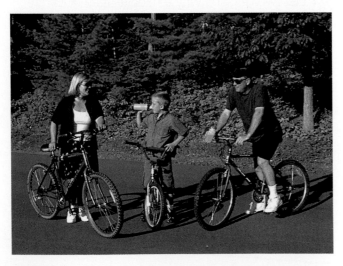

FIGURE 7-1   A family enjoying one another's company.

Another big decision is purchasing a home and learning how to manage that home. In the majority of homes today both partners work, and they will need to arrange their personal lives around their jobs. Early adulthood truly is a very busy and active time.

Early Adulthood Adjustments

During early adulthood, the body normally works efficiently. It remains at a high level of health for about the first 30 or 40 years of life. The body heals quickly through childhood, adolescence, and early and middle adulthood.

Health problems in early adulthood often accompany parenthood. Normal pregnancy, pregnancy with complications, and reproductive system disorders can occur in the adult woman. If an infant is born with birth defects or serious medical problems, parents may experience considerable stress and financial burdens. Other health problems can result from conditions related to automobile accidents and job-related injuries.

Many health professionals recommend taking certain **preventive health measures** to maintain a person's health and well-being and to prevent the development of health problems. For example, all persons should have a physical examination at least every 3 years. The early detection of diseases such as cancer, heart disease, and diabetes, as well as the effects of emotional stress, often leads to a better **prognosis** (outcome).

Preventive Health Measures for Women

The following tests may detect a disease in the early stages and are recommended preventive health measures for women:

- Have blood pressure checked at least every 2 years.
- Have an **electrocardiogram (ECG)** taken to detect any abnormalities of the heart.
- Check **cholesterol level** at age 45 and every year thereafter.
- Take a **bone density test** in middle adulthood to detect **osteoporosis**.
- Have a **colon** examination every 5 years beginning at age 50.
- Examine skin to check for skin cancer.
- Take a **thyroid-stimulating hormone (TSH) test**—to establish baseline function—by age 35 and then every 5 years thereafter.

- Have a **Pap smear** every 3 years to detect cancer and precancerous changes in the cervix.
- Do a monthly breast self-examination.
- Have a **mammogram** at least once before age 40.
- Have a pelvic examination every 3 years.
- Screen for a sexually transmitted disease (age and frequency of testing depend on the level of risk).

Preventive Health Measures for Men

The following tests may detect a disease in the early stages and are recommended preventive health measures for men:

- Have blood pressure checked every 2 years.
- Have a colon examination every 5 years after age 50.
- Take a **prostate** screening test—starting annually at age 50.
- Examine skin for cancer lesions every 2 to 3 years before age 50 and annually thereafter.
- Take a thyroid-stimulating hormone (TSH) test—to establish baseline function—by age 35 and then every 5 years thereafter.
- Do a monthly self-examination of the **testicles** starting in early adulthood.
- Have cholesterol tested to establish a baseline before age 30 and every 3 years after age 45.
- Screen for a sexually transmitted disease (age and frequency of testing depend on the level of risk).

The above tests are general recommendations made by health care providers and other authorities in the medical field. The main reason for these tests is to find the disease in the early stages in which treatment can be more effective.

Middle Adulthood

Society places great demands on a person in **middle adulthood**, or from 40 to 65 years of age. It is during this period that people are expected to be highly successful and productive as well as financially secure. If a woman had chosen in early adulthood to remain at home with her children, this may be the time when she decides to re-enter the workforce.

During the middle adult years, people often assess their accomplishments. Some may question how worthwhile their work or other achievements have been and seek a change. This change may take the form of a different lifestyle—a separation from their marriage partner, or a change in career or place of residence. Often during this stage of life, individuals are asked to take responsibility for care of their aging parents. The roles of parent and child often reverse once the parent is unable to manage all of his or her care. The phenomenon of daughters caring for their aging parents and their own children is so common that Dr. Elaine Brody has dubbed this middle generation the "Sandwich Generation": Boomer parents are pinched between raising their still-dependent children and carrying their parents over the threshold into late age.

Physically, those in their middle adult years will notice some changes. Their hair may turn gray or recede, and their eyesight may diminish and they may start wearing bifocals. Weight gain may occur as a result of a general slowing of their metabolism and inactivity. Hormonal changes that occur during **menopause**, when a woman's menstrual periods stop, may result in mood swings, changes in sleeping patterns, increased anxiety, or other physical symptoms, which can last to the mid-50s.

Middle Adulthood Adjustments

People in the middle adult years may have to make several major adjustments in response to a change in some area of their lives, as described next.

Family Relationships.   The middle years are generally the time when grown children leave the home. Parents who have been very involved in their children's lives may feel at a loss when this occurs (**empty nest syndrome**). As the children mature and gain independence, their own roles and responsibilities may become first priorities, and their ties with their family may become more secondary.

Another adjustment that can be either a positive or negative experience is when grandparents assume primary custody of their grandchildren. The children's parents, for various reasons, are not capable of assuming the responsibility of child-rearing, and the grandparents either take the grandchildren in or they go to a foster home. In the former situation, the grandparents are suddenly tied down to raising a child or children once again. This can also be quite a financial burden for the grandparents, many of whom are living on a limited income.

This is also a time when a single parent might be most troubled by the mixed emotions of his or her adolescent child or children. It is difficult to be the mediator without the support system of the other parent. Single parents may need to seek community support systems at this time. However, this can be a time when parents and children form close, adult relationships with each other. This also can be a time of freedom and creativity for parents, as they find they have more time to spend with each other and more time to develop their own mutual interests.

Regular Exercise.

It is important during the early and middle years of adulthood to become involved in a regular exercise program. Benefits of exercise include keeping one's weight down, increasing circulation, preventing bone and muscle loss, and being more physically fit. At any age, the unexercised body—although it may be free of symptoms of illness—will rust out long before it ever will wear out. Inactivity can make people old before their time. Just as inactivity accelerates aging, activity slows down the aging process. One of the best exercises is walking. Some other alternatives to walking are swimming, golfing, riding a stationary or moving bicycle, yoga, and dancing. If you are working in a home with a young or middle-aged adult, you should try to encourage the client to do some type of exercise within his or her limits.

Leisure-Time Activity.

In middle adulthood, individuals start doing more activities outside of the home, as leisure time is more plentiful than in early adulthood (Figure 7-2). How the person uses this extra time varies greatly, as much depends on where the person lives, the age of children still living at home, the financial situation, and individual interests. If there are still children at home, leisure-time activities usually evolve around them. Children are older and parents often become "taxi drivers," transporting their

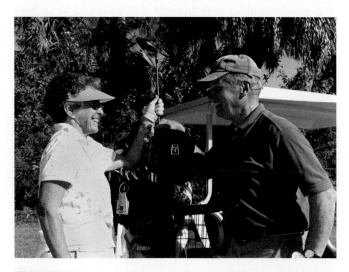

FIGURE 7-2 A middle-aged couple enjoying a day of golf.

children to all their activities or functions. If the children are gone, the couple may elect to do some traveling—maybe a cruise or car trip to see the country. Other couples or individuals might become involved in volunteer work. A favorite activity outside of the home in some areas of our country is playing card games such as euchre or bridge. Some individuals might elect to take short courses at a technical college in computers, photography, or gardening. The uses of computers and electronic media have opened many avenues for entertaining activities. Books and movies can now be downloaded and read or viewed in one's home, instantly. In general, individuals who keep themselves actively involved have better health outcomes than those who spend their time in front of the television set or using other media devices.

Illness and Disability in Early and Middle Adulthood

It is quite difficult for individuals with illnesses and disabilities in this age bracket to accept the fact that they need assistance from others to do their activities of daily living (ADLs) and in some cases may need financial assistance. They see other people their age engaged in full-time work, married, and having children, and they can become quite frustrated concerning their condition. In some situations, they are physically unable to have a sexual relationship, which can be quite depressing to a young person because intimacy with the opposite sex is an emotional need. Some individuals do rather well in accepting their limited abilities, whereas others do just the opposite. **Psychologists** (mental health specialists) tell us to try to center the attention of the despondent individual on his or her abilities rather than disabilities. This sometimes is easier said than done. As a home health aide, you will encounter some clients who are bitter, irritated, and angry because of their disabilities. At times, they may try to take their frustrations out on their caregivers.

It is easier for a person with a disability or special needs to remain physically and socially active today than it was years ago. With modern technology, a client can be transported in specially equipped vans or by the public transportation system. Many individuals now have motorized scooters or wheelchairs to assist them in their transportation needs (Figure 7-3). In some cases, cars are specially made to adapt to a person's specific disability, which makes it easier for the individual to enjoy the same activities as others in society. The majority of new restaurants and businesses are handicapped accessible and

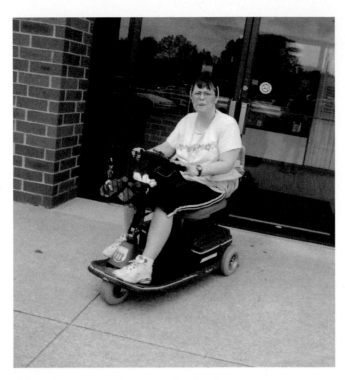

FIGURE 7-3   A motorized wheelchair can assist an individual with her transportation needs.

also offer special accommodations for toileting. Shopping malls and grocery stores sometimes have designated times for individuals with disabilities to shop. Occasionally stores will have extra help available to assist clients with their shopping needs. Many churches have special activities for individuals to attend, depending on their interests. Because of new laws and more public awareness, there are also more jobs and training programs available for individuals with special needs. An example of such an agency is the **Division of Vocational Rehabilitation (DVR)**. This agency can set up a training program for individuals with special needs and assist with the costs. The case manager or social worker is the individual who can assist the client in searching out these special programs or agencies.

If any of the clients you care for are mildly mentally impaired with Down syndrome, local communities often have places for them to work during the day for a small amount of money. These places are government funded and therefore have to meet certain government regulations. The goals of such facilities are to get individuals with disabilities out of the house, teach them a minor skill and good work habits, and offer them an opportunity to socialize with other individuals who have similar disabilities. The programs offered by such facilities

involve the individuals for about 8 hours a day, 5 days a week. As a home health aide, you may be assigned to care for these individuals when they are not at work, but need assistance with ADLs and cannot be left alone. As a home health aide you will need a great deal of patience and persistence in dealing with their various personality traits and reinforcing basic hygiene skills. The case manager or other family members will assist you in knowing how best to work with a specific client.

Emotional Needs of Clients with Disabilities

Two of the most important aspects of care of clients with disabilities or disabling conditions are to keep them physically and mentally active and to try to meet some of their emotional needs. These individuals have the same basic needs as a healthy individual of the same age.

In some areas of the country there are activities for individuals with special needs, such as the **Special Olympics**, in which your client may want to become involved. Your role is to encourage your client to participate and attend such functions. In most scenarios, the case manager initially will arrange for transportation and coordination of these activities. Your role will be to assist the client in getting ready to attend, including having the client dressed properly and having all the supplies needed with the client, such as medications, money, and toileting supplies. If the client plans to attend a special family event, you will need to see that the client's hair is clean and styled and that the client is dressed appropriately for the event. A family member or volunteer will transport the client to the event. Always check to see if the client has all supplies necessary for the time he or she will be gone. Your goal is to make it as pleasant as possible for the client and also the family members. Be sure the family members or volunteer know how to operate any special equipment and are instructed on any special care that the client may require.

WORKBOOK REVIEW

Go to the workbook and complete the review exercises and activities for Unit 7.

REVIEW

1. Name three causes of health problems in the early adult years.

   _____

   _____

   _____

2. List three adjustments that may need to be made during the middle adult years.

   _____

   _____

   _____

3. During what period of life does society expect the most from an individual?

   _____

   _____

   _____

4. Why are preventive health measures important?

   _____

   _____

   _____

5. The developmental tasks of early adulthood include which of the following?
   a. Focusing on improving oneself
   b. Developing close personal relationships
   c. Making career choices
   d. All of the above

6. The middle adult years are a time when adjustments are made due to which of the following?
   a. Grown children leaving home
   b. Aging parents who may need assistance with ADLs
   c. More leisure time available
   d. All of the above

7. The adult needs to exercise to
   a. improve circulation.
   b. prevent muscle loss.
   c. Keeping weight down.
   d. all of the above.

8. An x-ray of a woman's breast is called a(n)_____.

9. The _____ is used to detect cervical cancer.

10. _____ is the name of the test done to measure bone mass and to detect osteoporosis.

11. Family size is **increasing** or **decreasing** in the United States.

    _____

12. List six preventive health measures for men and women.

    _____

    _____

    _____

    _____

    _____

    _____

13. List two reasons for young adults to be frustrated if they are wheelchair-bound and rely on the home health aide for their ADLs.

    _____

    _____

Case Studies

14. John Kane, a 40-year-old paraplegic in a wheelchair, is to attend the wedding of his niece. His brother is going to pick him up at noon to take him to the wedding and reception. His brother has a van that has a lift to transfer John into the van. John has medication to take every day at 6 P.M. What are the responsibilities of the home health aide in getting John ready to go to the wedding?

15. You have been helping a 34-year-old man who is a paraplegic and who stays at home and says he is bored and depressed. What can you suggest to this client? List reasons why outside activities are important.

UNIT 8
Older Adulthood

KEY TERMS

accommodation
analgesics
antibodies
arteriosclerosis
arthroplasty
arthroscopy
atrophy
auditory
cataracts
cerumen
chronological age
conjunctiva

copious
dementia
depression
estrogen
floaters
functional age
glaucoma
hypothyroidism
immune system
integumentary system
intraocular pressure
iris

kyphosis
labia
melanoma
nocturia
orthopedic
osteoporosis
otosclerosis
Parkinson's disease
pelvic
pendulous
peripheral vision
phantom pain

presbycusis
progesterone
pupil
referred pain
sleep
sublingually
transurethral resection
 (TURP)
vertebrae

LEARNING OBJECTIVES

After studying this unit, you should be able to:

- Discuss the statistics regarding the older adult

- Name developmental tasks of the older adult

- List two signs of depression

- Discuss potential leisure-time activities for the older adult

- Describe physical changes in the body systems due to the aging process

- List ways to assist the home health aide to work with clients who have hearing loss or who have low vision

- Discuss sleep changes affecting the older adult

- Discuss the home health aide's responsibility in pain control measures for the client

- Discuss the role of the home health aide in medication administration

- Demonstrate the following:

 PROCEDURE 3   Caring for Hearing Aids

 PROCEDURE 4   Caring for an Artificial Eye

 PROCEDURE 5   Assisting the Client with Self-Administered Medications

The Aging Population

Old is defined as having lived or existed for a long time. *Old* and *aging* are relative to the individual person and that person's age at that time. Aging is a normal process for all individuals. Chronological age means how long a person has lived. The following classification defines aging (in years): old (65 to 74), middle-old (75 to 84), and old-old (85 and older). Whereas chronological age refers to how the person is functioning at a particular age, functional age means how well an individual is able to accomplish tasks of daily living.

Increase in Number

The U.S. population is aging. The proportion of Americans 65 years of age and older is expected to increase from 12% in 2005 to 20% in 2030. The number of people living to age 90 and beyond has tripled in the past three decades to almost 2 million and is likely to quadruple by 2050. This burst in numbers of the oldest-old puts extra pressure on elderly care programs, increases health costs, and depletes retirement savings, and tasks more Baby Boomers with the responsibility of caring for aging parents.

Those in the 90-plus age group often have one or more disabilities, challenges that affect even more individuals after age 95. There is a need to focus on being able to help people who are age 85 to 95 to live at home as long as possible and to live at home independently. Nursing home cost runs about $78,000 a year, most of it not covered by Medicare. The 90-plus rely on Social Security for almost half their income and on retirement pensions for about a fifth. Families who have an elderly relative living alone, and/or living far away, worry about the frightening possibility that they might fall and be left for hours or days, unconscious and undiscovered, with a bleed in the brain or developing illness such as pneumonia.

Increased life expectancy to well beyond 80 is the result of better public health measures, improvements in living conditions, and advances in medical care and technology. Today, 20% of the people over 65 are still employed and are working at least part-time. Some work because of financial need, whereas others do it because of their need to be contributing members of society.

Developmental Tasks of Older Adults

Individuals go through life facing many problems and achieving either success or failure. Examples of important steps in life are:

- Toilet training for the young child
- First day at day care
- First day at kindergarten
- First date for the teenager
- Marriage, separation, divorce
- Childbirth and child-rearing
- Retirement
- Loss of loved one

How a person confronts and solves problems earlier in life determines his or her behavior in later years. Successful problem solving leads to satisfaction and growth in one's life. This forms the foundation for happiness in older adulthood.

When a person has not successfully solved problems, this person may show signs of anxiety, depression, and inability for personal growth. Examples of developmental tasks of the older adult are:

- Adjusting to physical changes in one's body due to illness or the aging process
- Adapting to living alone
- Accepting the possibility of moving into an assisted-living facility
- Adjusting to new relationships with adult children and their offspring
- Adjusting to retirement and managing leisure time
- Adjusting to physical and emotional stress
- Dealing with the death of friends
- Accepting the approach of one's own death

Characteristics of Aging Well

Research and aging studies have revealed that the following habits are frequently seen in people who age well:

- Exercise three to five times weekly (Figure 8-1)
- Eat a low-fat diet
- Maintain ideal weight
- Do not smoke
- Consume alcohol in moderation
- Have a circle of friends with whom to socialize and see often
- Adequate finances to live comfortably
- Think positively

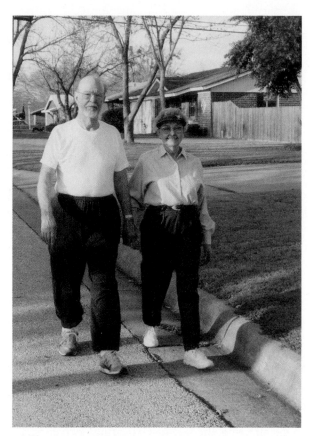

FIGURE 8-1 Exercise is an important part of aging well.

- Remain active, learning new things
- Establish conditions for good health—immunizations, medical intervention

Personalities do not really change over time. For example, someone characterized as a "mean old codger" was most likely that way when he or she was 25—age has nothing to do with it. And as we age, we still like to do things we did when we were younger. Older adults can still drive safely, run in the Senior Olympics, and remain interested in sex. Change is a constant in life and if one lives long enough, there is a lot of it! Think about the number of changes an older adult may experience: retirement, relocation, grandchildren and great-great-grandchildren, physical changes, and technological changes such as the computer. There are at least two common threads in older adults' lives: change and loss.

Depression

Physical changes that occur naturally as we age can make keeping up with change difficult. Sometimes change is loss: death of a spouse or friend, or loss of vision, or change of health status, for example. For a person of any age, these kinds of losses can be serious blows. For some older adults, they can be overwhelming. It may feel as if losses are coming faster than they can handle. The older adult grieves for each loss. Depression is a persistent sadness that makes it difficult to do day-to-day tasks. Depression in older adults can go undiagnosed for a variety of reasons. One reason is that physical illnesses can mask depression and depression, in turn, can look like a physical illness. Older individuals might deny they are depressed because they feel that admitting to the feelings of depression is a sign of weakness. Some people find it normal to talk about physical illness but not emotional pain. Depression has to be recognized before it can be treated. Depression may be shown in variety for ways: limited conversation, crying spells, insomnia and loss of appetite are just a few signs of depression.

Leisure-Time Activities

One of the secrets of keeping emotionally happy is being involved with other people and participating in leisure-time activities. There are many government, community, and church activities for older adults to become involved in without spending a great deal of money. For those individuals unable to drive or who do not have a car, a Senior Minibus can come to their door and transport them to get groceries, get a haircut, or go to the Senior Center for lunch. Many stores have special days on which they give seniors (55 or older) an extra percentage off of their purchases, plus a free snack. If one needs assistance in shopping, many stores will have extra help available to assist. This is also true when going to the movies. Senior Citizen Centers have scheduled activities all week, including exercise hour, crafts, and cards, and some of the larger ones even have water aerobics. The centers also facilitate occasional bus trips outside of the immediate area. Local school systems welcome the assistance of older adults to help with the reading and math programs. Many older adults still do some of the same activities they did when they were younger (Figure 8-2). Some travel extensively, seeing the world, whereas others might purchase a motor home and travel throughout the country. Many spend more quality time with their grandchildren or other family members than in busier times of life. A great deal depends on the older adult's financial status, physical health, and individual interests (Figure 8-3). Activities vary for individuals in both the 65 to 80 group and the 80 to 100+ group. The opportunity to keep involved is always available, so older adults just need to decide which direction they are going to take in their so-called Golden Years.

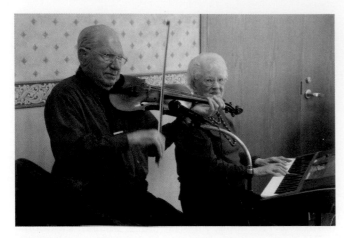

FIGURE 8-2 Using musical talent at a senior center.

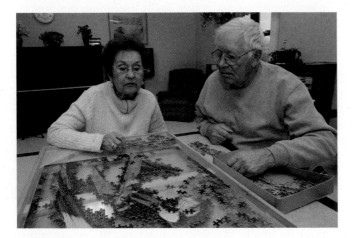

FIGURE 8-3 Putting a puzzle together.

Physical Changes Due to the Aging Process

Hearing Loss

A condition called **presbycusis** (gradual loss of hearing) is quite common in the elderly. Hearing ability gradually diminishes from the time a person is 40. Some hearing deficits cannot be helped by hearing aids, and the person's hearing is so poor that verbal communication is difficult. Following are tips you may find useful when working with a client who has hearing loss.

- Get the attention of the listener before speaking. Call the client by name before making a statement or ask a question. If your statement or question is misunderstood, then rephrase it rather than repeating the same words again.

- Keep the competing stimuli of background noise and distractions to a minimum. Turn off the radio or TV. Whenever possible, try to talk with the client on a one-to-one basis or in a small group rather than in a large group of people.

- Talk naturally or distinctly. Speak at normal levels. Speak a little more slowly and with a few more pauses. Many older clients cannot understand rapid speech.

- Use writing as a form of communication.

- Encourage the use of nonverbal communication such as lip movements, facial expressions, and gestures. Look at the listener when talking to the client. Try to stay within a few feet of the client with whom you are talking. Keep your hands away from your face.

- A sound system used for music, entertainment, or oral presentation should be adjusted so that base and lower tones are predominant, as some sounds are heard by clients with hearing loss whereas others are not. Hearing loss is greater for consonants than for vowels. For example, the S, Z, T, F, and G sounds are particularly difficult to discriminate.

Clients who are have hearing loss may have nerve damage affecting the **auditory** (hearing) nerve, or a disorder called **otosclerosis**. This condition occurs when the bones of the inner ear harden and sound waves no longer carry in the usual fashion (Figure 8-4). There is also an increase in **cerumen** (earwax) in the ears. The majority of clients with hearing loss do wear a hearing aid (Figures 8-5A and 8-5B). There are many different types of hearing aids; the most common are the following:

- In the canal
- Half-shell
- Behind the ear (Figure 8.5A)
- Full-shell (Figure 8-5B)
- Open fit

The most recent hearing aids are digital, whereas the older ones were analog. The cost of hearing aids varies widely—from several hundred to several thousand dollars. Clients should be encouraged to wear their hearing aids regularly and also take very good care of the aids. Some clients will have one hearing aid for each ear; others may have only one hearing aid. The style and model of hearing aid will dictate the type of batteries used. Because of the small size of most batteries, the lifetime of the batteries is short and they need to be replaced on a regular basis. See Procedure 3, Caring for Hearing Aids.

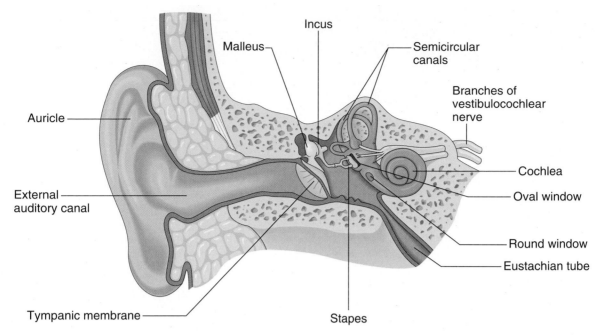

FIGURE 8-4 Internal view of the ear.

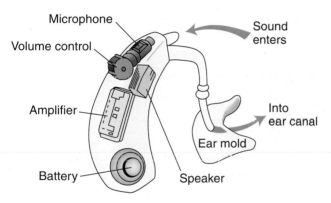

FIGURE 8-5A Behind-the-ear hearing aid. The ear mold is placed in the ear canal. The rest of the hearing aid is worn outside of the ear. Note the different parts of the hearing aid.

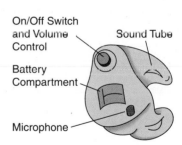

FIGURE 8-5B Full-shell hearing aid. This ear mold fits into the ear canal.

PROCEDURE 3 CARING FOR HEARING AIDS

Purpose

- To increase the hearing ability of the client
- To ensure the client's optimal use of the hearing aid(s)

Procedure

1. Wash your hands.
2. Assemble supplies:
   - cleaning tools
   - batteries (optional)
   - warm wet washcloth (optional)

(continued)

PROCEDURE 3   CARING FOR HEARING AIDS (continued)

3. Check the hearing aid for wax build-up and ensure the batteries are working. If there is wax build-up in the hearing aid, clean it with the tools that came with the hearing aid.
4. Replace the battery if necessary. Remove the protective foil from the new battery; wait for 2 minutes before inserting it to activate the battery. Take the hearing aid in your hand and open the battery door. Insert the battery so that you see the + symbol on the battery. Switch on the hearing aid by closing the battery compartment. It can take up to 15 second before it starts to work.
5. Check the inside of the client's ear for wax; if wax is visible, remove it with a warm wet washcloth.
6. Assist the client in inserting the hearing aid. Each hearing aid is individually programmed for the right ear or left ear. For the first step, identify right or left so you can insert the hearing aid into the correct ear (red = right; blue = left). Either have the client insert the tip of the hearing aid into the ear canal or insert it for the client. Carefully pull on the earlobe and push the hearing aid into the correct position.

Removing the Hearing Aid

1. To remove a hearing aid with a removal handle:
   a. Hold the removal handle between the thumb and index finger, and carefully pull the hearing aid up and out of the ear.
2. To remove a hearing aid without a removal handle:
   a. Put your thumb behind the earlobe and gently press the ear upward to push the hearing aid out of the canal. Grasp the protruding hearing aid and remove it.
3. Opening the battery compartment will turn off the hearing aid.

Helpful Hints

- Never immerse hearing aids in water. Do not wear when showering, bathing, or swimming.
- Protect hearing aids from heat.
- Whenever the hearing aid is not in use, leave the battery compartment open, so that any moisture can evaporate. Store hearing aids in a safe, dry, and clean place.
- Do not drop the hearing aid. Dropping onto a hard surface can damage the hearing aid.

Vision Changes

In older adults, the eyes appear to be farther back in the eye socket (sunken) and the eyelids seem to droop. The lids are no longer elastic and become baggy and wrinkled. The conjunctiva (membrane that lines the eyelids) becomes thinner and yellow. Fatty pads may form in this area of the eye. The glands produce less fluid. Sometimes the elderly call this "dry eye." The iris (pigmented part of the eye) fades or becomes irregular in shape (Figure 8-6). The pupil (lets light into the retina) becomes smaller, which means that less light is let into the back of the eye. Thus, the aging person has difficulty with night vision and perceiving the depth of objects. The fluid in the eye changes and clients may complain of floaters. These floaters are simply parts of the fluid that have broken off and are floating around in the eye. The term accommodation means the ability of a person to first see objects at a distance and then adjust sight to see something close-up, such as a newspaper. As a person ages, the lens of the eye loses this accommodation ability, and to compensate for this loss the individual may need to start wearing glasses with bifocal lenses. The older eye requires more light than the younger eye. To see clearly, the eye of a 65-year-old person needs more than twice as much light as that of a 20-year-old. A small amount of glare, which may hardly bother a younger person, may cause great difficulties for the older adult. Glare also may cause anxiety and inability to concentrate. The older eye does not adapt quickly to changes in light levels. Abrupt changes can be hazardous and may cause falls and other accidents. More than half of severe visual disabilities occur in people 65 and over. Legal blindness occurs most in this age group. Changes in

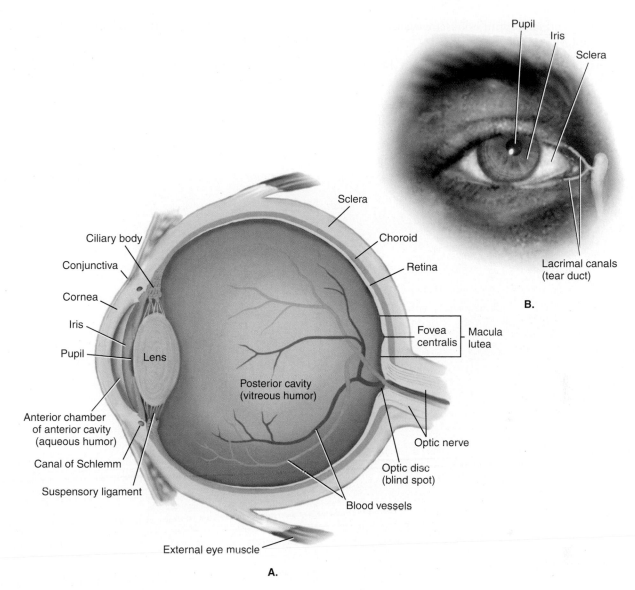

FIGURE 8-6 (A) View of the inner eye, (B) anterior view of the eye.

vision happen slowly, but older adults usually are aware of their vision changes. Following are tips you may find useful when working with a client who has difficulty seeing:

- Provide adequate light.
- Carefully adjust shades throughout the day to avoid glare from windows.
- Have the client wear sunglasses and wide-brimmed hats outside.
- Have a night-light on in bedroom at night.
- Be careful of where you place furniture. It is a common phenomenon that as older adults age they lose peripheral (side) vision. A common term used to describe this is "tunnel" vision.

- Use clocks, radios, watches, and telephones with large numbers.
- Contrasting colors make things easier to see. For example, doorways can contrast with the tablecloth, the chair seat can contrast with the floor, and personal items can contrast with a covering on the dresser top.
- Warm colors are easier to see—bright yellow, orange, and red.
- Avoid clutter. It is difficult to see when a space is crowded with items.
- If the client is blind, do not change anything in the home without asking the client.
- Have the client use a magnifying glass to read mail.

- Talking books and large-print books are available at the public library.
- Identify paper money by folding each type a different way for the client.
- Introduce yourself when you enter the home and then if necessary you can touch the client. Always tell the client when you are leaving.

- Give step-by-step instructions on what you want the client to do.
- When serving food, explain the location of each food and beverage item using the face of the clock: "Coffee is at 9:00; soup is at 3:00."

If the client has had an eye removed and has an artificial eye, refer to Procedure 4, Caring for an Artificial Eye.

PROCEDURE 4   CARING FOR AN ARTIFICIAL EYE

Purpose

- To ensure proper care of client's artificial eye
- To prevent infection or irritation of the eye socket

Procedure

1. Assemble equipment:
   - disposable gloves
   - storage container (optional)
   - cleansing solution such as baby shampoo
   - plastic container
2. Wash hands and apply gloves.
3. Tell the client what you plan to do.
4. Position yourself and all equipment to be on the same side as the client's artificial eye.
5. Remove the artificial eye by depressing the lower eyelid with your thumb while lifting the upper lid with your index finger. If the client can remove the artificial eye, let the client do it. Carefully take the eye and place it in a plastic container.
6. Carry the container to the sink. Place a washcloth or paper towel in the bottom of sink, as a precaution against breakage. Remove the eye from the container and gently rinse it with running water in the sink. A small amount of baby shampoo is often

recommended for cleansing the outside of the eye. Rinse the container and fill it with water.

7. Place the eye into the container. If the client's eye socket has drainage around it, wipe the outside off with clean warm washcloth. Assist the client to insert the eye into the socket. If the eye is moist, it will slide in easier. Position the notched edge toward the client's nose. You may need to depress the lower eyelid and replace the lid gently over the eye as it slips into the socket. If the eye socket is dry, artificial tears may be inserted into the eye socket.
8. If the client does not wish to have the eye inserted into the socket right away, the eye needs to be placed in water in a specially marked container.
9. Return all equipment and dispose of waste.
10. Remove gloves and wash hands.
11. Document procedure completion, your observations, and the client's reaction.

NOTE: An artificial eye is not routinely removed every day; some clients may leave the eye in for weeks without removing it. It is recommended that the client wear the artificial eye on a continuous basis.

Common Diseases of the Eye

Following are some common diseases of the eye in the older adult.

Cataracts. A person is diagnosed with cataracts when there is clouding of the lens of the eye (Figure 8-7). This diagnosis once meant a gradual, but steady, march toward blindness, which is not true today, because of advancement in treating this condition. This condition affects 60% of the senior population. Signs and symptoms of cataracts are (1) colors appear dull and hazy, (2) halos are seen around lights, (3) difficulty seeing while driving at night, and (4) increasing difficulty in reading. This condition can be

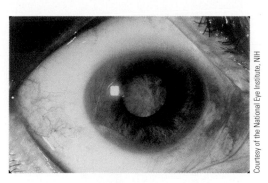

FIGURE 8-7 Cataracts—the lens is cloudy, thus interfering with the refraction of light rays.

easily repaired by 1-day surgery. After surgery, the client may need a ride home and someone to stay with him or her for 1 to 2 days. If there is not a friend or family member available, a home health aide may be employed to provide this service. The home health aide also may need to assist the client in putting eye drops in the eye. The client may not be able to read the label on the drops, and the aide will need to assist the client in reading the label—of the eye drop containers which will be colored-coded to prevent errors. After surgery, the client may no longer need to wear glasses, as he or she did before the surgery.

Glaucoma. Glaucoma is an insidious eye disease that has no noticeable symptoms until irreversible damage is done. Signs and symptoms of glaucoma may include (1) blurred vision, (2) severe eye pain, (3) headaches, (4) colored halos around lights, and (5) nausea and vomiting. It involves a loss of vision due to raised intraocular (inside) pressure, which damages the optic nerve. If untreated, glaucoma can cause blindness. Eye drops, laser surgery, and an operative procedure are methods used to help prevent further damage. In some cases oral medication may also be prescribed.

Dry Eye. Dry eye is insufficient lubrication (tears) to keep the eye comfortable. Symptoms of dry eye are (1) stinging or burning of the eye, (2) scratchiness, (3) stringy mucus in or around the eye, and (4) excess tearing. Dry eye is treated by eye drops called artificial tears. They lubricate the eyes and help maintain moisture. Artificial tears are available without a prescription—many brands are available.

Digestive System Changes

As a person ages, the ability to taste diminishes due to the fact that the taste buds on the back of the tongue are less sensitive to taste sensations. The natural teeth are usually replaced with dentures or the person may lack some teeth, which makes chewing food more difficult. The salivary glands produce less saliva, which causes problems in breaking down certain foods and makes the older person thirstier. The sense of smell is decreased, so food does not smell as good as it once did. Some older individuals have problems with an inefficient gag reflex and choke readily on thin liquids. The older adult's digestive process is also affected due to less production of digestive juices. These changes can cause a person to have decreased appetite and thirst. It is no wonder that good nutrition is difficult for older adults, especially those over 90. Following are tips to assist you in helping the older client eat a proper diet; these tips might help improve the nutritional status of your client:

- Cut food in smaller pieces.
- Offer liquids often during the day.
- Encourage the client to season his or her food with spices and herbs, rather than salt.
- Use food thickeners or buy liquids that are pre-thickened, as individuals choke less on thicker liquids.
- Use nutritional liquid protein supplements.
- Discourage foods that are high in fat, which are difficult to digest.
- Encourage good oral care before meals and have clients wear their dentures.

Urinary System Changes

The size of the bladder and kidney decreases and muscle control diminishes. Because of these changes, the person needs to urinate more often and starts having problems such as nocturia (night urination), frequent urination, incontinence, and leaking.

Immune System Changes

The immune system starts to decline as we grow older. Antibodies, which are like soldiers fighting off invading microorganisms, are not as plentiful in the older adult as in the younger adult. Because of this decline in antibodies, the immune system fails to recognize and destroy diseased cells. This may be the reason for the increase in cancer cells as the person grows older. The antibodies do not respond as quickly in the older adult, and thus that person does not recover from infections as fast. Older adults need to be encouraged to be immunized against influenza, pneumonia, whooping cough, and shingles because of their deficient immune systems.

Musculoskeletal Changes

As one grows older, one's muscles become weaker and sometimes atrophy (waste away). There is a change in joints and other supportive structures. There is reduced flexibility plus stiffness, particularly in the morning. After the age of 55, a few joints may need replacement because of stiffness and pain. Minerals in bones decrease, which makes the bones more vulnerable to fractures. Pelvic (hip bone), long bone, wrist, and back fractures are the most common. The older person walks with shorter steps, is more cautious about taking steps, and has a wider leg stance to achieve better balance. When an individual has knee pain or damage from an earlier injury, the first surgery done on the knee is usually an arthroscopy (arthro, joint, and scopy, scope). This is a minor surgery in which the orthopedic specialist repairs the knee joint without a surgical incision using a scope to see the inside of the knee. This surgery will help the person for a few years, but if the knee is badly damaged a more extensive surgery called a knee arthroplasty (replacement of joint) will need to be done. An individual who has had an arthroplasty will need assistance for about 6 weeks after the surgery. Often a home health aide is assigned for a short time to care for the client. If the hip needs to be replaced, it is called a hip arthroplasty.

Kyphosis. As a person ages, the padding between some of the vertebrae (small bones of the spinal column) shrinks, which causes the vertebrae to bend forward. This condition is called kyphosis (Figure 8-8).

Osteoporosis. Osteoporosis is often referred to as the *silent disease* because bone loss occurs without any signs or symptoms. Osteoporosis is characterized by a decrease in bone mass due to the decline in the female hormone estrogen, which helps maintain bone strength. As estrogen levels decrease, bones become more porous and fragile. More than 40% of women over the age of 50 will suffer a fracture in their lifetime due to this condition. Although women are at the highest risk for osteoporosis, it can affect men as well. Oftentimes the condition becomes apparent when one experiences a disabling bone fracture from a bump or fall. The test used to diagnose this condition is called a bone density test. Exercise and proper diet can be helpful in prevention of osteoporosis.

Reproductive System Changes

Females have reproductive changes due to lowered levels of estrogen and progesterone (hormones). Pubic hair

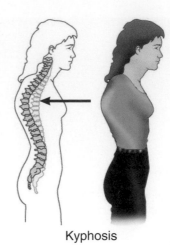

Kyphosis

FIGURE 8-8 Kyphosis—note the forward curvature of the spinal column.

loss is common, and the labia (lips) shrink. The uterus is reduced in size and there is less lubrication of the cervix. These changes make the female more vulnerable to infection and irritation. Occasionally, an older woman may get an infection of the vagina, which is very difficult to treat, and often the drainage is copious (large amount) and very odorous. The breasts lose their elasticity and become pendulous (hanging loosely). The nipples become flat and smaller. Cancer of the breast, ovaries, and uterus are common cancers of the female.

The male has reduced testosterone hormones and reduced seminal fluid production. As a result, he may have a reduced desire for sexual relations. The testicles will atrophy and thus reduce the production of sperm. The prostate gland enlarges, which can cause problems with urination such as dribbling, frequent urination, and urinary tract infections. In some cases, medication can aid in the reduction of the size of the prostate gland. If medications do not work, a surgery called a transurethral resection (TURP) (surgery) may be indicated.

Integumentary (Skin) System Changes

As a person ages the skin, or integumentary system, becomes thinner and sometimes paper thin like tissue paper. The person no longer has a fatty layer under the skin in many parts of the body. This affects the ability of the body to regulate its temperature. The older adult's legs may lose their hair and also become shiny and blue due to poor circulation. Age spots occur on various places on the body. If a skin lesion appears either black or brown with

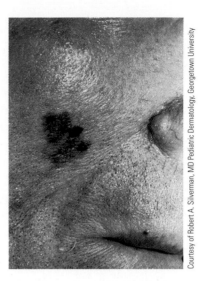

Courtesy of Robert A. Silverman, MD Pediatric Dermatology, Georgetown University

FIGURE 8-9   Melanoma—malignant type of skin cancer.

an irregular border, this may be a sign of **melanoma** (malignant skin cancer; Figure 8-9). Hair growth decreases in some areas on the body and increases in other areas. Men often become bald, but have increased hair in their ears and eyebrows. Women have increased facial hair. Pubic hair also changes, and loss is common due to hormonal changes in the body. The sense of touch diminishes, and older adults can burn themselves and not even feel it. There is a lack of oil production and the skin becomes dry and tears easily. The older adult's fingernails become more brittle and the toenails thicken and become difficult to cut.

Endocrine System Changes

There is less production of hormones by the endocrine glands in various systems. Because of less hormone production there is an increase in diabetes and **hypothyroidism** (thyroid deficiency) in the older adult.

Respiratory System Changes

There is reduced elasticity of the lungs and diminished breathing capacity as the person ages. Because of these changes, the person may have problems with the exchange of oxygen and carbon dioxide. Secretions of the lung usually become thicker, especially if the person smokes. There is greater incidence of cancer of the lung, pneumonia, and emphysema in the older adult.

Circulatory System Changes

Many changes take place in the circulatory system in the older adult. The arteries become harder, are less elastic,

and fill up with plaque. The veins lose their ability to expand and contract. The valves lose their effectiveness, and the heart cannot pump blood through the body without a great deal of effort. There is a greater incidence of diseases such as **arteriosclerosis** (hardening of the arteries) and congestive heart failure in the older adult.

Nervous System Changes

As a person ages, circulation of the blood to the brain decreases and there is a gradual reduction of brain cells. Transmission of messages from one part of the body to another does not work as well as it once did. It just takes a little longer for older adults to accomplish a task. Their intelligence does not change, unless they have a form of **dementia** (loss of memory). There is a greater incidence of diseases such as dementia and **Parkinson's disease** (a degeneration of nerve cells in the area of the brain that controls muscle movement).

Changes in Sleep Patterns

Sleep is a period of continuous or intermittent unconsciousness in which physical movements are decreased. Generally, as we age, sleep is of shorter duration but the same amount. In other words, we often sleep as many hours as we did when we were younger, but each period of sleep lasts a shorter length of time. It is common for people to be less physically active as they grow older and thus require less sleep. Additionally, the bladder gets smaller, so the need to urinate becomes more frequent during the night. These factors can often leave the older adult feeling as if he or she never gets a good night's sleep. Although the home health aide knows these changes are normal, the aide should listen and observe carefully because disrupted or poor sleep patterns can be a sign of adverse drug reactions or, possibly, depression. Reassurance given to the older adult about the amount of sleep he or she is getting may help.

Pain

As a person ages, the ability to feel pain diminishes. The older adult may have slight pain in the right lower abdomen and not think it is serious because it is only a dull ache. On the other hand, that same pain in a younger person would be severe. The individual would know to seek medical help because the pain, accompanied by nausea, would be a sure sign of appendicitis. This makes the older adult more vulnerable for undiagnosed illness and injury. A home health aide needs to be alert to any behavioral change that might indicate the client is in pain.

A few signs and symptoms to look for are increased vital signs (blood pressure usually goes up when a person is in pain), sweating, facial grimacing, holding or squeezing a particular part of the body, nausea or vomiting, and crying, moaning, or just not talking. If a person has dementia, it is the home health aide who will pick up a few clues that the client is having pain, as the client may not be able to express this in words.

Some clients will always complain of some discomfort or pain in some part of their body. They seem to dwell on their discomfort all the time. These clients most likely do have chronic pain due to arthritis or other diseases, and because of their constant complaining, the home health aide often ignores their complaints. When a change does occur with this type of client, it often goes unrecognized because of the client's previous behavior. How people perceive pain is highly individual, and involves heredity, stress, anxiety, fear, depression, previous experience, and general health. Motivation also plays a huge role—and helps explain why a person who is gravely injured in a car accident can ignore his own pain to save his buddies, whereas someone who is depressed may feel incapacitated by a minor sprain.

When a client does complain of pain, a home health aide should ask the following questions:

1. Where is the pain? Ask the client to be as specific as possible—not just the right leg, but where on the right leg.

2. When did it start?

3. Describe the pain—is it dull, viselike, sharp, cramping, stabbing, knifelike?

4. Have you had this type of pain before—if so, what helped to relieve the pain?

5. Did you do something prior to the pain starting; (e.g., kneel in your garden pulling weeds)?

6. Is the pain constant or does it come and go?

7. Using a pain intensity scale, can you rate your pain (Figure 8-10)?

When documenting the client's pain, it is permissible to use the client's own words in describing his or her pain.

There are also different types of pain. One type is called **referred pain**. An example of this is a person who has pain in the lower leg, but once x-rays are taken, the source of the pain is identified as a hip joint that needs to be replaced. The pain radiated from the person's hip to the lower leg. **Phantom pain** is the sensation of pain a person may feel in an amputated limb. The client will complain of pain in the missing limb because nerve endings are still active. This pain is real, and the client may need to take painkillers to relieve it. Acute pain has a sudden onset, a well-defined and easily identifiable cause, and runs a short course (e.g., pain from a sprained ankle). Chronic pain has a source that is hard to find, lasts a long time, and often causes fatigue and depression in clients (e.g., back pain or headaches).

Nursing actions to relieve pain vary. The most common treatment is with drugs. There are mild pain relievers or **analgesics** such as aspirin or Tylenol available over the counter, and stronger pain relievers such as Vicodin available by prescription. Currently in the United States, the painkiller Vicodin is the most prescribed drug for pain relief.

Painkillers are usually administered before the pain becomes too intense. Each client will have in his or her care plan what medication should be taken to relieve pain. The majority of drugs are ordered "prn," which means they are given only when the client has pain. There is also a time limit on the orders, such as "Percodan q 4 hours for severe pain prn." This means that the client can have this medication every 4 hours if she or he is in pain.

Other nursing measures that might reduce pain are a back massage, rest and relaxation, walking, pleasant music, or reading. Meditation, hypnosis, and tai chi are old ways of dealing with pain and are often successful. Cognitive behavioral therapy, which is offered at many

Pain Intensity Scale										
0	1	2	3	4	5	6	7	8	9	10
(no pain)					(moderate pain)				(worst possible pain)	

FIGURE 8-10 Pain levels—have the client use this scale to rate his or her pain.

pain-management programs, teaches clients to challenge their negative thoughts about their pain and substitute more positive behavior. Clients may find themselves in a vicious circle of more pain, more anxiety, more fear, more depression. The aide needs to interrupt that circle.

Guided imagery, in which a client imagines something relaxing, for example, floating on a cloud, also works in part by diverting attention away from the pain, as does mindfulness meditation.

The type of pain medication is prescribed according to the intensity of the pain. Pain is rated on a scale of 0 to 10, with 0 being no pain and 10 being the worst pain imaginable. Pain levels and corresponding medications are as follows:

Mild to Moderate (1–3): Over-the-counter medication, such as Tylenol (acetaminophen), Advil, or Aleve (naproxen).

Moderate to Severe (4–6): If one of the above medications does not work, an opioid medication is prescribed. Opioids are the strongest pain-relieving medication available. They include Vicodin (acetaminophen and hydrocodone) and Ultram (tramadol).

Severe (7–10): For severe pain that is not relieved with one of the above, a stronger opioid, such as morphine, oxycodone, hydromorphone, methadone, or levorphanol, may be ordered. There are many ways to receive pain medication: orally (pill, capsule, liquid), locally (ointment or patch applied to the skin), rectally (suppository), intravenously (IV; injection into a vein), subcutaneously (subQ; injection directly under the skin), or intramuscularly (IM; injection directly into muscle).

Medication

Today, the majority of older adults take some form of medication. At one time, people took medicine just to treat a disease they already had. Today, many medications are given to older adults to prevent diseases. Examples are aspirin to prevent blood clots and cholesterol-lowering drugs to prevent heart problems. There are different types of medicines, such as prescription drugs, nonprescription drugs (e.g., aspirin, laxatives, cough medicine), and vitamin supplements and dietary supplements such as Saint-John's-wort, ginseng, or glucosamine and chondroitin. If the client takes one or more of the these, they should all be written on the care plan because they are considered to be a type of medicine. If the client has any allergies, or

if the client has had a problem taking a medicine before, that also should be noted. The medication record should indicate what each medicine is for and if it is prescribed by a health care provider. Recent changes in pharmacy laws allow pharmacists to prepackage a client's medicines in individual or daily doses, which assists in reducing errors in medication administration. If the client is taking antibiotics, be sure the client takes the complete 10- to 14-day course even if he or she feels better and wants to stop; the client must take them until they are all gone. Because of the expense of drugs, some clients might elect to take half a dosage; if so, this needs to be documented and reported. Don't mix alcohol or hot drinks with medication administration. They change the effect of the drugs and may destroy the ingredients. Encourage the client to use a special medication reminder container. This will be a handy reminder if the client cannot remember whether she or he took the medication. If the client needs to divide the pill or capsule, it is better to use a special cutter to get a more accurate cut (Figure 8-11). If the client wants to crush the pill for easier swallowing, check with the case manager to see if it is permissible. If the client is taking any herbs, vitamins, or other over-the-counter medications, make sure the case manager is aware of this.

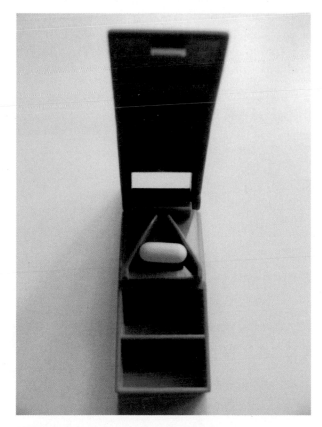

FIGURE 8-11 A simple pill cutter that is used rather than a knife to divide a pill.

These may cause serious reactions with some prescription medications.

Always be on the alert for drug reactions because they are common occurrences with the older adult. As a home health aide, you might be the first person to notice one or more of the following signs of a drug reaction:

- Tendency to bruise more easily
- Skin rashes
- Diarrhea
- Constipation
- Heartburn
- Dizziness
- Nausea and vomiting
- Fever
- Extreme fatigue
- Change in behavior

Some drugs are not eliminated from the body of an older adult as they might be in a younger person, resulting in drug build-up. Given with every prescription bottle today or attached to a bottle when it is refilled is a list of possible side effects of that particular drug. Save these papers just in case you need them for a quick reference. Encourage the client to stay with the same pharmacy so that all of the client's records will be in one place. Check the expiration dates on the bottles; do not give a medicine after the date on the bottle—it may not work as well. Do not share the client's medicine with another person in the household. It is not uncommon for the wife to take her husband's medication, for example, but this is not safe. It is wise to tell the older client not to take medications in the dark, but rather in a well-lit room. If you see the prescription bottle is running low, request a refill for the client. Most pharmacies have a call-in system, so all you need to do is call in and the medicine will be ready for pick-up. Some pharmacies might even deliver the drugs for a nominal fee. If your client refuses to have his or her prescription refilled or refuses to take his or her medicines because of financial reasons, do report this to the case manager. The case manager may be able to find funding to assist the client in purchasing required medications.

When a client has an appointment with his or her health care provider, it is wise to bring along a record of all the medicines the client is taking and the dosage. Have the client keep a list of drugs he or she is currently taking and the dosage, including prescription, nonprescription, or any herbal supplements. This list of medications can then be brought to the appointment with the health care provider. Figure 8-12 is an example of a list of medications form that can be used in the client's home.

Although home health aides do not administer medication because they are not licensed to do so, aides are allowed to do the following for the client:

a. Check the client's medication schedule and remind the client when medicine is due. The case manager

Date	Name of My Medicine	How Much Do I Take	When Do I Take It	What Do I Use It for
Example	Ibuprofen	1 tablet 400 mg	3 times a day after meals	Arthritis
	Ferrous Sulfate	2 tablets	Once a day	Anemia

FIGURE 8-12   Example of a list of medications form.

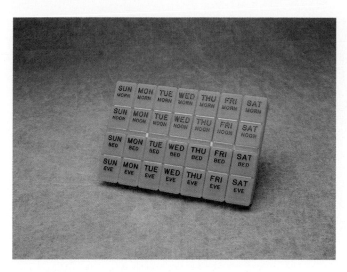

FIGURE 8-13 Special medication container.

or pharmacist may prepare your client's medication in special containers that have all the medication needed for a specific time interval (Figure 8-13).

b. Assist clients in checking to see if the dosage of medicines is correct.

c. Bring the medicine containers or prefilled medication containers to the client.

d. Shake the liquid medicines if necessary before opening the bottle for the client.

e. Read the label on the medication to see if it is to be taken with food or on an empty stomach.

f. Open the container or bottle and observe the client removing the capsule or liquid from the bottle.

g. Check to make sure the correct method of taking the medication is followed. For example, some medications are taken with juice or milk instead of water. Others are taken on an empty stomach, still others with food.

h. Check to see if the eyes are clean before the client inserts eye drops into the eyes.

i. Check the ears to see if there is any visible earwax before the client inserts eardrops.

j. Encourage the client to take the medications as ordered.

k. Bring water and a stirring stick to the client to mix powdered medication such as Metamucil, as this drug needs to be mixed immediately before administration or it will become thick or solid, making it impossible to swallow.

l. Perform any monitoring activities required, such as checking the pulse, the blood pressure, or the blood sugar, before the drug is taken. Pulse needs to be taken before certain heart medications can be taken, for example.

m. Note how much medication is left in the container. Follow instructions for getting the prescription refilled.

n. Assist the client to a comfortable position to take the medication.

o. Leave the medication within easy reach of the client. Remind the client to take the nighttime dose in a well-lit room.

p. Place sleeping and pain medication bottles in a safe place after each use.

q. If a client is taking once-a-day medication, the client should be encouraged to take the medication at the same time every day.

r. If a client takes a pain medication or insulin injections, the exact time the client takes it needs to be documented.

s. If a client refuses to take his or her medication, that should be charted and also the reason for not taking it. The case manager should be notified.

t. Place nitroglycerin tablets within the client's reach at all times. When the client has chest pain, the client needs to place these tablets under the tongue immediately. Nitroglycerin tablets are given **sublingually** (under the tongue) and should not be swallowed, as the gastric juices will destroy the effects of the drug.

u. If a client has questions about the prescribed medication, encourage the client to ask the case manager. The client should be knowledgeable about medications that he or she is taking.

Special Precautions for a Client with Low Vision

The aide must take special care in assisting clients who are blind or have low vision with their medications. Be sure that medications are coded so that the client can find the correct bottles when they are needed. Medications for the client who is blind must be kept in exactly the same spot so that an error will not be made. Special arrangements should be made by the pharmacist or case manager in setting up the coding.

Refer to Procedure 5, Assisting the Client with Self-Administered Medications.

PROCEDURE 5   ASSISTING THE CLIENT WITH SELF-ADMINISTERED MEDICATIONS

- The following information should be made available to the aide by the case manager and clearly written down:
  - Name of each medicine
  - What each medication is for
  - Description of medicine—color, form
  - Time(s) of day or night when each medicine is to be taken. Some medications are given 3 times a day (tid), usually before (ac) or after (pc) each meal. Others may be ordered 4 times a day (qid) or every 6 hours (q6h). A medication taken every 6 hours could be given at 6 A.M., noon, 6 P.M., and midnight.
  - How long the medicine should be taken
  - Whether the medicine should be taken with food or other liquid
  - Possible side effects
- The home health aide should be informed of common reactions to medications so the case manager can be called if side effects appear.

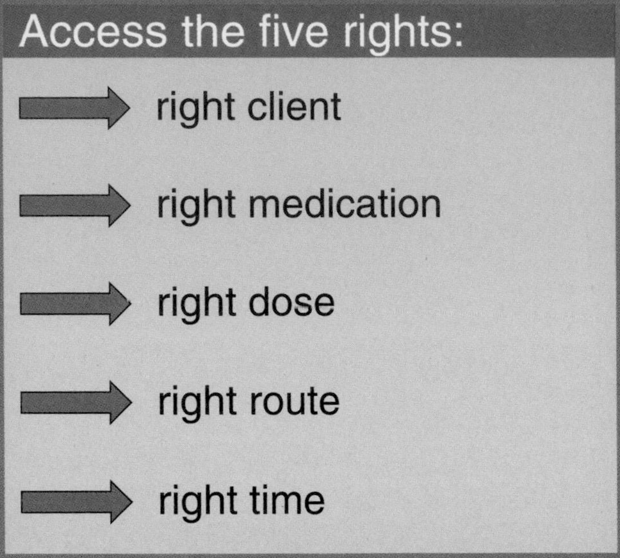

Access the five rights:

➡ right client

➡ right medication

➡ right dose

➡ right route

➡ right time

FIGURE 8-14   Five Rights in Medication Administration.

Purpose

- To relieve pain, to help the body fight infections, to prevent diseases, and to treat diseases
- To encourage the client to take the prescribed medication at the right time, in the right dose, in the right amount, and in the right manner (Figure 8-14)

Procedure

1. Assemble supplies and wash hands:
   - medication sheet
   - medication(s)
   - glass of water, yogurt, or applesauce
2. Take the supplies to where the client is sitting.
3. Place the client in comfortable position.
4. Tell the client it is now time to take the medication(s).

5. Open the prefilled medication container(s) or open the bottle(s) of medication.
6. Have the client take the medication out of the prefilled container or pour it from the bottle(s).
7. If the client makes an error in taking or pouring the medication from the bottle, tactfully remind the client that an error has occurred. Have the client reread the label.
8. Have water available to help the client swallow the medication. If the client is having difficulty in swallowing the medication, the medication can be mixed with yogurt or applesauce.
9. Stay with the client until the client swallows the medication(s).
10. Return medication containers to their storage place.
11. Document the medication/s taken.

WORKBOOK REVIEW

Go to the workbook and complete the review exercises and activities for Unit 8.

REVIEW

1. Chronological refers to which of the following?
   a. How old a person is
   b. How well an individual is able to accomplish tasks of daily living

2. Which of the following are common problems for older adults?
   a. Adjusting to loss of one's spouse
   b. Adapting to living alone
   c. Adjusting to chronic illness
   d. All of the above

3. Aging brings about specific changes in breathing due to
   a. thinner chest walls.
   b. diminished breathing capacity.
   c. thinner lung secretions.
   d. all of the above.

4. Which of the following would be helpful to someone with visual problems?
   a. Providing adequate lighting
   b. Speaking louder
   c. Providing finger foods for snacks
   d. Reading to the person

5. The older adult may have trouble chewing food due to which of the following?
   a. Less saliva in mouth
   b. Poor teeth
   c. Dentures
   d. All of the above

6. Which of the following would be helpful when working with an older adult with hearing loss?
   a. Speaking slowly and clearly
   b. Facing the client when speaking
   c. Avoiding background noise or music
   d. All of the above

7. Individuals with osteoporosis are at risk for
    a. blood clots.
    b. fractures.
    c. strokes.
    d. heart attack.

8. If a client complains of pain, list four questions you should ask the client.

    _____

    _____

    _____

    _____

9. T F   In the aging process, the sense of smell decreases, as well as the flow of saliva.

10. T F   An analgesic is a drug that relieves pain.

11. T F   Another name for earwax is cerumen.

12. T F   Cataracts is a disorder that affects the lens of the eye.

13. T F   Antibiotics are taken only until the symptoms of the infection are no longer present.

14. T F   Glaucoma can cause blindness if left untreated.

Case Studies

15. On Thursday you arrive at the home of a longtime client. The client is surprised to see you, and asks, "Why are you working on Sunday?" You realize that this client has not been herself lately. What do you do?

16. You are to give Gail Thompson a shower and range-of-motion exercises for the knee that she just had surgery on. Gail complains of pain in her knee and refuses a shower and her exercises. She does have pain medication ordered. She has not had a shower since returning from the hospital. How would you proceed?

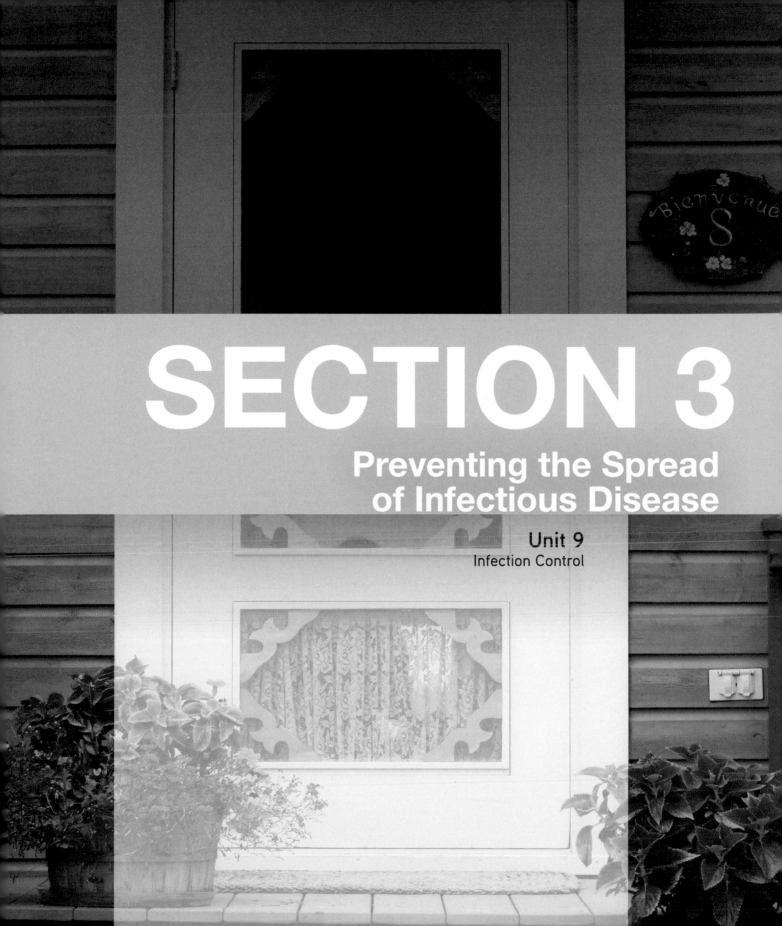

SECTION 3
Preventing the Spread of Infectious Disease

Unit 9
Infection Control

UNIT 9
Infection Control

KEY TERMS

acquired
  immunodeficiency
  syndrome (AIDS)
airborne
antibiotic-resistant
bacteria
bedbugs
biohazard
Clostridium difficile
  (C-diff)
conjunctivitis
contact precautions
contaminated
disinfection
droplet precautions
ELISA

fungi
germs
hepatitis A, B, C
herpes zoster (shingles)
human immunodeficiency
  virus (HIV)
immunizations
incident report
incubation period
infection
infectious disease
inflammation
isolation
jaundice
Kaposi's sarcoma

methicillin-resistant
  Staphylococcus aureus
  (MRSA)
microorganisms
nosocomial infection
Occupational Safety and
  Health Administration
  (OSHA)
pathogens
personal protective
  equipment (PPE)
Pneumocystis carinii
  pneumonia
portal of entry
protozoa
reservoir

rickettsiae
source
standard precautions
sterile
susceptible host
transmission-based
  precautions
tuberculosis
U.S. Centers for Disease
  Control and Prevention
  (CDC)
vancomycin-resistant
  enterococcus (VRE)
virus

LEARNING OBJECTIVES

After studying this unit, you should be able to:

- Name three different types of microorganisms

- List signs and symptoms of
  an infection

- Distinguish between an infection and an
  inflammation

- Explain the links of the chain of infection

- Explain the differences between disinfection and
  sterilization

- Describe the actions of the home health aide
  related to infection control practices

- List the ways infectious diseases are spread

- Name the single most effective precaution to prevent the spread of infections

- List five examples of when aides must wash their hands

- Describe standard precautions and when they are used

- Describe the three types of transmission-based precautions and when they are used

- List five requirements of OSHA and the CDC that affect home health aides

- List signs and symptoms and nursing care for a client with tuberculosis

- Discuss three types of hepatitis and the differences between them

- Discuss how a person can become infected with HIV

- Describe the three different stages of HIV/AIDS

- Discuss symptom-specific nursing care for clients with AIDS

- Demonstrate the following:

  PROCEDURE 6   Handwashing

  PROCEDURE 7   Gloving

  PROCEDURE 8   Applying and Removing Personal Protective Equipment

Infectious Disease

An **infection** is the invasion of body tissue by disease-producing organisms. An **infectious disease** is one that is readily communicable or easily passed on to others (contagious).

Signs of a client having an infection are fever and chills, fatigue, loss of appetite, discharge from infected areas, redness, pain or tenderness, nausea or vomiting, diarrhea, or a skin rash. An **inflammation** of a body part may have similar signs, but an inflammation does not have a pathogen (germ) in the area (Figure 9-1). An example of an inflammation is the reaction that takes place in a person who sprains an ankle. The ankle will be swollen, reddish, painful, and warm to the touch—these are called the classic signs of an inflammation. Infectious diseases can be spread through various routes: airborne, carried by animals and insects, contact (or carried by humans), prenatal from mother to fetus, in food, or carried by soil and water.

The Chain of Infection

The first step in the chain of infection is that there is a **pathogen** or **germ** (Figure 9-2), which is called the causative agent. The second step in the chain is that the germ must have a place to live and thrive—this is called the **reservoir** or the **source**. The next step is for the germ to leave the reservoir and be transmitted to another host. This is called the mode of transmission, or the method by which the pathogen moves from one place to another. In order for the germ to enter a body, the germ must have a **portal of entry** such as a break in the skin, or through the blood (such as HIV). The germ has a better chance

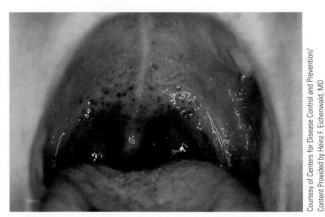

Courtesy of Centers for Disease Control and Prevention/ Content Provided by Heinz F. Eichenwald, MD

FIGURE 9-1   Redness, swelling, heat, and pain are signs of inflammation. A sore throat is an excellent example of painful inflammation.

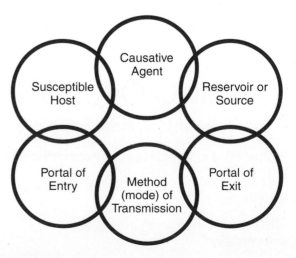

FIGURE 9-2   The chain of infection.

of multiplying and surviving if the client (host) is weak. Instead of the term *weak*, the term susceptible host is used. An example of a susceptible host is a client in the later stages of cancer who suddenly develops a condition called herpes zoster (shingles; Figure 9-3). The primary sign of shingles is a painful itching rash that occurs over the body, following along the nerves of the body. The virus that causes shingles is quite common, but a normal, healthy individual is able to prevent the virus from entering and multiplying in the body.

If a client develops an infection while being hospitalized, this type of infection is called a nosocomial infection. There is less chance for this type of infection to occur if a client is discharged early from the hospital.

The purpose of infection control is to disrupt the chain of infection. Breaking one link is all that is needed to prevent the spread of infection (Figure 9-4).

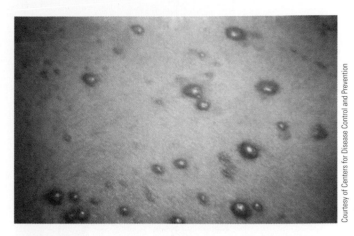

Courtesy of Centers for Disease Control and Prevention

FIGURE 9-3   A rash in a client with shingles. The blisters are intact, so the client is infectious.

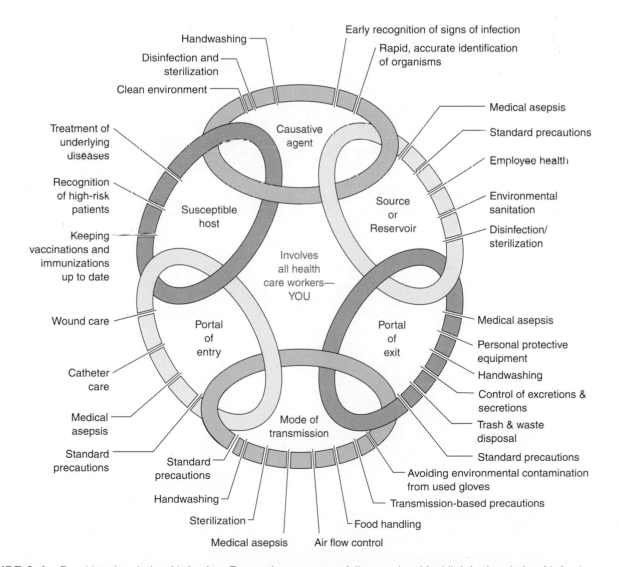

FIGURE 9-4   Breaking the chain of infection. Preventive measures follow each critical link in the chain of infection.

Causes of Infectious Diseases

Microorganisms are so small that they can be seen only under a high-powered microscope. There are beneficial microorganisms and microorganisms that can cause disease. The microorganisms that are capable of causing disease are called *germs* or *pathogens*. The time between the entry of germs into the body and the appearance of the first sign of disease is called the **incubation period**. Strong, healthy people are more able to fight off pathogens than are weak or unhealthy people (Figure 9-5).

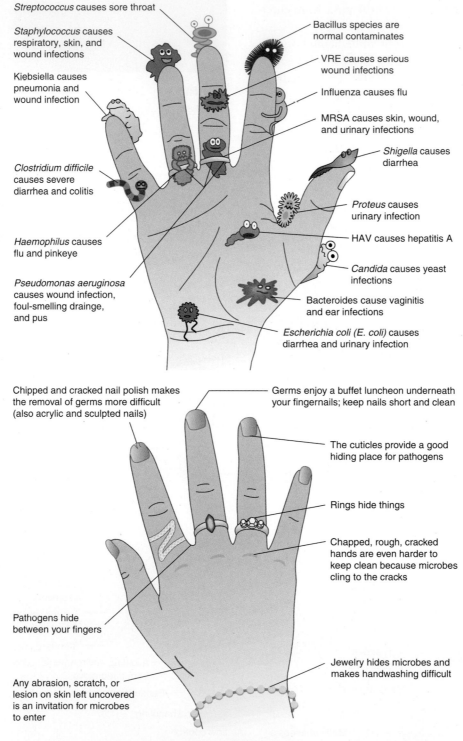

Streptococcus causes sore throat

Staphylococcus causes respiratory, skin, and wound infections

Klebsiella causes pneumonia and wound infection

Clostridium difficile causes severe diarrhea and colitis

Haemophilus causes flu and pinkeye

Pseudomonas aeruginosa causes wound infection, foul-smelling drainge, and pus

Bacillus species are normal contaminates

VRE causes serious wound infections

Influenza causes flu

MRSA causes skin, wound, and urinary infections

Shigella causes diarrhea

Proteus causes urinary infection

HAV causes hepatitis A

Candida causes yeast infections

Bacteroides cause vaginitis and ear infections

Escherichia coli (E. coli) causes diarrhea and urinary infection

Chipped and cracked nail polish makes the removal of germs more difficult (also acrylic and sculpted nails)

Germs enjoy a buffet luncheon underneath your fingernails; keep nails short and clean

The cuticles provide a good hiding place for pathogens

Rings hide things

Chapped, rough, cracked hands are even harder to keep clean because microbes cling to the cracks

Pathogens hide between your fingers

Any abrasion, scratch, or lesion on skin left uncovered is an invitation for microbes to enter

Jewelry hides microbes and makes handwashing difficult

FIGURE 9-5 Examples of how a worker's hands can transfer germs.

Ways to Kill Germs	Description	Use
Disinfection	The use of chemical products—such as mouthwash, disinfectants, alcohol, Lysol, and bleach—to kill pathogens.	Household items Clothes Hands Thermometers
Sterilization	The application of dry or steam heat (e.g., boiling water) under controlled conditions.	Baby bottles and nipples Dishes and utensils
Pest control	Use of chemicals and other means to rid areas of pests.	Rats, mice Flies, bedbugs Fleas, mosquitoes

FIGURE 9-6   Germs can be destroyed by applying infection control techniques.

There are many different types of microorganisms. Bacteria are microscopic organisms that multiply rapidly. Protozoa are tiny one-cell microorganisms. Bacteria and protozoa can live for a long time and continue to multiply in air and water. Many types of bacteria and protozoa exist, but only a few cause diseases. Viruses are microorganisms that can live only by feeding on living cells. Most viruses are capable of causing infections. Diseases caused by viruses include influenza, colds, human immunodeficiency virus (HIV), and hepatitis. Fungi include two groups of organisms—yeast and molds—that live normally in the body. Under certain conditions they can cause diseases such as athlete's foot (tinea pedis), ringworm (tinea capitis), thrush, or vaginitis (*Candida albicans*). Yeasts and molds are known as opportunistic parasites. When the human immune system is depressed and unable to protect the body, these organisms can invade the body and cause severe infections. Another example of a microorganism that can cause a disease and lives on lice, ticks, fleas, mites, and other insects is rickettsiae.

Practicing good infection control techniques is the best defense against the spread of germs (Figure 9-6). If there is a possibility of the presence of germs (pathogens) on an article, the article is considered contaminated. Articles that are free of all living organisms are sterile. The process of sterilization completely destroys microorganisms on objects. Many sterile supplies, such as gauze dressings, applicators, and instruments, come prepackaged in paper for convenience. They must be opened, handled, and used in a special way so that they will not become contaminated. Disinfection is the process of destroying disease-producing organisms by using chemicals. For example, if a home health aide uses a stethoscope on one client, the diaphragm of the stethoscope must be disinfected or wiped with an alcohol sponge before using it on another client. This will prevent the spread of germs from one client to another.

Controlling the Spread of Infectious Disease

Almost everyone practices some form of infection control in daily living. Some of the most common practices are:

- Handwashing
- Bathing, brushing teeth, shampooing hair
- Changing clothing regularly
- Cleaning bathroom sink, tub, bowl, and floor (Figure 9-7)
- Cleaning kitchen, washing dishes
- Vacuuming and mopping floors
- Laundering clothing and bed linens
- Cleaning from the cleanest area to the dirtiest area
- Covering your nose when coughing or sneezing
- Flushing the toilet after each use
- Using a separate towel and washcloth for each person in the household; if wet, letting towels and washcloths air-dry before reuse
- Keeping tabletops and countertops clean and dry

When illness is present, added care must be taken to prevent the spread of germs. An ill person's body is weak and cannot resist other germs. The person's body is so busy fighting one illness that it cannot fight off new germs. The person's immune system is depressed.

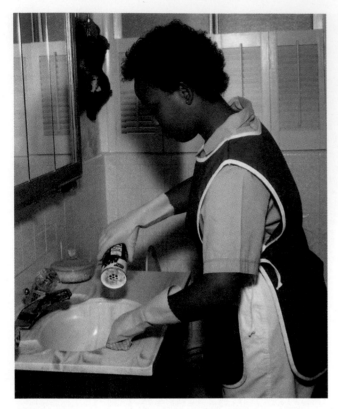

FIGURE 9-7   Cleaning the bathroom on a regular basis helps in the control of infections.

Most germs grow and reproduce very rapidly. They easily spread disease from one part of the body to another. Germs can spread from one person to another by direct contact. An example is when a person coughs and you are within a few feet of the person—germs can escape from the person's mouth and you may breathe in these germs. Germs can be spread when others touch contaminated objects or surfaces and then spread the contaminant to others. This is called spreading germs by indirect contact. Tissues used by the client should be placed in a paper bag at the client's bedside. Dressings or bandages from open cuts or wounds must be double-bagged in plastic and then discarded. Careful cleaning of the client's room is important in stopping the indirect spread of germs.

Immunizations

Artificial defenses called **immunizations** protect against specific pathogens. Immunizations against viruses are provided by vaccines. Zostavav is a vaccine that is used to prevent shingles in older adults. Pneumococcal Vaccine Polyvalent is used to prevent pneumonia in older adults.

Health care workers who have direct contact with clients are advised to get a hepatitis vaccine.

Agency Requirements

Two government agencies are very involved in preventing the spread of infections and diseases while delivering care. Guidelines for working with clients with infectious diseases are issued by the **U.S. Centers for Disease Control and Prevention (CDC;** www.cdc.gov) and **Occupational Safety and Health Administration (OSHA;** www.osha.gov). In order to be accredited, a home health care agency must follow these guidelines. A few of the guidelines that affect the home health aide directly are as follows:

1. The employer must provide the home health aide with training on working with protective care equipment (e.g., gloves, goggles, and mask).

2. The employer must provide the home health aide with necessary protective equipment when caring for a client who has an infectious disease.

3. The employer must provide immunization against hepatitis B with no cost to the home health aide.

4. The employer must provide tuberculosis testing yearly with no cost to the home health aide.

5. The employer must provide training in **biohazard** waste and what to do if the possibility of exposure exists.

The guidelines also state that if the home health aide accidentally pricks a finger with a needle or other sharp instrument that is contaminated, this must be reported to his or her agency immediately. The home health aide is also required to fill out an **incident report**. On this report the home health aide states (1) how the accident happened, (2) where it happened, (3) details about the injury or accident, (4) if there were any witnesses, and (5) the date and time it happened.

Guidelines from these two government agencies are constantly being updated. It is the responsibility of the home health care agency to keep home health aides aware of changes that affect how they need to care for their clients. New diseases constantly appear—for example, in the year 2014, there as a severe EBOLA epidemic. In the past 30 years, there have been 35 new infectious diseases worldwide. The U.S. death rate from infectious diseases, which dropped in the first half of the 20th century and then stabilized, is now double what it was in 1980.

Infection Control Measures

A home health aide has a duty to protect clients from unnecessary harm. In addition to keeping the home environment clean and following everyday infection control practices, the aide also should be in good physical health. An aide who is ill risks carrying germs into the client's environment.

The home health aide's hands are the most common means of carrying infection. To control the spread of germs and to protect the aide and client, the aide's hands must be washed frequently. Do not give germs a free ride—wash your hands frequently either with alcohol-based hand cleaner or soap and water; refer to Procedure 6, Handwashing. The hand cleaner you use should be at least 60% alcohol. Handwashing should be performed as follows:

- On arrival at the client's home
- Before and after each client contact
- Before preparing food
- Before and after each meal
- After blowing the nose or sneezing
- After using the bathroom
- After handling soiled items such as linens, clothing, or garbage
- Before putting on gloves and after removing gloves
- After contact with items contaminated with blood, feces, or other body fluids

---

PROCEDURE 6   HANDWASHING

Purpose
- To prevent the transfer of disease-producing organisms from person to person or place to place

Procedure
1. Collect the items needed for handwashing and bring them to the sink:
   - soap (bar or liquid; liquid is preferred)
   - soap dish—optional
   - towel (paper towels preferred)
2. Use a clean paper towel to turn on the water and adjust the temperature. Wet hands with the fingertips pointing down (Figure 9-8).
3. Apply soap—either liquid or bar.
4. With fingertips pointing down, lather well. Rub your hands together in a circular motion to generate friction (Figure 9-9). Wash carefully between your fingers, on the palms, and on the back of the hands, and rub your fingernails against the palm of the other hand to force soap under the nails. Keep washing for 15 seconds. Be sure to clean under the fingernails (Figure 9-10).

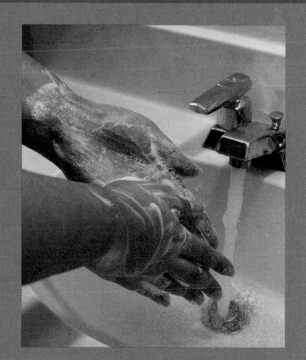

FIGURE 9-8   Wet hands, apply soap, and rub hands to cause lather. Keep hands pointed down so that water does not run up the arms.

(*continued*)

PROCEDURE **6**   HANDWASHING (*continued*)

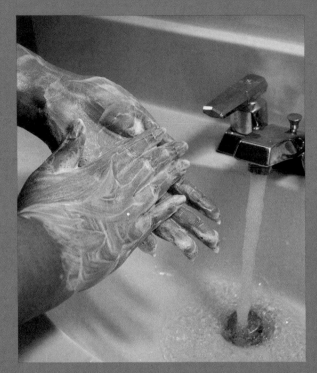

FIGURE 9-9   Use friction between the hands to clean well.

5. With fingertips still pointing down, rinse all the soap off. Be careful not to lean against the side of the sink or touch the inside of the sink because germs are present on these surfaces.
6. With a clean paper towel or clean hand towel, dry your hands. Use a clean paper towel to turn off the faucet (Figure 9-11). Do not turn off the faucet with your clean hands because the faucet handles are contaminated.
7. Discard the paper towel in the wastebasket.

NOTE: Cloth towels can spread germs when reused.

Alcohol-Based Hand Rub

8. Apply product to the palm of one hand. Rub the hands together, covering all surfaces of the hands, until the hands are dry.
9. Apply hand lotion if hands are dry or chapped.

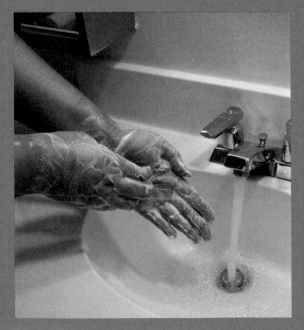

FIGURE 9-10   Always clean your fingernails.

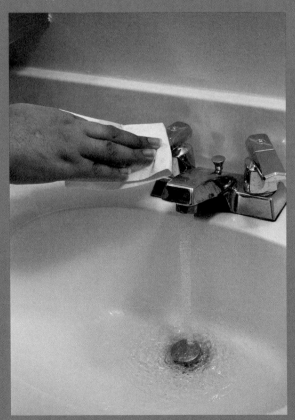

FIGURE 9-11   Turn off the faucet with a dry paper towel.

The aide should keep in mind that handwashing is the most important procedure involved in controlling the spread of disease.

Standard Precautions

We cannot tell if people have an infectious disease just from looking at them. Therefore, certain measures must be taken to prevent the spread of infection. These measures are called standard precautions and must be used at all times for all people, regardless of the client's condition or diagnosis. Standard precautions are designed to protect the home health aide and the client. Standard precautions provide guidelines for handwashing, personal protective equipment (PPE) use (gloves, gowns, masks, goggles), client care equipment, environmental care, linen handling, and safe needle use. See Figure 9-12 for specific guidelines.

Although the use of special or standard precautions is important to prevent the spread of infection to, or from, a client, keep in mind how odd it must feel to a client to be cared for by a person wearing barriers. Most of us are used to health professionals and paraprofessionals using gloves, gowns, or masks. However, to a person who is feeling isolated or depressed, these protective barriers may increase their feelings of loneliness and sadness. Your tone of voice, what you say, and the gentleness of your touch thus become even more important.

Other Wastes

- Dispose of sharps—needles, razor blades, and other sharp items—in a puncture-proof, leak-proof container near the point of use. Do not recap or handle needles before disposal. The container should be labeled with the biohazard symbol and color-coded red (Figure 9-13A, B).
- Dispose of wastes in plastic bags.
- Wipe up blood spills immediately. Use gloves and a solution of 1 part bleach to 10 parts of water.

Transmission-Based Precautions

Transmission-based precautions are precautions taken in addition to standard precautions. They are used when the pathogen that is causing the infection is highly contagious. There are three types of transmission-based precautions, depending on how the organism is spread from one person to another. The first type is airborne, which is used when caring for a client with tuberculosis, chickenpox, or measles. The reasoning behind the extra precautions is that the organism is very small and can stay in the air for a longer period. Thus, the extra precautions deal with how the air is handled in the client's room and within the ventilation system. It is the responsibility of the home health care agency to deal with the home ventilation and air-exchange system. The second type is called droplet precautions. These extra precautions are used when caring for a client who has an infectious disease such as influenza and the microorganism can spread by coughing, sneezing, or talking. The home health aide must wear a mask when caring for the client. When taking the client out of the home, the client must also wear a mask. Contact precautions are special measures that need to be taken if the client has an infection such as conjunctivitis (pinkeye), impetigo, or a staphylococcal wound infection. These diseases are highly contagious. Extra measures that need to be taken are (1) wear gloves at all times, (2) wash hands with soap before and after applying gloves, (3) wear a gown or apron when entering the room and doing direct client care, (4) limit the client's contact with others, and (5) take special care when disposing of all equipment and supplies that come in contact with the client. Contaminated items such as bloody dressings must be placed in a specially marked red bag or container with the biohazard symbol (Figure 9-13A, B).

Antibiotic-Resistant Organisms

The most popular method used to treat an infection is with an antibiotic. Occasionally, a pathogen or microorganism is not killed by an antibiotic; this is an antibiotic-resistant pathogen or microorganism. Two organisms that are seen in home health care that are resistant to antibiotics are methicillin-resistant *Staphylococcus aureus* (MRSA) and Vancomycin-resistant Enterococcus (VRE). Although standard precautions are the same for clients with hepatitis and HIV, there are extra precautions that should be taken for MRSA and VRE clients. When caring for clients with VRE or MRSA, the home health aide should wear gloves whenever providing any personal care to these clients, not just when expecting to come into contact with bodily substances.

Clostridium difficile (C-diff)

A healthy colon is lined with bacterial flora—hundreds species of bacteria. Many are beneficial, but some are not. When a person uses antibiotics to treat an unrelated infection, an imbalance in the flora may occur, as antibiotics do not discriminate good bacteria from bad. This imbalance of flora in the colon allows the *Clostridium difficile (C-diff)* germ to grow and multiply, producing

STANDARD PRECAUTIONS FOR INFECTION CONTROL

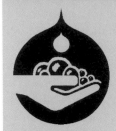

Wash Hands
Wash after touching **blood, body fluids, secretions, excretions,** and **contaminated items.** Wash immediately **after gloves are removed** and before applying gloves.

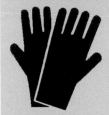

Wear Gloves
Wear when touching **blood, body fluids, secretions, excretions,** and **contaminated items.** Put on **clean** gloves just **before touching mucous membranes** and **nonintact skin.** Change gloves between tasks and procedures on the same client after contact with material that may contain high concentrations of microorganisms. Remove gloves promptly after use, before touching noncontaminated items and environmental surfaces.

Wear Mask and Eye Protection or Face Shield
Protect mucous membranes of the eyes, nose, and mouth during client care activities that are likely to generate **splashes** or **sprays** of **blood, body fluids, secretions,** or **excretions.**

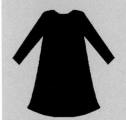

Wear Gown
Protect skin and prevent soiling of clothing during procedures that are likely to generate **splashes** or **sprays** of **blood, body fluids, secretions,** or **excretions.** Remove a soiled gown as promptly as possible and wash hands to avoid transfer of microorganisms to other people or environments.

Client Care Equipment
Handle used client care equipment soiled with **blood, body fluids, secretions,** or **excretions** in a manner that prevents skin and mucous membrane exposures and contamination of clothing.

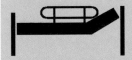

Environmental Control
Follow procedures for routine care, cleaning, and disinfection of environmental surfaces, beds, bedside equipment, and other frequently touched surfaces. Double-bag soiled disposable items (e.g., adult briefs). If blood gets on the floor or other surfaces, wash the area with a solution of 1 part bleach to 10 parts water.

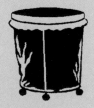

Linens
Handle, transport, and process used linens soiled with **blood, body fluids, secretions,** or **excretions** in a manner that prevents exposures and contamination of clothing. A large plastic bag or garbage bag can be used to discard soiled linens.

FIGURE 9-12   Standard precautions guidelines.

(continued)

Biohazards
Prevent injuries when using needles, scalpels, and other sharp instruments or devices; when handling sharp instruments after procedures; when cleaning used instruments; and when disposing of used needles.
Do not remove used needles from disposable syringes by hand, and do not bend, break, or otherwise manipulate used needles by hand. Place used disposable syringes and needles, scalpel blades, and other sharp items in puncture-resistant sharps containers located as close as practical to the area in which the items were used. When the container is full, return it to your agency; do not throw it in the regular trash or garbage can.

FIGURE 9-12 (continued)

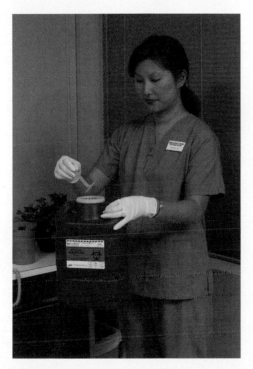

FIGURE 9-13A Place sharps in specially marked container after use.

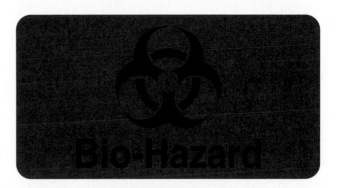

FIGURE 9-13B Biohazard symbol.

toxins that can damage the colon. Signs and symptoms of this infection are severe diarrhea and abdominal pain.

The client with a communicable disease may be placed in **isolation**. This means that the client is kept away from others in the household. Isolation helps prevent family members and the home health aide from getting the client's germs. If the family members want to participate in the client's care, they also will have to use personal protective equipment.

PROCEDURE 7 GLOVING

Purpose

• To prevent the spread of infections

NOTE: Gloves come in various sizes. Be sure you use the correct size of gloves, because if the glove is too small, it will break or tear easily; if the glove is too large, germs can enter easily. Gloves are made from different materials. If a home

health aide is allergic to certain types of glove materials, hypoallergenic gloves can be used.

Procedure

1. Wash your hands.
2. With your dominant hand, pull out one glove and slide it onto your other hand.

(continued)

PROCEDURE 7 GLOVING (*continued*)

3. With the gloved hand, pull out another glove and slide your dominant hand into it.
4. Interlace your fingers to make the gloves comfortable and adjust the top of the gloves to stay flat.

Removal of Contaminated Gloves

1. Use your dominant hand to grasp the opposite glove on the palm side, about 1 inch below the wrist (Figure 9-14).
2. Pull the glove down and off so that it is removed inside out and keep hold of that glove with the fingertips of the gloved hand (Figure 9-15).

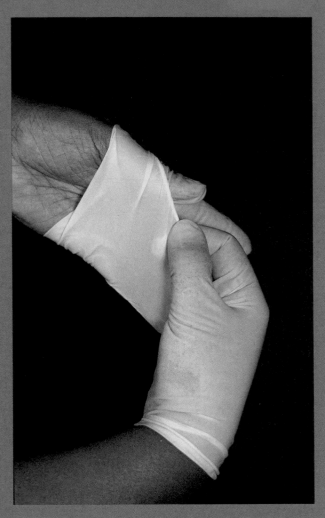

FIGURE 9-15 Pull the glove down and off, inside out.

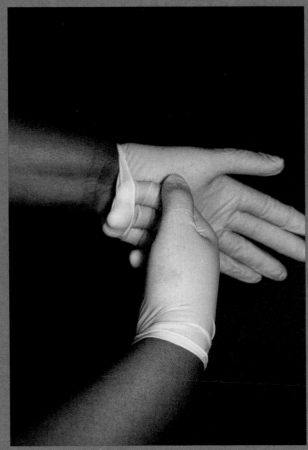

FIGURE 9-14 To remove gloves, grasp the glove on the palm side.

3. Using your ungloved hand, insert the fingers into the inside of the remaining glove and pull it down and off, inside out, so that the glove you are holding with your fingertips is now inside the glove that you are taking off (Figure 9-16).
4. Drop both soiled gloves together into the waste receptacle (Figure 9-17).
5. Wash your hands.

(*continued*)

PROCEDURE 7 GLOVING (*continued*)

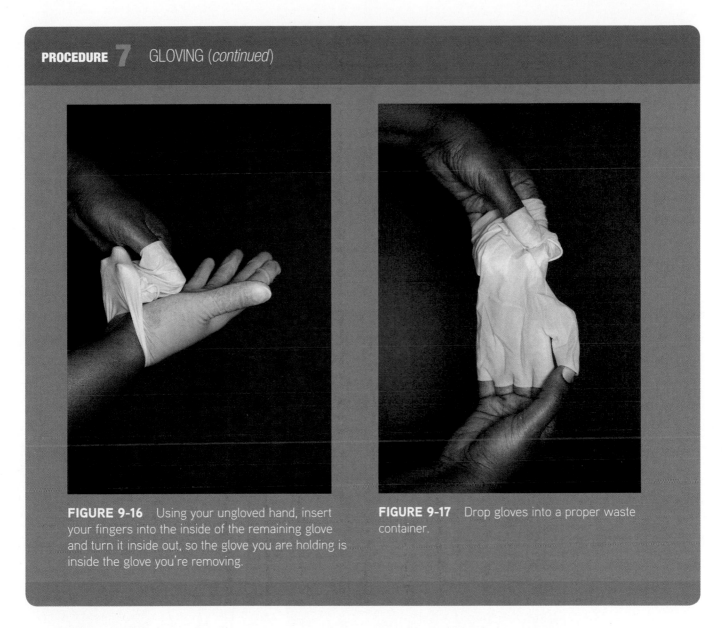

FIGURE 9-16 Using your ungloved hand, insert your fingers into the inside of the remaining glove and turn it inside out, so the glove you are holding is inside the glove you're removing.

FIGURE 9-17 Drop gloves into a proper waste container.

Standard precautions provide guidelines for wearing personal protective equipment such as gowns and masks. Wearing gloves and masks prevents the spread of germs and prevents the contamination of the aide's clothing. The home care agency will provide the aide with specific personal protective equipment. Refer to Procedure 7 Gloving and Procedure 8 Applying and Removing Personal Protective Equipment.

PROCEDURE 8 APPLYING AND REMOVING PERSONAL PROTECTIVE EQUIPMENT

Purpose

- To prevent contamination of the aide's clothing
- To reduce the transmission of germs

Procedure

1. Assemble personal protective equipment (Figure 9-18).
2. Wash your hands.

(*continued*)

PROCEDURE 8 APPLYING AND REMOVING PERSONAL PROTECTIVE EQUIPMENT (*continued*)

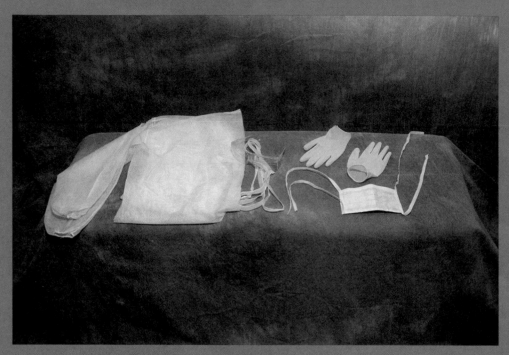

FIGURE 9-18 Protective barriers used in standard precautions: gloves, disposable gown, goggles, and disposable mask.

3. Unfold and open the gown so that you can slide your arms into the sleeves and your hands come right through. Slip the fingers of both hands inside the neckband of the gown and grasp the two strings at the back and tie into a bow, not a knot, so that they can be undone easily after the procedure is completed. Reach behind you, overlap the two edges of the gown so that your uniform is completely covered, and then secure the waist ties (Figure 9-19A, B).

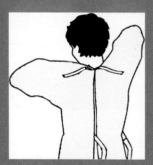

FIGURE 9-19B Slip your hand inside, under the neckband, and adjust it to fit. Tie the neck ties. Then reach behind, overlapping the edges of the gown so your clothing is completely covered, and tie the waist ties.

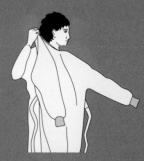

FIGURE 9-19A Unfold the gown, then slip your arms in and pull it up to your shoulders.

4. Apply the mask and adjust the mask over your nose and mouth. Tie the top strings first and then the bottom strings. Your mask must always be dry, so that droplets are not absorbed into the paper of the mask. If the mask becomes wet, you must replace it.

5. Apply goggles or face shield if at risk for splashing.

PROCEDURE 8 APPLYING AND REMOVING PERSONAL PROTECTIVE EQUIPMENT (*continued*)

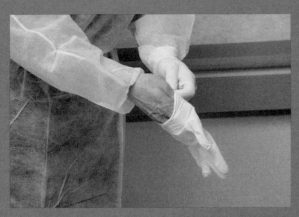

FIGURE 9-20 Pull the gloves over the cuff of the gown.

6. Apply gloves. Stretch the glove cuff over the gown sleeves at the wrist (Figures 9-20 and 9-21).

REMEMBER: Your moisture-resistant gown is only worn once and is then discarded in a container for contaminated waste.

Removing Contaminated Gown and Mask

1. Undo the waist ties of your gown.
2. Remove gloves.
3. Remove protective eyewear.
4. Remove gown. Untie gown at neck and waist. Remove from shoulder. Fold and roll gown down in front into a ball, so the contaminated area is rolled into the center of the gown (Figure 9-22). Dispose of the gown in the appropriate waste container.
5. Remove mask. Undo your mask, bottom ties first, then top ties. While holding the top ties, drop the mask into an appropriate waste container.
6. Wash hands.

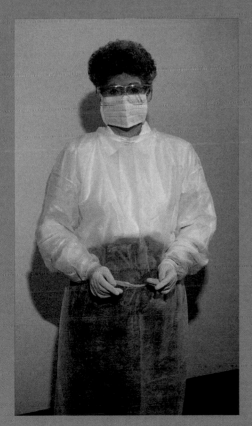

FIGURE 9-21 Properly masked, gloved, and gowned aide.

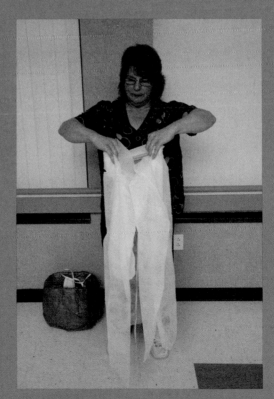

FIGURE 9-22 Fold the gown inside out and dispose of it in a proper waste container.

Isolation is more difficult to arrange in the home than it is in a hospital. Ideally, isolated clients should have their own bathroom. However, when this is not possible, the home health aide will have to clean and disinfect the sink and toilet area each time the client uses it. Disposable dishes, equipment, or tissues should be used whenever possible. The client should use a separate set of dishes and utensils than is used by the family. Combs, brushes, toilet articles, towels, and washcloths used by the client should not be used by others. Keeping these items separate helps prevent the indirect spread of infection.

All contaminated materials from the client's room must be discarded by placing them in a double plastic bag or in a covered garbage container. The client's linens and clothing must be washed separately from other family laundry. The client's dishes must be washed separately or placed in a dishwasher. After the isolation period is ended, any items used by the client should be discarded or disinfected. It is important to destroy all germs on the items used before returning them to general family use.

Bedbugs

Bedbugs are parasites that can be found anywhere in a home (Figure 9-23A). They are tiny, flat, and clear or white in appearance. They hide in the seams of clothing and furnishings. They may hide in cracks and cervices in mattresses, bed frames, pictures, door casings, and other areas. They can survive in both hot and cold climates. They bite and cause a painful, rash-type area on the skin (Figure 9-23B). If bedbugs are noted, a professional exterminator will be called to eliminate them. If you suspect bedbugs in a home, inform the case manager immediately.

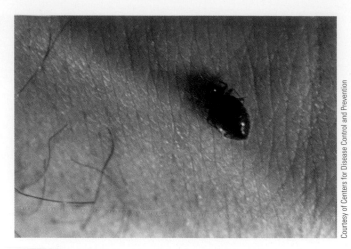

Courtesy of Centers for Disease Control and Prevention

FIGURE 9-23B The bedbugs bite and cause a painful rash on the skin.

Tuberculosis

Tuberculosis (TB) is an airborne disease, which means that it is spread by droplets in the air released from deep within the lungs when a TB sufferer coughs. Anyone sharing a poorly ventilated room with an individual with TB can contract the disease. TB is more likely to occur in clients with weak immune systems, such as people with HIV or terminally ill clients. The incidence of TB is on the rise. Individuals who live in crowded spaces, have poor nutrition, are substance abusers, are under a high amount of stress, or lack medical care are good candidates for this disease.

When an aide is assigned to care for a client with TB, the aide will need to use standard precautions, especially when handling the client's sputum and nasal secretions. A special mask, if required, will be provided by the home care agency to wear while caring for a client with TB. Another important aspect of care is making sure to remind the client to take medication as prescribed. *The medication must be taken on schedule; otherwise, the effects of the drugs will be decreased.* TB can be cured if caught in the early stages and if the client takes the medication as ordered, usually for 6 months. If the client does not take the medication as prescribed, be sure to notify the case manager.

The home health aide also will need to be checked yearly by having a TB skin test or a chest x-ray. The signs and symptoms of TB come on rather slowly. It is common for an individual to have TB for a long time before the signs and symptoms become evident or full blown. The first signs of TB are cough with green or yellow mucus, weight loss, slight fever, and pain in the chest, back, or kidney. Night sweats, shortness of breath, and spitting up large amounts of pus-colored sputum develop as the disease progresses. Treatment usually consists of medications and rest.

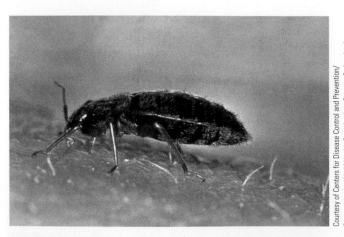

Courtesy of Centers for Disease Control and Prevention/ Donated by the World Health Organization, Geneva, Switzerland

FIGURE 9-23A The bedbug is tiny and clear in appearance before it has eaten.

Hepatitis

Hepatitis is a viral infection that mainly affects the liver. Classic signs and symptoms of this liver disease are jaundice (yellowing of the skin and whites of the eye), (Figure 9-24), fatigue, abdominal pain, loss of appetite, and nausea. There are many different types of hepatitis, depending on the name of the virus causing the infection. The three main types are hepatitis A, B, and C.

Hepatitis A. The cause of this mild type is the hepatitis A virus (HAV). It is usually spread from person to person by feces, salvia, and contaminated food. Signs are jaundice, fever and nausea, dark urine, and loss of appetite.

Hepatitis B. This is a more serious type of hepatitis and could lead to complications that may cause liver cancer or cirrhosis of the liver. These complications may be fatal to the client. The virus that causes this condition is called hepatitis B virus (HBV; Figure 9-25). This virus may be found in the blood and body fluids, including urine, tears, semen, vaginal secretions, and breast milk. The disease is spread through sexual contact, contamination by needle sticks, and the use of contaminated personal care items (e.g., razors, nail clippers, toothbrush). Many individuals who are infected with the virus may not know it because the signs at first are silent. The only way one might know is through a blood test. Thus, the infected person can pass it on without knowing it. The primary signs of the infection are flu-like symptoms. Eventually, jaundice will become apparent and clients will develop other symptoms such as dark urine and light-colored stools. The disease can be treated with a variety of medications.

The home health aide may get vaccinated to prevent acquiring the virus. This vaccine is divided into three injections over a 6-month period. The Engerix-B Vaccine is recommended for health workers.

Hepatitis C. Hepatitis C is caused by hepatitis C virus (HCV). This is a chronic disease that remains in the bloodstream, eventually destroying the person's liver. This disease is the leading cause of liver transplants in the United States. The disease occurs when blood and body fluids from an infected person enter the body of a person who is not infected. The virus is spread through shared needles of intravenous drug users, needle-stick injuries at work, or from a mother to an infant while in utero, if the mother is infected. After 6 to 8 weeks of the initial infection, the client may suffer symptoms similar to those of the flu. These signs and symptoms include joint pain, nausea, vomiting, muscle aches, and fatigue. After this stage, the client may be symptom-free for a period. Eventually, the liver will be destroyed, and if a transplant does not take place, the client will die.

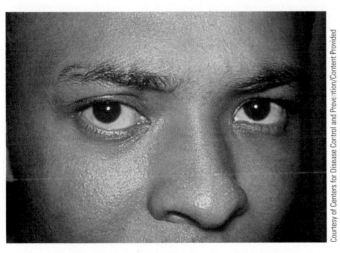

FIGURE 9-24 Jaundice is a yellowing of the skin and whites of the eyes caused by hepatitis and other conditions.

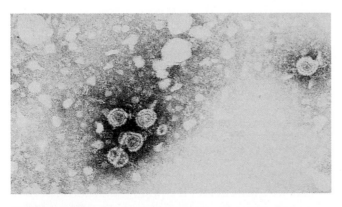

FIGURE 9-25 Electron micrograph of hepatitis B virus.

Courtesy of Centers for Disease Control and Prevention/Content Provided by Dr. Thomas F. Sellers; Emory University

AIDS

Acquired immunodeficiency syndrome (AIDS) is a chronic, severe immunologic disorder caused by the human immunodeficiency virus (HIV). This virus interferes with the body's ability to fight the organisms that cause disease. HIV is a sexually transmitted disease. It can also be spread by contact with infected blood, shared needles, or from mother to child during pregnancy, childbirth, or breast feeding. It can take years before HIV weakens the immune system to the point that the person has AIDS. The acute infection phase is the shortest stage of HIV infection. The first signs are flu-like illness 3 to 6 weeks after being infected with the virus. Then, for 7 to 10 years, the symptoms disappear. The immune system during this time gradually becomes weaker. This is called the chronic stage. A blood test called the CD4 count is done to monitor the

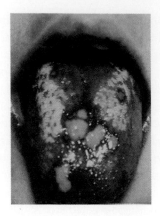

FIGURE 9-26   White patches on the tongue are evidence of the fungus disease called thrush.

progress of the disease. A few signs and symptoms that a client may display once the CD4 count gets lower are fatigue, swollen lymph glands in the neck and groin, night sweats, weight loss, dyspnea, chronic diarrhea, yeast infections of the mouth (Figure 9-26) and vagina, and easy bruising and bleeding of the skin. Because of the client's weakened immune system, the client is very susceptible to other infections throughout life. A rare form of skin cancer can occur in the later stage, which is called **Kaposi's sarcoma** (Figure 9-27). Other later signs are dementia, brain cancer, and *Pneumocystis carinii* **pneumonia**. Death usually follows within 2 to 3 years after the appearance of these symptoms, if not treated.

A diagnosis of HIV is made through a blood test. The most common test is the antibody or **ELISA** test, which detects HIV antibodies in a person's blood.

At this time, HIV is considered to be the most dangerous of the sexually transmitted diseases (STDs). Before 1981, HIV was unknown in this country. Today,

HIV is widespread not only in the United States, but worldwide. Africa, Haiti, and some parts of Asia have a high incidence of the disease. The drug Truvada can be given to prevent HIV, but the cost of the drug is between $11,000 and $14,000 a year. There is no cure for HIV/AIDS once the virus is in the body, but a variety of drugs can be used in combination to control the virus. Each of the classes of anti-HIV drugs blocks the virus in different ways. Medications are started when certain lab values exist, and multiple medications will be used. Side effects of these drugs include:

- nausea, vomiting, diarrhea
- abnormal heart beat
- shortness of breath
- skin rashes
- weakened bones
- bone death, particularly in hip joint

Drug therapy should be combined with a healthy lifestyle such as regular exercise, a healthy diet, and avoidance of cigarettes and illegal drugs to protect the immune system.

Children with HIV need special attention and care. Often the scenario is that one or perhaps both parents are HIV positive and will eventually die. The child is then left without any parental care. When caring for a child with HIV, be very observant for signs that may indicate an infection, such as fever, vomiting, and diarrhea. It is better that the child has plastic or washable toys, as stuffed toys can hold dirt and hide germs that can make a child sick. Try to keep the child away from sandboxes and animals. Do the utmost to keep the child from contracting any type of infectious disease, as this could kill the child, as his or her immune system is very depressed.

Caring for the Client with AIDS

The emotional and physical support of caregivers, family, and friends is crucial in helping those with AIDS lead as normal a life as possible, for as long as possible.

One of the major concerns of the U.S. Department of Health is to provide proper care for the AIDS client while protecting health care workers. At this time, the Centers for Disease Control and Prevention (CDC) indicates that one cannot get HIV from casual social contact (e.g., shaking hands, hugging, coughing, sneezing, or kissing), contact with tears of an HIV-positive individual, or from the perspiration of an HIV-positive individual.

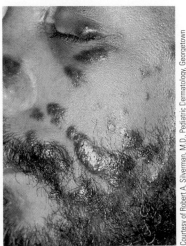

Courtesy of Robert A. Silverman, M.D., Pediatric Dermatology, Georgetown University

FIGURE 9-27   Typical skin lesions of Kaposi's sarcoma.

What a Home Health Aide Can and Should Do

When working with a client with AIDS, it is important to know that many misconceptions about the disease exist. The home health aide should learn the facts about AIDS, use standard precautions when performing client care, and remain nonjudgmental of the client, regardless of how the disease was contracted. A home health aide must never reveal to friends, neighbors, or anyone else the nature of a client's illness. That is considered an invasion of privacy, and the client can file a complaint with the State Department of Human Rights if such information is revealed by the agency or the aide.

The home health aide should create a comfortable and pleasant environment for the client. Figure 9-28 shows a sample care plan for the client with AIDS.

WORKBOOK REVIEW

Go to the workbook and complete the review exercises and activities for Unit 9.

Sign/Symptom	Care to Provide	Purpose
Weakness/tiredness	High-calorie diet with in-between meal high-protein snacks	To provide protein nutrition and to slow muscle deterioration
Fever	Sponge baths; give additional fluids by mouth; cover with blankets during chill periods	To lower the temperature and to prevent complications; to keep client comfortable
Night sweats	Sponge baths; frequent clothing and linen changes; give additional fluids	To provide comfort, prevent dehydration, and prevent skin breakdown
Cough	Observe and record patterns and changes; offer cough medicine if prescribed	To make the client comfortable and to obtain relief from strain
Dyspnea	Record and report abnormal breathing; place in sitting position; give oxygen as ordered	To provide adequate oxygen
Skin lesions	Keep client from scratching—be sure fingernails are short; wear gloves when working with client with lesions	To prevent infections and further skin problems
Dry hair and hair loss	Use mild shampoo and hair conditioner	To prevent scalp irritation
Mouth lesions	Provide saline or diluted mouthwashes; brush teeth gently; check to be sure client can swallow without difficulty; avoid spicy and acidic foods	To prevent spread of lesions in the mouth and maintain adequate nutrition
Diarrhea	Encourage fluid intake and if rectal area becomes red, apply a lanolin cream to the area	To maintain fluid balance; to prevent skin breakdown
Impaired immune system (when client is very susceptible to other infections)	Give shower or bath; do not allow visitors who have infections, such as colds	To prevent infection and to assist in client protection
Unstable emotional responses	Be aware of client's feelings as well as your own; offer emotional support and be kind	To create an atmosphere of mutual trust

FIGURE 9-28 Sample care plan for client with AIDS.

REVIEW

1. List the times when the home health aide's hands should be washed.

2. List five ways that diseases can be transferred from one person to another.

   _____

   _____

   _____

   _____

   _____

3. Name three different types of germs that can cause diseases.

   _____

   _____

   _____

4. A disease-producing microorganism is called
   a. contaminated.
   b. contagious.
   c. a vector.
   d. a pathogen.

5. All home health aides should use standard precautions when caring for all clients. Standard precautions include which of the following?
   a. Wearing gloves when handling body substances
   b. Wiping up blood spills with a solution of bleach and water
   c. Wearing goggles and gloves if required to prevent contact with the client's infectious substances
   d. All of the above

6. List four components of the chain of infection.

   _____

   _____

   _____

   _____

7. List four common signs and symptoms of an infection.

   _____

   _____

   _____

   _____

8. Fill in the blank: _____ is the practice used to prevent the spread of harmful germs from a person, place, or thing to another person, place, or thing.

9. Match the type of transmission-based precaution in Column I with the correct definition in Column II.

   Column I

   _____ 1. droplet precautions

   _____ 2. airborne precautions

   _____ 3. contact precautions

   Column II

   a. used to prevent the spread of germs through the air

   b. used to prevent the spread of germs transmitted by sneezing or coughing

   c. used with wound infections

10. An infection that develops when a client is hospitalized is called a(n) _____ infection.
    a. facility
    b. acquired
    c. nosocomial
    d. delayed

11. An effective method of preventing the spread of infectious diseases in the home is
    a. isolating client from family.
    b. soaking clothes in bleach.
    c. handwashing.
    d. hanging clothing of clients outside on clothesline.

12. Before using a stethoscope, the aide wipes the earpieces with alcohol. This is an example of
    a. disinfection.
    b. sterilization.
    c. cross-infection.
    d. contamination.

13. List two ways HIV can be transmitted from one person to another.

    _____

    _____

14. HIV primarily attacks what body system?
    a. Respiratory
    b. Circulatory
    c. Immune
    d. Nervous

15. List five signs or symptoms of AIDS in the later stage.

    _____

    _____

    _____

    _____

    _____

Case Studies

16. Your client, Mrs. Jones, is positive for human immunodeficiency virus. After assisting her with a bath, you notice several droplets of blood on the bathroom floor. You make a determination that the blood is a result of Mrs. Jones's menstrual flow. What steps should you take to clean up the blood on the bathroom floor?

17. You have been assigned to a new client, and on your first visit to the home you notice that the kitchen is very dirty. The floors are dirty and sticky, and dishes are piled in the sink. The counters are filled with papers and look like they have not been wiped down in some time. Why is a dirty kitchen a health risk to your client? What steps could you take to organize the workload of keeping the kitchen clean?

18. You are assigned to help your client, who has an open skin lesion, with a bath. Do you need to wear gloves while assisting her with her bath? Under what conditions would you be required to wear gloves when giving care to the client? Give specific examples of three procedures where you would be required to wear gloves.

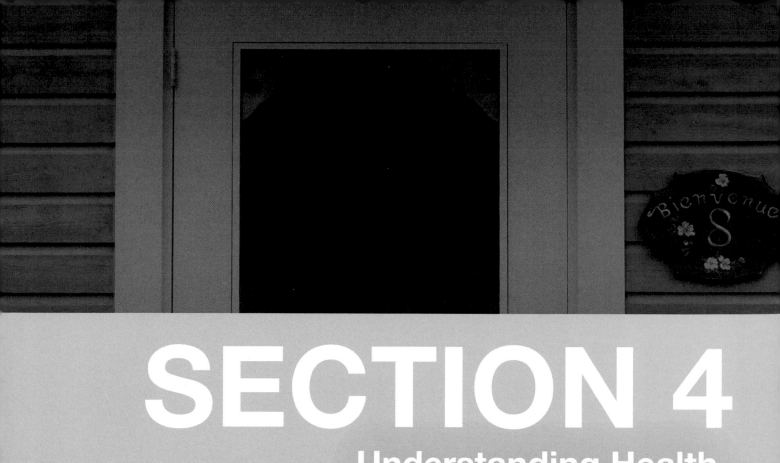

SECTION 4
Understanding Health

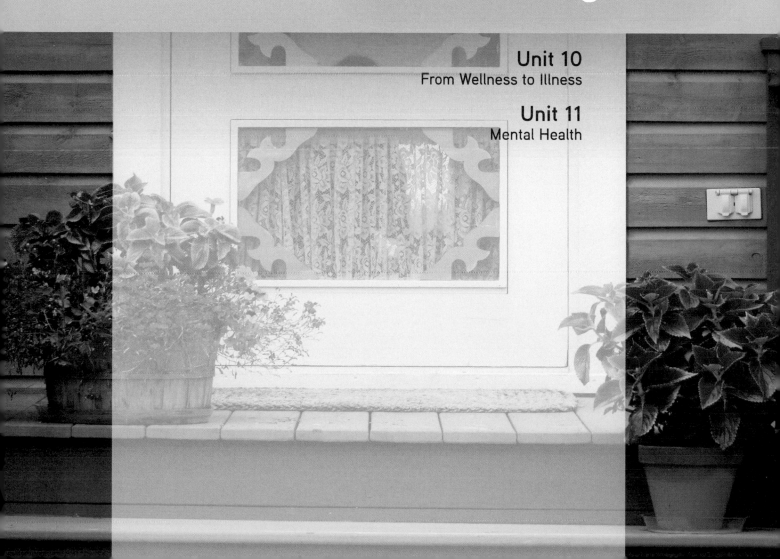

Unit 10
From Wellness to Illness

Unit 11
Mental Health

UNIT 10
From Wellness to Illness

KEY TERMS

afebrile
apical
apnea
blood pressure
brachial
bradycardia
Celsius/centigrade scale
Cheyne-Stokes
contracture
diastolic

digital thermometer
disability
dyspnea
exhalation
Fahrenheit scale
febrile
hypertension
hyperthermia
hypotension
hypothermia

inhalation
orthostatic hypotension
palpate
pulse
respiration
sign
sphygmomanometer
stertorous
symptom
systolic

tachycardia
temporal artery
temporal artery
  thermometer (TAT)
tympanic ear
  thermometer
vital signs

LEARNING OBJECTIVES

After studying this unit, you should be able to:

- Discuss wellness

- Make a distinction between an emotional disorder and an internal disorder

- Define disability

- Explain why vital signs are measured

- List factors that affect vital signs

- Identify abnormal and normal temperature ranges

- Measure body temperature using different types of thermometers

- Identify various sites for feeling a pulse

- Explain the normal range of pulse for different age groups

- Describe characteristics of normal and abnormal pulses

- Describe characteristics of normal and abnormal respirations

- Describe the normal rate for respirations in an adult

- Describe the normal and abnormal ranges for blood pressure

- Name the pieces of equipment used to take blood pressure

- Describe the two-step method of taking blood pressure

- List requirements for accuracy in measuring height and weight

- Distinguish between the different levels of consciousness

- Discuss nursing care that needs to be done for clients who are unconscious

- Discuss hypothermia and hyperthermia

- Demonstrate the following:

  PROCEDURE 9 Taking a Tympanic (Ear) Temperature

  PROCEDURE 10 Taking an Oral (Mouth) Temperature (Digital Thermometer)

  PROCEDURE 11 Taking a Temporal Artery Temperature

  PROCEDURE 12 Taking a Radial Pulse

  PROCEDURE 13 Taking an Apical Pulse

  PROCEDURE 14 Counting Respirations

  PROCEDURE 15 Measuring Blood Pressure

  PROCEDURE 16 Measuring Weight and Height

The Remarkable Body

Bodies come in all shapes and sizes. There are records of men who have been as tall as 9 feet and as short as 26 1/2 inches. These statistics are interesting because they show the tremendous contrasts possible within the human body. Just as there are contrasts in size, there are other individual differences. Heredity is the passing of traits from parents to their children. Heredity can determine height, weight, general appearance, skin color, talents and abilities, basic physical wellness, and many other things. All children get half of their heritable material from each parent. However, some traits are more dominant than others. This explains why some children are more like one parent than the other.

Another factor that helps determine body size, shape, and wellness is environment. Environment is the sum total of the circumstances, conditions, and surroundings affecting the development of an organism. Some environmental factors that may affect growth are nutrition, financial conditions, climate, number of children in the family, and the parents' ages and occupations. The child who is born healthy with good hereditary characteristics is likely to start life as a well person. If the child grows up in a healthy environment where he or she is well fed, clothed, sheltered, respected, and loved, the child will continue to be well physically and mentally. An identical twin with the same heritable material would not be as likely to develop into a well person if the twin were raised in an unhealthy environment. Many argue about which is more important, heredity or environment. One side believes that good heredity can overcome poor environment. The other side claims that good environment can rescue a child with poor heredity. It is clear, however, that both contribute to a person's development. Ways to control heredity are limited; however, environment can, to some extent, be controlled.

Imagine how hard it would be if, each second of the day, you had to consciously perform every body function. Most people take their bodies for granted as long as everything seems to be in good working order. Think of all the activities constantly occurring and all of the things that could go wrong. Maintaining a state of wellness seems miraculous.

The human body is remarkable because it can continue to work when some of its parts break down. Damaged brain cells cannot be "repaired," but there are so many brain cells that new ones can be trained to take over. Many body structures are in "pairs." A body has two arms, two legs, two kidneys, two eyes. In the well body all of the parts work together.

What happens when one of a pair becomes diseased? In the case of kidneys, one can be removed surgically and the other will take over the work. The person with only one kidney must be more careful with diet and generally take more health precautions than the average person, yet a person can return to a state of wellness with even one kidney. The human body and mind are able to adapt. The home health aide's efforts are important in helping a client adapt physically, mentally, and emotionally. Human beings have often been compared to machines. When functioning perfectly, the body operates as smoothly as a well-oiled machine. The human body, however, is much more efficient than any machine. Unlike a machine, the human body often can repair itself; for example, new skin can grow over a wound. When the body functions at its peak efficiency with all of its parts working like a finely tuned engine, it is in a state of wellness.

The body is a complex organism. It is made up of millions of cells, which are the smallest structural units of the body. Many cells make up a tissue, and tissues make up organs (Figure 10-1). Organs act together in making the total body function. All of these separate units interact within the body in systems. There are nine body systems, each one performing a necessary function in the body (Figure 10-2).

Internal Health

Wellness is the normal state of the human body. Illness occurs when the body machinery is not working properly. This may be caused by external factors or it may result from an internal disorder (abnormality). Internal problems occur when some part of the body is not working correctly. Accidents and environmental hazards are examples of external causes of illness.

Some external environmental factors that may affect people's health are air and water. Particles or organisms present in the air and water can enter the body and cause illness. People who have asthma and lung disorders have great difficulty breathing when the air quality is poor. Coal miners may breathe in coal dust, which harms the lungs. These particles can seriously damage the respiratory system. Viruses are external organisms carried through the air in water droplets. When they enter the nose or mouth they can cause infectious diseases. Flu, the common cold, and measles are examples of virus infections.

Illness, an accidental injury, a birth defect, or the normal sensory losses of aging may be the cause of a disability. A disability may involve impaired mental or emotional functioning or involve an impaired body function, such as eyesight or ambulation (walking). The Americans with Disabilities Act (a national law protecting the rights of people with disabilities; see www.dol.gov) defines a person with a **disability** as someone who:

- Has a physical or mental impairment that substantially limits one or more major life activities
- Has a record of such an impairment
- Is regarded as having such an impairment

Because the home health aide will be caring for clients who are ill or disabled or who are recovering from an illness, it is important for the aide to understand the basic principles and terms related to disorders and diseases and to their treatment.

Internal Disorders

Internal disorders may happen at any age. However, they are more likely to occur as the body grows older and becomes more prone to breaking down. Usually young people recover more quickly from accidents and diseases because their body tissues and cells repair and grow at a faster rate. It takes longer for recovery in older persons because the growth rate of new cells is slower. The circulatory system often becomes less efficient as people age. Heart disease, stroke, diabetes, and hypertension are major physical disorders of the older adult.

Emotional Disorders

An internal disorder that can happen at any age is an emotional breakdown. Many times, a person who normally functions well suffers an emotional breakdown when external stress becomes too great. Illness, pain, and physical trauma put stress on the body and the person's emotions. On the other hand, physical care such as proper nutrition, exercise, companionship, and relief from pain can do much toward lifting depression and relieving mental stress.

Emotional and physical health depend on one another. Emotional illness may sometimes cause a physical illness. For example, a client who believes that there is poison in the food will refuse to eat. This can lead to severe malnutrition. Physical illness can bring on emotional problems, too. Some clients seem more able to cope with illness than others. A person who is ill or suffering from a disability caused by an accident, illness, or aging has to cope with an increase in physical and emotional pain as well as many losses. The individual who is ill experiences a decrease in physical and emotional energy, an increase in physical discomfort, and perhaps chronic pain.

Observing Signs and Symptoms

In later units, individual medical conditions are discussed. For each condition, the home health aide will be told the signs and symptoms that may arise during the illness. The aide must be able to recognize, record, and report significant signs and symptoms. A **sign** is a change that can be observed or measured. Signs of emotional stress might include wringing of the hands and unusual or sudden changes in behavior. Signs of a physical change

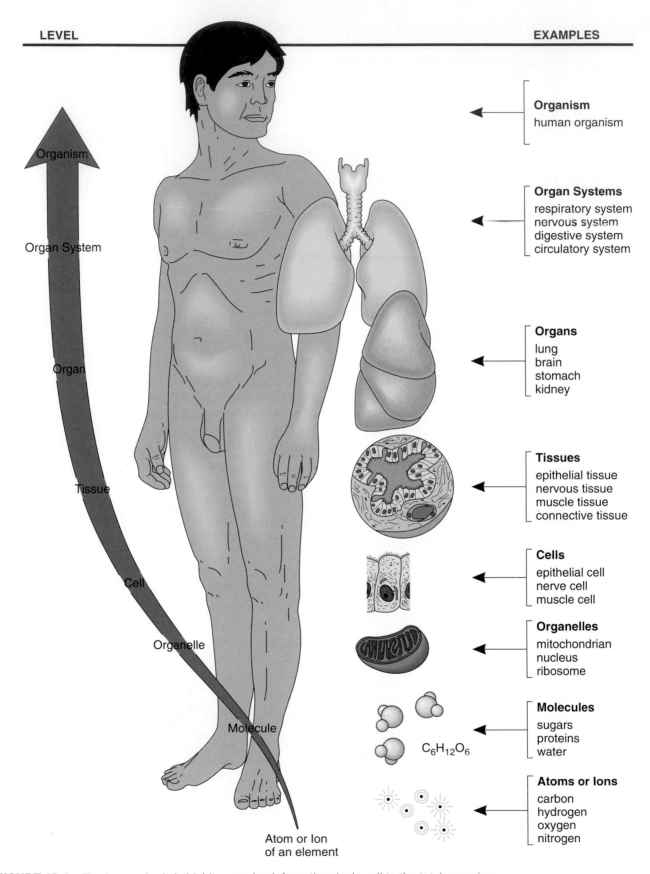

LEVEL

EXAMPLES

Organism

Organ System

Organ

Tissue

Cell

Organelle

Molecule

Atom or Ion
of an element

Organism
human organism

Organ Systems
respiratory system
nervous system
digestive system
circulatory system

Organs
lung
brain
stomach
kidney

Tissues
epithelial tissue
nervous tissue
muscle tissue
connective tissue

Cells
epithelial cell
nerve cell
muscle cell

Organelles
mitochondrian
nucleus
ribosome

Molecules
sugars
proteins
water

$C_6H_{12}O_6$

Atoms or Ions
carbon
hydrogen
oxygen
nitrogen

FIGURE 10-1 The human body is highly organized, from the single cell to the total organism.

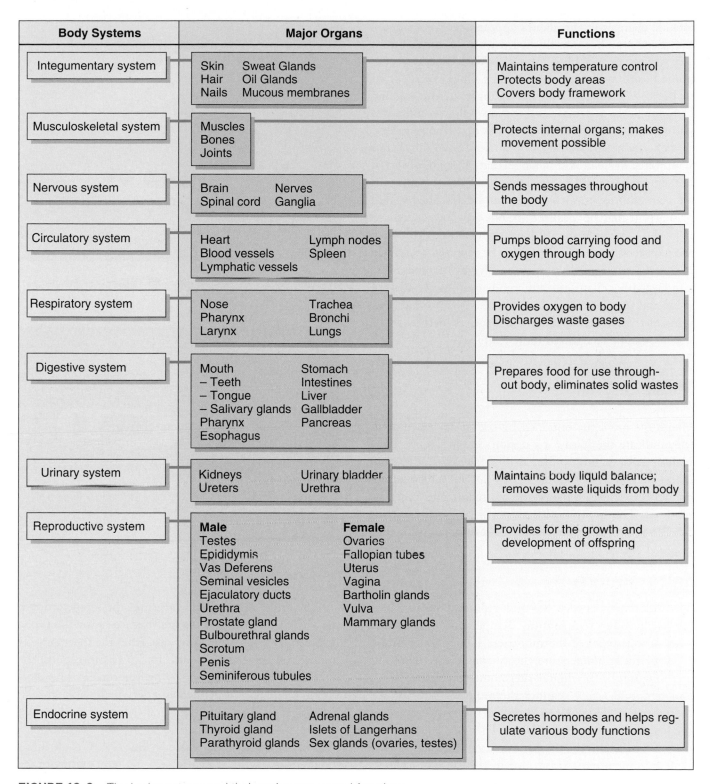

Body Systems	Major Organs	Functions
Integumentary system	Skin Sweat Glands Hair Oil Glands Nails Mucous membranes	Maintains temperature control Protects body areas Covers body framework
Musculoskeletal system	Muscles Bones Joints	Protects internal organs; makes movement possible
Nervous system	Brain Nerves Spinal cord Ganglia	Sends messages throughout the body
Circulatory system	Heart Lymph nodes Blood vessels Spleen Lymphatic vessels	Pumps blood carrying food and oxygen through body
Respiratory system	Nose Trachea Pharynx Bronchi Larynx Lungs	Provides oxygen to body Discharges waste gases
Digestive system	Mouth Stomach – Teeth Intestines – Tongue Liver – Salivary glands Gallbladder Pharynx Pancreas Esophagus	Prepares food for use throughout body, eliminates solid wastes
Urinary system	Kidneys Urinary bladder Ureters Urethra	Maintains body liquid balance; removes waste liquids from body
Reproductive system	**Male** **Female** Testes Ovaries Epididymis Fallopian tubes Vas Deferens Uterus Seminal vesicles Vagina Ejaculatory ducts Bartholin glands Urethra Vulva Prostate gland Mammary glands Bulbourethral glands Scrotum Penis Seminiferous tubules	Provides for the growth and development of offspring
Endocrine system	Pituitary gland Adrenal glands Thyroid gland Islets of Langerhans Parathyroid glands Sex glands (ovaries, testes)	Secretes hormones and helps regulate various body functions

FIGURE 10-2   The body systems and their major organs and functions.

include changes in the client's appearance. For example, the client may become flushed, turn pale, break into a heavy sweat, or turn blue (cyanotic). With experience, the home health aide learns which signs should be reported to the case manager. Irregular eating patterns, swelling of lower limbs (edema), and a deep yellow complexion (jaundice) are also physical signs that may be observed.

A home health aide also should be alert to the client's symptoms. **Symptoms** are changes that cannot be observed but are experienced by the client. Examples of symptoms are pain and discomfort. A pain can be described as dull or sharp. It may be localized (in one area) or generalized (all over). The aide should have the client describe how the pain feels so that the pain can be reported accurately to the case manager. As a home health aide becomes more familiar with a client, the aide can better observe signs of stress and pain. After the aide has seen the normal reactions of the client, deviations (change), which could be serious, can be recognized more readily.

Vital Signs

Vital signs are signs obtained by use of an instrument; they indicate the status of a person's life functions. They include temperature, pulse, respiratory rate (TPR), and blood pressure (BP). Vital signs must be measured accurately. Changes outside the normal range must be reported. The home health aide will be given exact instructions as to when to take these measurements for each assigned client.

Temperature

The difference between the heat produced and the heat lost is the body temperature. Temperature is measured with various types of thermometers. The most common types of thermometers are the tympanic ear thermometer (Figure 10-3), digital thermometer (Figure 10-4), and temporal artery scanner thermometer (an infrared thermometer designed to measure the temperature of the **temporal artery**; Figure 10-5). The **tympanic ear thermometer** measures the temperature from the blood in the tympanic membrane (eardrum) in the ear. The value is close to the core body temperature. To obtain an accurate reading, gently place the disposable cover over the probe and gently insert it in the ear canal. Press the button to activate the thermometer. Within a few seconds, the temperature will be displayed on the screen. See Procedure 9, Taking a Tympanic (Ear) Temperature.

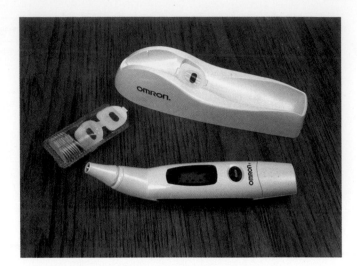

FIGURE 10-3 Tympanic (ear) thermometer.

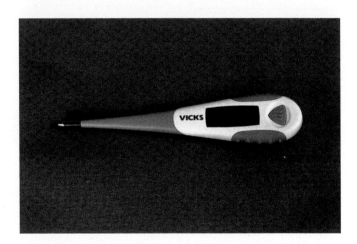

FIGURE 10-4 Digital thermometer.

The **digital thermometer** measures the temperature in the client's mouth. Sheaths are used to cover the probe before and are discarded after use. After the thermometer has been in the client's mouth for 20 to 60 seconds, the temperature will be displayed on the screen. The thermometer is battery operated and very reasonable in cost. See Procedure 10, Taking an Oral (Mouth) Temperature (Digital Thermometer).

The **temporal artery thermometer (TAT)** is an infrared thermometer designed to measure temperature of the skin surface over the temporal artery, a major artery of the head. The temporal artery is positioned close to the skin surface to provide the access needed to take an accurate measurement. It is easy to use because the artery is located at the front of the forehead. This type of thermometer is easier and gentler than other types of measurement

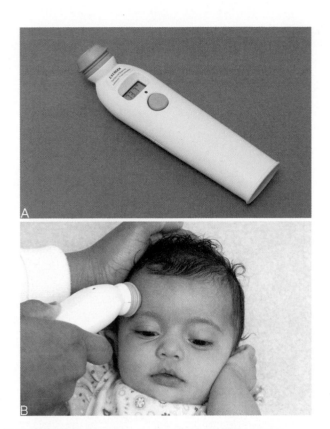

FIGURE 10-5   Using a temporal artery thermometer. (A) Temporal artery thermometer, (B) slide thermometer across the forehead.

devices because it is truly non-invasive and quick. This thermometer is battery operated. See Procedure 11, Taking a Temporal Artery Temperature.

Body temperature varies from person to person. When a person's body temperature is above normal, that is, over 100°F orally (mouth), the client is said to have a fever. Another term for fever is febrile. If a person's temperature is in the normal range, the term afebrile is used. Fever is a sign of a disease, not a disease in itself. When a person or child has a fever, this indicates that the body is reacting to an infection. Fever can cause the immune system to start fighting the infection and producing more white blood cells. A normal healthy person can tolerate a fever for a short period without any complications.

A person's body temperature varies throughout the day. It is lower in the morning and higher in the afternoon, when the body has been more active. Certain factors can raise a person's temperature, such as exercising, being outside in warm weather, or wearing too many clothes. Figure 10-6 shows the normal body temperatures taken by various methods.

A person's temperature can be measured using the Celsius or centigrade scale (0°C for freezing and 100°C for boiling), or the Fahrenheit scale (32°F for freezing and 212°F for boiling).

	Oral	Temporal	Tympanic
Average Temperature	98.6°F/37°C	97.6°F/36.5°C	99.6°F/37.5°C
Range	97.6–99.6°F (36.5–37.5°C)	97.4–100.1 F (36.3–37°.8C)	98.6–100.6°F (37–38.1°C)

FIGURE 10-6   Temperature variations in the same person.

PROCEDURE 9   TAKING A TYMPANIC (EAR) TEMPERATURE

Purpose

- To measure the client's body temperature
- To check the temperature to note any significant change

Procedure

1. Gather the equipment needed:
   - ear thermometer and disposable probe
   - recording device
   - disposable gloves

(continued)

PROCEDURE 9 TAKING A TYMPANIC (EAR) TEMPERATURE (*continued*)

2. Wash your hands thoroughly and put on gloves.
3. Tell the client that you plan to take a temperature in the ear.
4. With thermometer in hand, place a new probe on the thermometer (Figure 10-7).
5. Turn the thermometer on (Figure 10-8).
6. For an adult, pull the top of the ear up and back (Figure 10-9); for a child under 2, pull the earlobe down and back (Figure 10-10) and gently insert the probe into the ear (Figure 10-11).
7. Press the top button as you insert the probe into the ear.

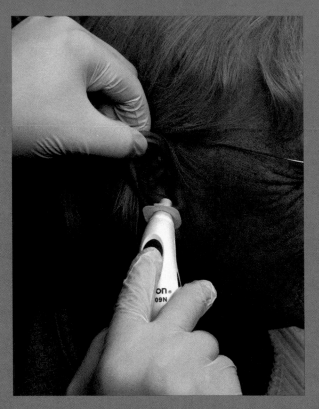

FIGURE 10-9 For an adult, pull the top of ear up and back.

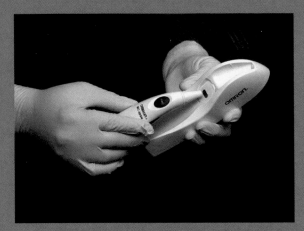

FIGURE 10-7 Applying a clean probe to the tympanic thermometer.

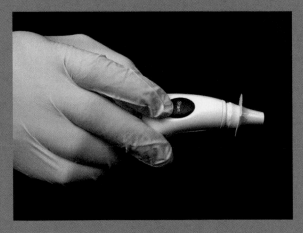

FIGURE 10-8 Press the button to turn the thermometer on.

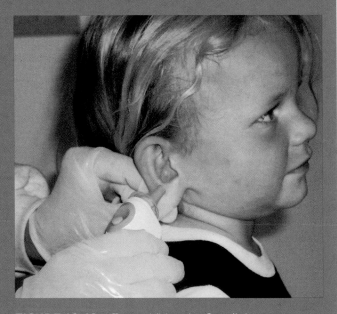

FIGURE 10-10 For a child under 2, pull the earlobe down and back.

(*continues*)

PROCEDURE 9 — TAKING A TYMPANIC (EAR) TEMPERATURE (*continued*)

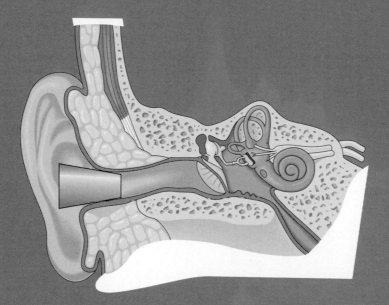

FIGURE 10-11 Inserting the probe into the ear.

8. Listen for a beep, which will only take a few seconds, then remove the probe from the ear.
9. Read the temperature indicated on the thermometer screen (Figure 10-12).
10. Remove the probe cover and discard.
11. Record the reading.
12. Remove gloves and wash your hands.

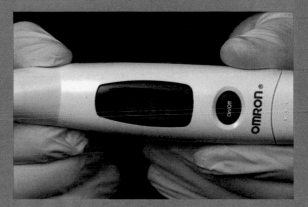

FIGURE 10-12 Screen showing the temperature of the client.

PROCEDURE 10 — TAKING AN ORAL (MOUTH) TEMPERATURE (DIGITAL THERMOMETER)

Purpose

- To obtain an accurate reading of the client's temperature
- To check the temperature to note any significant change

Procedure

1. Gather the equipment needed:
   - thermometer and sheath cover
   - recording device
   - disposable gloves

(*continues*)

PROCEDURE 10   TAKING AN ORAL (MOUTH) TEMPERATURE (DIGITAL THERMOMETER) *(continued)*

2. Wash your hands and put on gloves.
3. Apply sheath cover over the end of the thermometer (Figure 10-13).
4. Insert the probe tip well under the client's tongue. Turn the thermometer on. Place the tip of the thermometer sublingually into a heat pocket (Figure 10-14).
5. Ask the client to close the mouth and wait 10 to 20 seconds.
6. Listen for the beeps and remove the thermometer.

7. Remove the sheath cover and discard.
8. Turn the thermometer off.
9. Record the temperature.
10. Remove gloves and wash your hands.

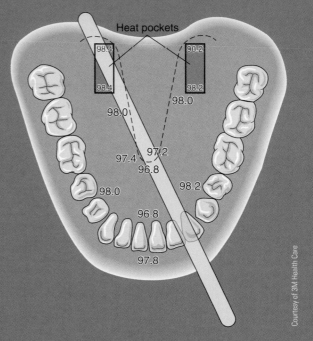

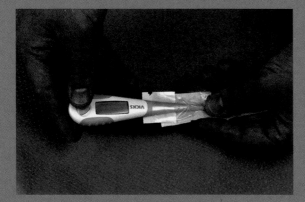

FIGURE 10-13   Apply the plastic sheath over the tip of the thermometer.

FIGURE 10-14   Place the tip of the thermometer sublingually into a heat pocket.

Courtesy of 3M Health Care

PROCEDURE 11   TAKING A TEMPORAL ARTERY TEMPERATURE

Purpose

- To obtain the client's temperature reading.
- To check the temperature to note any significant change.

NOTE: Measure only the side of the head exposed to the environment. Anything covering the area to be measured (hair, hat, wig, bandage) would insulate the area, resulting in falsely elevated readings.

   If there is perspiration on the forehead, take the temperature behind the earlobe. First push away any hair, exposing the area. Then, slide the thermometer on the neck around the earlobe. This method is often used on infants, as their foreheads may be wet with perspiration.

Procedure

1. Gather the equipment needed:
   - thermometer
   - disposable gloves if there may be contact with blood, body fluids, or open lesions. (Gloves are not necessary unless required by agency policy or potential exposure to body fluids.)

(continues)

PROCEDURE 11   TAKING A TEMPORAL ARTERY TEMPERATURE (*continued*)

- probe covers (optional) and alcohol wipes
- recording device

2. Wash your hands.
3. Apply probe cover or clean the tip of the thermometer with an alcohol wipe.
4. Holding the thermometer as you would a pencil, press the probe of the thermometer against the center of the client's forehead between the eyebrow and the hairline. Push the switch to the "ON" position with your thumb. Keep this button depressed.

5. Slide the thermometer straight across the forehead, not down the side of the face. Release the button and remove the thermometer from the forehead. Note the reading on the digital display.
6. Wipe the tip of the thermometer with an alcohol wipe or dispose of the probe.
7. Record the temperature.

Pulse and Respiratory Rates

Two other vital signs that a home health aide is required to take and record are the pulse and respiratory rates. These two readings are usually taken one after the other. After taking the pulse, the client's arm is held in the same position and the respirations are counted. It is better if the clients do not realize that respirations are being counted because they may change their respirations if they know they are being observed. The results are more accurate if the client thinks that only the pulse rate is being checked.

Pulse.   The pulse is the force of the blood pushing against the artery walls. Movement of the blood through the arteries is initiated by the heart's contraction. Thus, the pulse rate should be the same as the heart rate. The pulse may be felt at any of the sites shown in Figure 10-15. The most common site for checking the pulse is the radial artery, which can be felt inside the wrist on the thumb side. Procedure 12 demonstrates how to take a radial pulse. Procedure 13 demonstrates how to take an apical pulse. Pulse rates differ depending on the age, sex, size, and physical condition of the client (Figure 10-16). The normal adult pulse rate is between 60 and 100 beats per minute. A slow heartbeat is called bradycardia. A fast heartbeat is called tachycardia. Pulse readings show the rate, rhythm, and volume of blood pulsing through the artery. Rate is the times per minute. Rhythm is the evenness or regularity of the beat. An irregular pulse may indicate skipped heartbeats or changing rhythm patterns. Volume is the fullness of the beat. It can be described as strong, full, or weak; if it is very weak, the term thready is used.

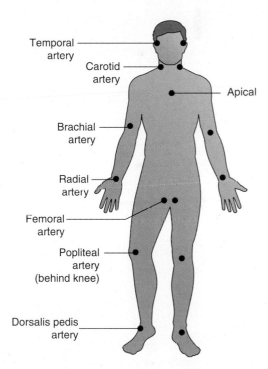

FIGURE 10-15   The pulse may be felt at any of the places shown.

Average pulse rates		
Adults	60–100	beats per minute
Children over 6	70–110	beats per minute
Children under 6	80–120	beats per minute
Infants	100–140	beats per minute

FIGURE 10-16   Average pulse rates.

PROCEDURE 12   TAKING A RADIAL PULSE

Purpose

- To measure, record, and observe the character and rate of the client's pulse
- To report changes

Procedure for Determining Pulse Rate

1. Gather the equipment needed:
   - wristwatch with a second hand
   - recording device
2. Wash your hands.
3. Tell the client that you are going to check the pulse rate. Ask the client to help by remaining quiet and still while you are counting.
4. Have the client sit in a comfortable chair or lie in bed with arms resting gently on the chest.
5. Place the tips of your first two fingers lightly on the pulse site. The radial pulse on the inner wrist is most often used (Figure 10-17). **NOTE:** Do not use your thumb to feel the client's artery. Using the thumb can result in an inaccurate reading.
6. Count the pulse beats for 1 full minute.
7. Record the pulse rate, regularity, and strength. Also record the time the pulse was taken.

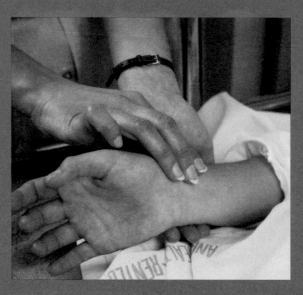

FIGURE 10-17   Locate the pulse on the thumb side of the wrist with the tips of your fingers.

PROCEDURE 13   TAKING AN APICAL PULSE

Purpose

- To obtain an accurate pulse rate
- To determine the regularity and strength of the pulse

Procedure

1. Gather the equipment needed:
   - stethoscope
   - watch with a second hand
   - alcohol wipes
2. Explain the procedure to the client.
3. Clean the stethoscope diaphragm and earpieces. Note: If you are using a stethoscope you used on a previous client, you will need to clean the diaphragm of the stethoscope. If you, the home health aide, have your own stethoscope, you do not need to clean the earpieces each time.
4. Place the stethoscope earpieces in your ears.
5. Place the stethoscope diaphragm (Figure 10-18A) over the apex of the client's heart, 2 to 3 inches to the left of the breastbone, below the left nipple (Figure 10-18B).
6. Listen carefully for the heartbeat. It will sound like "lub-dub."
7. Count the louder sound (lub) for 1 complete minute and record. A quiet environment will help you to hear the beats.
8. Record the pulse.

(continues)

PROCEDURE 13 TAKING AN APICAL PULSE (*continued*)

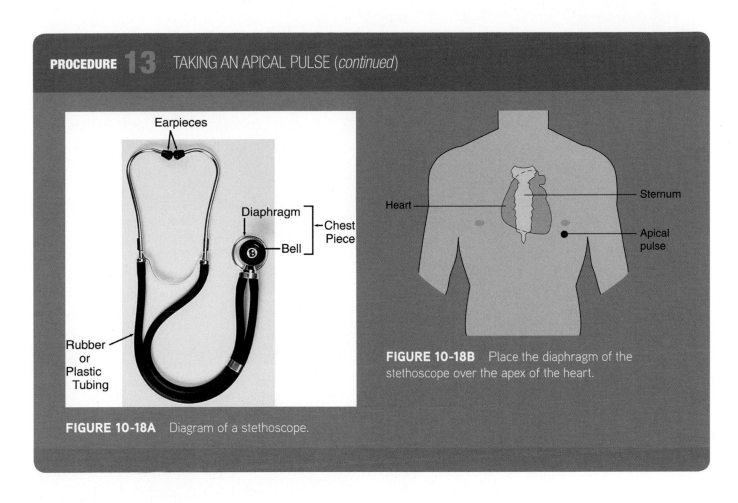

FIGURE 10-18A Diagram of a stethoscope.

FIGURE 10-18B Place the diaphragm of the stethoscope over the apex of the heart.

Apical-Radial Pulse

Taking the radial and apical pulse rates at the same time is done to see if one is the same as the other. For optimal comparisons you need two people for this procedure. A family member or the client's friend may be recruited to assist the home health aide with the procedure.

1. Perform the same beginning and ending procedures as in Procedures 12 and 13.

2. One person palpates (feels) the radial pulse and the other person counts the apical pulse at the same time. One aide is usually the timer and says "start," and then after 60 seconds, the aide says "end."

3. Compare the results and record the numbers on a notepad.

4. Document both pulse rates, for example:

Apical pulse = 100 @ 10:00 AM
Radial pulse = 92
Pulse deficit: 8 (100 − 92 = 8)

Respiration. Respiration is the sum total of processes that exchange oxygen and carbon dioxide in the body. However, respiration is most commonly known as breathing. The act of one inhalation and one exhalation is counted as one respiration. The character of respirations is described as regular or irregular; labored, difficult, shallow, or deep; and noisy or quiet. Respirations that sound like snoring are called stertorous. Difficult or labored breathing is called dyspnea. Sometimes respirations stop for a few moments. This absence of breathing is called apnea. The normal rate of respirations for adults is 16 to 20 per minute. In adults, respiration rates of 25 or more are called accelerated. Weak respirations, which are characterized by only slight chest movements, are described as being shallow. Breathing characterized by many large breaths is described as being deep. Cheyne-Stokes is a term used to describe respirations that are very rapid and then stop and then start again. This type of breathing pattern occurs prior to the client's death. Procedure 14 demonstrates how to count respirations.

PROCEDURE 14   COUNTING RESPIRATIONS

Purpose

- To count the rate and observe the character of respirations

Procedure

1. Gather equipment needed:
   - wristwatch with a second hand
   - recording device
2. After the client's pulse has been taken, leave the fingers in position on the wrist. By doing this, the client is not aware that you are counting respirations. One rise and fall of the chest counts as one respiration. Count the number of respirations during a full 1-minute period.
3. Note how deeply the client breathes. Also check the regularity of the rhythm pattern. Note the sound of the breathing.
4. Record the number of respirations occurring in 1 minute. Record the character of the client's breathing.
5. Report changes from the client's usual way of breathing.
6. Wash your hands.

Blood Pressure. Blood pressure is measured in two parts—systolic and diastolic—by using an instrument called a sphygmomanometer (Figures 10-19). Blood pressure is the amount of force the blood exerts against the walls of the arteries as it flows through them. It is expressed in numbers, with the higher number (systolic) representing the pressure while the heart is beating, and the lower number (diastolic) representing the pressure when the heart is resting between beats. The systolic number is always stated first and the diastolic second; for example: 134/72 (134 over 72); systolic = 134, diastolic = 72. Normal blood pressure for an adult is 120/80, although it may vary depending on age, sex, emotional state, fitness, and weight. Blood pressure at or above 140 mm Hg (The mm is millimeter of mercury—the units used to measure blood pressure) systolic and 90 mm Hg diastolic is considered high blood pressure. Blood pressure is taken by the use of an aneroid sphygmomanometer (an instrument with a cuff, rubber bulb, and dial gauge for recording pressures; Figure 10-19) and a stethoscope (listening device that magnifies sound). The cuff should be the right size for the client's arm; otherwise, an incorrect reading may be obtained. Cuffs come in various sizes: child, normal adult, and extra-large.

When a person has a blood pressure that is higher than normal range, the person has **hypertension**; when it is below normal range, the person has **hypotension**. Blood pressure doesn't stay the same all the time. It is lower during sleep and rises upon awakening. Blood pressure rises

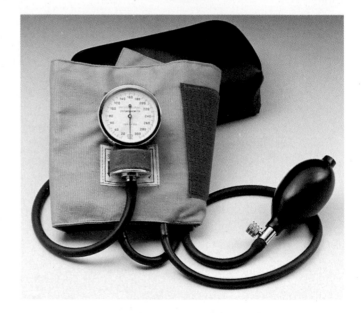

FIGURE 10-19   Aneroid sphygmomanometer.

with excitement, stress, activity, and age. If the number stays above normal most of the time, the person is at risk for serious health problems. During this time, high blood pressure can damage the heart, blood vessels, kidneys, and other parts of the body. A very high blood pressure reading can be extremely dangerous and is often life threatening. Blood pressure monitoring is essential to control this health condition. High blood pressure can lead to kidney failure, heart attack, and strokes. Hypertension is sometimes called the "silent killer" because a person can have high blood pressure and not know it. Hypertension is treated with diet, exercise, reduction of stress, and medications.

Occasionally, you may need to measure a client's blood pressure when the client is lying down, and again when the client is sitting up. The health care provider may order you to do it this way because the client may have a condition called **orthostatic hypotension**. When the person changes position, the person's blood pressure falls rapidly. Refer to Figure 10-26 for blood pressure classifications.

PROCEDURE 15   MEASURING BLOOD PRESSURE

Purpose

- To take blood pressure using the two-step method
- To accurately report and record blood pressure readings

Procedure

1. Gather equipment needed:
   - sphygmomanometer
   - stethoscope
   - alcohol wipes
2. Wash your hands.
3. Explain to the client what you plan to do. Have the client sit or lie in a comfortable position with one arm extended at the same level as the heart. The palm should be upward. The arm should be in resting position. The arm should not be dangling by the hip because you may get an inaccurate reading. Locate the **brachial** pulse (Figure 10-20).

4. Pick up the stethoscope. Clean the earpieces with alcohol wipes. Place the stethoscope around your neck.
5. Place the cuff on the client's arm, at least 1 inch above the elbow (Figure 10-21). Make sure the cuff is evenly positioned around the arm and then tighten it so it fits snugly. If the cuff is marked with an arrow, place the cuff so that the arrow points over the brachial artery.
6. Attach the dial gauge to the top of the cuff so you can read it (Figures 10-22, 10-23).
7. **Palpate** the radial pulse.
8. Explain to the client that as the cuff inflates, she or he will feel tightness in the arm that may be slightly uncomfortable. Begin to inflate the cuff by pumping the cuff with one hand while using the fingers of the other hand to feel for the radial pulse. Notice when you no longer feel the radial pulse. Deflate the cuff and wait 15 seconds.

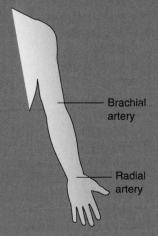

FIGURE 10-20   Location of brachial and radial arteries.

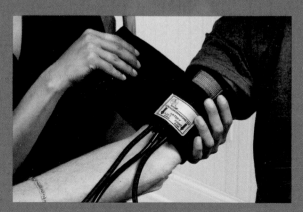

FIGURE 10-21   Apply the cuff snugly to the area at least 1 inch above the elbow.

(continues)

PROCEDURE **15**   MEASURING BLOOD PRESSURE (*continued*)

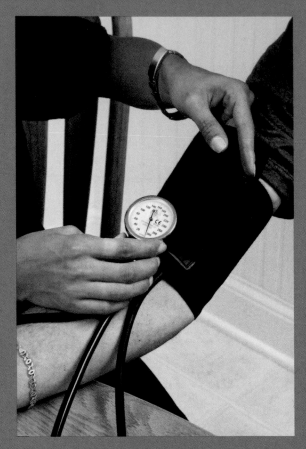

FIGURE 10-22   Attach the gauge to the top of the cuff.

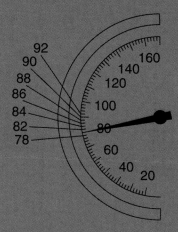

FIGURE 10-23   The aneroid scale.

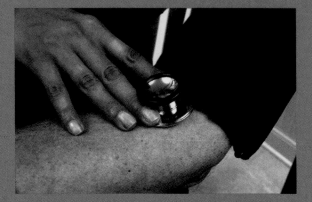

FIGURE 10-24   Notice the placement of the fingers over the diaphragm to ensure a firm fit to the skin.

9. Place the earpieces of the stethoscope in your ears and place the diaphragm over the brachial artery (Figure 10-24).
10. Inflate the cuff 30 mm Hg beyond the point at which you last felt the pulse.
11. Deflate the cuff at an even rate of 2 to 4 mm Hg per second. Turn the valve counterclockwise to deflate the cuff.
12. Note the point on the scale where you heard the first sound. This is the systolic reading. You should hear this sound near the point where the radial pulse disappeared.
13. Continue to deflate the cuff. Note the point where the sound disappears or becomes muffled; remember this number. This is the diastolic reading.
14. Deflate the cuff completely and record the blood pressure.
15. Record the reading in even numbers, for example, 134/78 or 102/64 (Figure 10-25).
16. If you are unsuccessful in obtaining a blood pressure reading after the first attempt, move to the client's other arm and try again, repeating the same procedure. (A second reading taken immediately, in the same arm, would probably be inaccurate and the client would become uncomfortable.) Never guess. If a blood pressure is hard to take or

(*continues*)

PROCEDURE **15**   MEASURING BLOOD PRESSURE (*continued*)

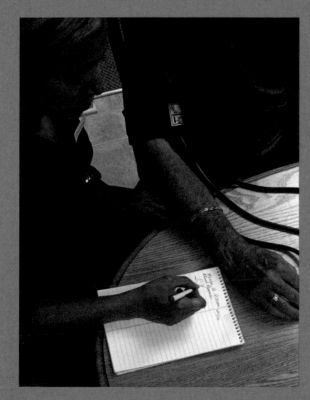

FIGURE 10-25   Record your reading right away. If a repeat procedure is necessary, wait at least 1 minute.

you are not sure, tell the case manager. Record the reading.

17. Wash your hands.

NOTE:

- If you are taking the blood pressure of a stroke client or a client who has had a mastectomy, use the unaffected arm only.

- If your client is having home dialysis (as part of a kidney treatment), or is receiving intravenous (IV) fluids, take the blood pressure on the unaffected arm.

- Do not inflate the cuff unnecessarily high.

Classification of Blood Pressure (BP)

Category	SBP mmHg		DBP mmHg
Normal	<120	And	<80
Prehypertension	120–139	Or	80–89
Hypertension, Stage 1	140–159	Or	90–99
Hypertension, Stage 2	≥160	Or	≥100

Key: SBP = systolic blood pressure   DBP = diastolic blood pressure

FIGURE 10-26   Blood pressure reading guidelines.

Courtesy of National Heart, Lung, and Blood Institute. May 2003

Height and Weight.   Occasionally it is necessary to obtain a client's height. You will need a tape measure to do this. Have the client stand to take the measurement. Be sure the client is standing as straight as possible and that the client is not wearing shoes. Another task that may need to be done monthly, weekly, or daily is weighing a client. Weight changes can make a difference in medical prescriptions, and often you may need to report daily to the case manager any change in the client's weight. For instance, some medication amounts are determined by the weight of a client, and a sudden weight loss would require a lesser dose. See Procedure 16, Measuring Weight and Height.

PROCEDURE 16 MEASURING WEIGHT AND HEIGHT

Purpose

- To determine if any weight gain or loss has occurred
- To measure height in the lying or standing position

Procedure for Weight

If the client is bedridden and cannot stand to be weighed, the agency can bring a chair scale into the house. If the client is mobile, weight can be checked daily or weekly on a bathroom scale (Figure 10-27A) or wheelchair scale (Figure 10-27B). Guidelines are as follows:

1. The client should be weighed at the same time of day.
2. The client should be wearing the same amount of clothing each time.

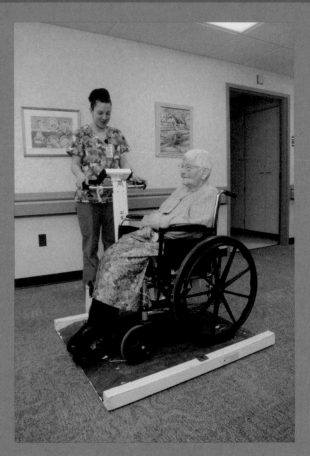

FIGURE 10-27B Assistive living facilities use a wheelchair scale to weigh clients who cannot stand. The aide weighs the wheelchair first and then weighs the client and subtracts the weight of the wheelchair to obtain the client's weight.

3. The scale should be checked to see if it is balanced correctly.
4. Record and document weight.

NOTE: Height is not a common measurement for the elderly. As individuals age, there is some "settling" and a loss of height of perhaps an inch or two. If you need to take the height of an immobile client, you need a tape measure and a pad and pencil.

Procedure for Height

1. Have the client positioned in bed flat on his or her back with the arms and legs straight.

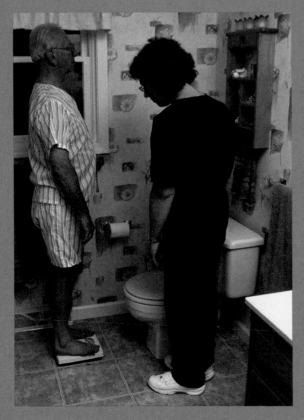

FIGURE 10-27A Weighing client using a portable bathroom scale.

(continues)

| PROCEDURE **16**   MEASURING WEIGHT AND HEIGHT (*continued*) |

2. Make a small pencil mark at the top of the client's head on the sheet.
3. Make a second pencil mark even with the bottom of the heels.
4. Using the tape measure, measure the distance between the two marks.
5. Record the height on the paper and then on the client's chart.
6. If the client can stand, have the client stand with his or her back to the wall. Mark the

wall with a small pencil mark on top of the client's head. The client should not wear shoes.
7. Measure from the floor to the small pencil mark with a tape measure.
8. Record the height on paper and then on the client's chart.

Levels of Consciousness

In most cases, a home health aide will be assigned to care for clients who are conscious. Consciousness is the normal state of awareness. Conscious people are responsive and know who and where they are. Normal consciousness varies in intensity throughout the day.

Have you had the experience of going into another room to look for an item, only to forget what it was when you got into the room? Have you ever been talking to someone and at some point lost the purpose of the conversation? These examples show that different levels of consciousness exist. While doing routine work, thoughts may wander and daydreaming may occur. At other times, a person may be extremely aware of and sensitive to surroundings and events (Figure 10-28).

Sleep is a temporary state of unconsciousness. Other types of unconsciousness are due to a body malfunction or an injury. Fainting is an example of a temporary loss of consciousness. The blood supply to the brain is decreased;

the person feels dizzy and may black out. When the head is lowered, the blood rushes back to the brain and the faintness disappears.

The deeply comatose client is totally helpless, and the home health aide must follow the care plan instructions carefully. The client's bed should be comfortable and kept clean and dry. The client should also be given frequent mouth care. Two of the greatest potential problems for a comatose client are pressure sores and contractures. Contracture is the abnormal shortening of muscle tissue. When contractures occur, the muscles become inelastic and fixed. The hands may curl into tight fists and become locked into that position. The arms and legs also become stiff. In some cases, the entire body curls into the fetal position. Exercising the client's limbs can help prevent contractures. Exercises done to prevent contractures and the loss of motion in the joints are called range-of-motion exercises.

A comatose client must have special care. Figure 10-29 indicates the special needs of the unconscious client and how to meet those needs.

Level	Physical Signs and Client Reactions
Alert	Client is aware of the environment and responds promptly and appropriately to verbal, auditory, and visual stimuli.
Drowsiness	Client can answer questions but is confused and fades in and out of sleep.
Stupor	Client is restless and can only be aroused by continuous stimulation. Responds to bright lights and loud sounds, and can locate painful site.
Coma	Client responds only to painful stimuli, if at all. In a deep coma, all responses are lost. Must be turned and repositioned or will remain in one position. Client is incontinent.

FIGURE 10-28   Levels of unconsciousness.

Care Required	Frequency	What to Do
Mouth care	Every 2 hours	Wipe tongue, lips, gums, and teeth with mouth swab. Lubricate lips with lip balm. Wipe away saliva as it dribbles from the mouth.
	When client vomits	Turn client to side at first sign of vomiting. Catch vomitus in a bowl or basin held to the side of the mouth. Wipe mouth with a damp cloth.
Eye care	Every 2 hours	Cover eyelids with soft cloth moistened in water.
Repositioning	Every 2 hours	Turn from back to side, and side to front, etc. (This prevents pressure sores from forming.)
Range-of-motion (ROM) exercises	As ordered	Exercise all of the client's body parts if permitted. (Keeps blood circulating, prevents contractures, and prevents loss of motion in joints.)
Body massage with lotion	Every 2 hours	Rub skin firmly but gently. Rub in a circular motion around bony prominences.
Care of bowel and bladder drainage	Every 2 hours	Check perineal area and bed linens to see if they are clean and dry. If client has not voided for 8 hours, report it. If client has not had bowel movement for 2 days, report it.
Accident prevention	At all times	Put up half rails or place chairs beside bed to prevent falls. Observe for signs of vomiting and keep saliva wiped away; client may choke or inhale fluids into the lungs. Keep blankets and pillows away from the client's nose and mouth to avoid smothering.
Room ventilation	Open windows or vent	Keep temperature between 66–70°F, keep drafts from client. Open windows or vents to circulate air. A small fan may help circulate air.
Tender loving care (TLC)	At all times	Talk to the client as if the client were conscious. Client may be able to hear and understand. (Communication gives client a link with reality.) Use gentle touch often; hold the client's hands and run your fingers across the client's forehead.

FIGURE 10-29   Meeting the special needs of the unconscious client.

Hyperthermia and Hypothermia

Hyperthermia (heatstroke) and **hypothermia** (abnormally low internal body temperature) are two conditions that may occur when the environmental conditions are extreme and the person's skin is unable to regulate body temperature, a situation not uncommon among the elderly and children.

Hyperthermia

Older people are more likely to die from heat-related causes than younger persons. Chances of experiencing heatstroke are increased by a weak or damaged heart, hypertension, circulatory problems, diabetes, being overweight, infection or fever, drinking alcohol, or a previous stroke.

Hyperthermia Signs and Symptoms

1. Lack of energy
2. Mild discomfort
3. Lack of appetite
4. Dizziness
5. Muscle cramps
6. Diarrhea, nausea

7. Chest pain

8. Excessive weakness

9. Severe mental changes

10. Breathing problems

11. Vomiting

12. Dry skin (no sweating)

An older person may be reluctant to run an air conditioner or a fan because of the cost. He or she may not want to keep open a window due to fear of crime, or may be unable to manage opening a window that is stuck or painted shut. For the client's and your own safety, try to gently convince the client to open a window while you are there. If the client is afraid, be sure to close it again before you leave. Be sure to encourage your client to drink plenty of fluids on very hot days.

If any client, older or younger, shows many of the previously listed signs or symptoms and has an elevated body temperature due to heat, take the following steps:

1. Loosen clothing.

2. Place the client in a semi-sitting position, with the head slightly elevated to the body.

3. Bathe the head and body in cool water to lower the body temperature.

4. Give sips of cool water or ice chips to suck on.

5. Call for medical assistance whenever you suspect a person is suffering from hyperthermia.

Hypothermia

Hypothermia is a condition marked by an abnormally low internal body temperature, usually 95°F (35°C) or under. This decrease in body temperature is due to exposure to a cold environment. Infants are at risk because of immature temperature control. The risk factors to the elderly are increased due to chronic illness, poverty, and some medications.

Hypothermia Signs and Symptoms

1. A change in appearance or behavior during cold weather

2. Uncontrollable shivering or lack of shivering

3. Slow and sometimes irregular heartbeat, shallow or very slow breathing

4. Weak pulse, low blood pressure

5. Confusion, disorientation, or drowsiness

6. Pain in the extremities

7. Slurred speech

8. Lack of coordination, sluggishness

9. Stiff muscles

10. Low indoor temperatures and other signs that the person has been in a cool or cold room

You may visit a home that has little or no heat due to a lack of money for gas or oil, a lack of wood for a wood-burning stove, or no heating system in the home. If the client is experiencing money problems that have caused the heat to be turned off or is unable to cool the home, be sure to let your case manager know. Most communities have emergency money available for utilities that can be given to individuals or families in need.

To warm a person whom you suspect of having hypothermia, take the following steps:

1. Take the person's temperature. If it is below 95°F (35°C) call for help.

2. Wrap the person in a warm blanket, quilt, towels, or extra clothes. Make sure that you cover the head and neck.

3. Use hot water bottles or electric heating pads on the person's abdomen (never on a high setting or with water too hot). Do not place hot water bottles on the feet. Do not rewarm extremities and the core (trunk of body) at the same time.

4. If the person is alert, give small quantities of warm (not hot) food or a sweet, warm drink—but nothing alcoholic.

5. Do not rub the person's limbs.

6. Call for medical assistance whenever you suspect the person is suffering from hypothermia.

WORKBOOK REVIEW

Go to the workbook and complete the review exercises and activities for Unit 10.

REVIEW

1. When counting a client's pulse rate, which of the following is correct?
   a. Place your thumb over the client's artery.
   b. With your fingers, use light pressure on the wrist on the thumb side.
   c. Count the beats over any vein.
   d. Check the artery on the right side of the wrist.

2. You have just recorded a blood pressure as 130/72. The bottom number stands for the
   a. systolic pressure.
   b. diastolic pressure.
   c. mercury pressure.
   d. pulse deficit.

3. The top number of a recorded blood pressure stands for the
   a. systolic pressure.
   b. diastolic pressure.
   c. mercury pressure.
   d. pulse deficit.

4. Blood pressure above normal is called
   a. hypotension.
   b. hypothermia.
   c. dyspnea.
   d. hypertension.

5. Which of the following would be a sign that the aide can see?
   a. Headache
   b. Sore thumb
   c. Swollen thumb
   d. Pain in the ear

6. Which of the following would be a symptom that the client would tell you?
   a. White patches in the mouth
   b. Dark-colored urine
   c. Nausea
   d. Vomitus

7. Normal respiration rates are _____ per minute.
   a. 12–24
   b. 10–16
   c. 16–20
   d. 60–80

8. A person with a disability is someone who
   a. has a physical or mental impairment that substantially limits one or more major life activities.
   b. has a record of an impairment.
   c. is regarded as having an impairment.
   d. all of the above.

9. Which of the following are signs of hyperthermia?
   a. Dry skin and breathing problems
   b. Uncontrollable shivering and weak pulse
   c. Cool, dry skin
   d. Chills

10. T   F   A person who is unconscious should be repositioned and given a back rub every 2 hours.

11. T   F   For accurate measurement of weight, it is best to weigh the client at the same time every day and with the same amount of clothing on.

12. T   F   When taking an apical pulse, place the diaphragm of the stethoscope 1 to 2 inches below the right nipple.

13. T   F   A temperature of 102°F would be an example of a fever.

14. T   F   An example of tachycardia is a pulse of 80 beats per minute.

15. T   F   The absence of breathing for a short period of time is called dyspnea.

16. T   F   A temporal artery thermometer scans a client's temperature by sliding a probe over the client's forehead.

Case Studies

17. On a cold day in January you visit a client whom you see twice a week for postpartum care. You notice that the apartment feels cold when you walk in. The mother is lethargic, cannot concentrate on a conversation with you, and her speech is slurred. The baby's skin is cool to the touch, and she is stiff and has a weak pulse. What do you suspect the mother and child are suffering from? List the steps you would take to help the mother and baby.

18. It is a hot, summer day when you visit your elderly client Mr. Banks, who lives in a large, public housing complex. The housing complex he lives in is known for having a high crime rate, where the elderly are particularly vulnerable. He rarely leaves his apartment and refuses to open a window. When you arrive for today's visit you notice that his face is flushed and his skin is warm and dry to the touch. He is feeling weak and complains of chest pains when he greets you. His pulse is irregular, and his temperature is elevated to 101°F. What do the signs and symptoms indicate? Would you call for medical assistance? Why or why not?

UNIT 11
Mental Health

KEY TERMS

adjustment

anxiety disorder

bipolar disorder

cognitive

compulsions

delusions

depression

emotion

external stimulus

hallucinations

internal stimulus

mental disorder

obsessions

optimist

pessimists

post-traumatic stress
disorder

psychology

psychosis

schizophrenia

stress

LEARNING OBJECTIVES

After studying this unit, you should be able to:

- Identify several common emotions

- Identify how a physical response can result from an emotional reaction

- Discuss the tasks of personality development defined by Erikson

- Define mental illness

- Define delirium, psychology, stress, mental health, and adjustments

- Differentiate between external and internal stimuli

- Describe the characteristic behavior of a client with schizophrenia

- Describe two common moods seen in clients with mood disorders

- Explain the differences between an obsession and a compulsion.

- Identify the major signs of depression

Mentally Healthy Individuals

Psychology is the science of human behavior. It is the study of the way the mind works and how emotions and feelings affect human behavior. Just as no two bodies are exactly alike, no two minds react in the same way. Adjustment is the change a person makes in behavior to deal with a situation. A person is mentally healthy if he or she can see reality as it is, respond to its challenges, and develop a reasonable strategy for living. A mentally healthy person has compassion or feelings for other people. A mentally healthy person can accept the limitations and possibilities of reality. When chronic illness occurs, a well-adjusted person may feel stressed, even overwhelmed at times. A well-adjusted person is able to handle the daily problems of living, taking bad times in stride and coping with crises. The well-adjusted person has a good self-image and can be flexible when meeting new or difficult obstacles. It takes less time for a well-adjusted person to recover from a difficult situation. People can adjust easily to some situations and not to others. A person does not have to be strong all the time. The mentally healthy person is able to make life work in a way that is both personally and socially acceptable.

To understand basic psychology, it is necessary to review the nervous system. The brain acts as the body's communication center. All messages (called stimuli) from the five senses are carried to the brain, where they are received and acted on. There are both internal and external stimuli. For example: The stomach is empty, so the nerve endings in the stomach send a message to the brain. The brain translates the impulses, and the individual thinks, "I'm hungry," and looks for food. This is an internal stimulus. On the other hand, on entering a room where food is being cooked, a person might smell a pleasant aroma or see an attractive piece of fruit. The sight and smell of the food can stimulate the nerve endings and the person might think, "I'm hungry," and eat the food even though it was not mealtime. This is an external stimulus.

Internal stimuli cause automatic or unconscious reactions within the body. External stimuli come from outside the body and bring about a conscious reaction. Psychology relates to both internal and external stimuli. In some conditions, chemical imbalances within the body or brain and nerve cell damage can cause changes in behavior. In other cases, environmental conditions may have a direct effect on emotional health.

Emotions

The stages in the development of one's personality are determined over an individual's life span. There are critical time frames when cognitive (being able to reason and make judgments) functioning, and motor skills are being developed that allow one to feel a sense of achievement or failure. According to Erikson, social and cultural influences are significant during an individual's growth and development phase. A person must successfully master each period in order to develop a positive image. If a person does not successfully master each phase, then negative feelings occur (see Figure 11-1).

Physical Stage	Year of Occurrence	Tasks to Be Mastered
Oral-sensory	Birth to 18 months	To learn to trust–Trust vs. Mistrust
Muscular-anal	18 months–3 years	To recognize self as an independent being from mother–Autonomy vs. Shame and Doubt
Locomotor	3–6 years	To recognize self as a family member–Initiative vs. Guilt
Latency	6–12 years	To demonstrate physical and mental skills–Industry vs. Inferiority
Adolescence	12–20 years	To develop a sense of individuality as a sexual human being–Identity vs. Role Confusion
Young Adulthood	20–35 years	To establish intimate personal relationships with a mate–Intimacy vs. Isolation
Adulthood	35–50 years	To live a satisfying and productive life–Generativity vs. Stagnation
Maturity	50 plus	To review life's events and examine how they have influenced the development of a unique individual–Ego Integrity vs. Despair

FIGURE 11-1 Tasks of personality development according to the stages defined by Erikson.

Emotions are common to all people and are neither good nor bad. An **emotion** is a strong, generalized feeling. The way a person shows emotion may be healthy or unhealthy. There is a wide range of acceptable levels of emotional behavior. Well-adjusted people most often use emotions in a healthy way to serve their purposes; they can control emotions so as not to harm themselves or others. There are a wide range of emotions that are regarded as normal, including fear, anger, grief, and others. Whether emotional behavior is healthy depends on whether a person can express these emotions in a manner that is socially acceptable.

Emotions may cause physical reactions. Anger and fear sometimes cause the heart to beat faster, respirations to increase, and chemical changes to occur within the body. The mouth may become dry; the person may become pale and may start to shake. Such physical changes are common and usually of short duration. Emotions can trigger the release of hormones and produce unusual results. For example, it is not unusual for those experiencing a shocking or traumatic event to find that they are physically capable of functioning at unusually high levels of strength and energy.

Individuals develop a pattern of emotional response. This may be a hereditary characteristic, although environment also can influence mental health. Some babies, for instance, seem calmer and happier than others. The social environment of a family can influence whether a baby's early experiences are pleasant or unpleasant. As years pass, the child's successes and failures in daily life influence the child's emotional patterns. The child who is healthy and who is given tender, loving attention from birth has a good chance of growing up to be well adjusted.

The type of emotion (pleasant or unpleasant) that a person feels most of the time is referred to as his or her disposition. A disposition is the usual mood of an individual. An **optimist** probably feels more pleasant emotions, and therefore has a brighter outlook, than a pessimist. The aide who has a cheerful outlook may transfer this pleasant mood to the client. Words, tone of voice, actions, and facial expression show how a person looks at life. This often exposes the person's inner feelings. **Pessimists** may be just as well adjusted as optimists but their viewpoints differ. Pessimists tend to take a negative view of situations. A classic example showing the difference between an optimist and a pessimist is to consider a glass filled half-way with water. An optimist would be more likely to regard the glass as half full, whereas the pessimist may regard the glass as half empty.

People have mood changes or emotional cycles. It is normal to feel high or low from time to time. In some

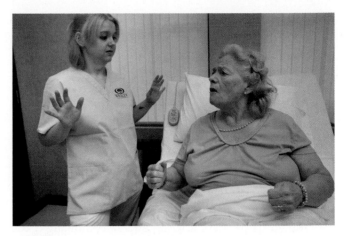

FIGURE 11-2   Aide reacting to an angry client.

people, this mood swing is more noticeable than in others. Emotional cycles can be affected by the time of day, the season of the year, and the weather. An emotionally healthy person can function in both high and low emotional cycles. For example, some people are happiest and function best early in the day. Others, who are sometimes called "night people," are more alert in the evening hours. Some people find that the season affects their feelings. Some dislike the winter and feel down; others dislike the summer months.

Mentally healthy people learn to make their emotions work for them. One can deal with negative emotions in a positive way. When a home health aide feels angry with a client, the aide cannot have a tantrum. Strong outbursts of emotion are not acceptable while on duty. Sometimes anger must be expressed, but it should be done in a way that is constructive. A home health aide must not only deal with her own emotional needs, but must also be aware of the emotional needs and reactions of the client. This requires a great deal of self-control and self-discipline. The home health aide must be sensitive to the emotions of the client. Clients are often frightened and worried about their health. The home health aide must be kind and understanding and think of the client's needs first. Illness can cause temporary changes in the client's personality. This often requires the client to make many adjustments. It takes time to accept the physical changes caused by a disease. The home health aide must be willing to allow clients to express their emotions (Figure 11-2). The well-adjusted aide will be able to endure the client's strong emotional feelings without becoming a part of them.

Stress

Stress is defined as a mentally or emotionally disruptive influence or upsetting condition that occurs in response to adverse external stimuli. Stress may be seen as anger, depression, silence, outbursts, crying, sadness, jealousy, and frustration, to name a few of the symptoms. If stress occurs too fast and too often, even normal individuals have a problem dealing with it. The home health aide must realize that the client and family members are undergoing great stress at the time of illness. Conditions that can cause stress are called stressors. Examples of possible stressors when a family member is ill are costs of medical care; prescription drug costs; costs of extra medical equipment; watching a family member in pain; having to schedule someone to be with the ill family member 24 hours a day, 7 days a week; and not knowing if the family member will improve with care. Visitors and extended family members may also raise the level of stress. Family members are not accustomed to having a home health aide in their home. The aide must recognize that all family members have different personalities and deal with stress in various ways.

It is interesting to note that older adults have more stress-free days than younger adults. Older adults deal better with their stressors. Older adults seem to say, "Hey, it's not worth getting upset about small things."

There are definite stressors recognized in the life cycle. Younger people worry about tension in relationships, middle-aged people are burdened by demands put upon them, and older adults face health and financial problems.

Handling stress effectively is an important component of mental health and is essential for avoiding both physical and mental illness. Stress can make the body more vulnerable to physical illnesses such as colds, ulcers, headaches, and high blood pressure. In severe and prolonged cases, stress can lead to emotional illness.

Although no one can avoid stress all the time, steps should be taken to either eliminate the stressor or to diminish its negative effects. Regular exercise and adequate sleep will help to strengthen the body's resistance to stress. Relaxation is another useful technique to diminish stress and may include participation in hobbies, quiet meditation, or some other activity that an individual enjoys. It is often helpful to talk about stressful situations with a trusted friend. If these measures are not enough, it may be necessary to consult with a professional.

Mental Disorders

Emotions play an important role throughout our lifetime. Although there is a broad range of feelings that are considered normal reactions to everyday life, other feelings or behaviors may signal a problem that requires medical attention. A person is said to have a **mental disorder** if he

or she is having difficulty functioning satisfactorily in society as a result of changes in thoughts, behavior, personality, or emotion. A mental disorder can be temporary or permanent and can affect people of all backgrounds and economic levels. Mental disorders can be caused by physical or chemical changes in the brain, genetics, and social and psychological factors. Mental illness is never caused by a character weakness. Most people with mental illness require special treatment from a mental health professional. The most common treatments used today are drug therapy, talk therapy (or "counseling"), or a combination of both. There are different kinds of mental disorders. A few of the more common ones are anxiety disorders, post-traumatic stress disorder, delirium, obsessive-compulsive disorder, schizophrenia, and bipolar disorder.

Anxiety Disorders

Individuals with **anxiety disorder** can live a fairly normal life, but they are always worrying. They are constantly worrying about their marriage, their job performance, their past mistakes, and future problems. This disorder can cause tension, irritability, and difficulty sleeping. It is not uncommon for this type of individual to be prone to panic attacks. During a panic attack, this person may display shortness of breath, pounding heart, and light-headedness. These individuals do have insights into their problems, but are unable to quit worrying.

Post-traumatic stress disorder is a form of anxiety disorder. This condition develops after a traumatic event, and is seen often in soldiers returning home from war or in rape victims. Since soldiers have been returning from the Middle East, incidence of post-traumatic stress disorder has dramatically increased. The Veterans Health Service has expanded its mental health units to help these men and women. These individuals repeatedly relive the event either by remembering details about the event or through recurrent nightmares. If not treated, individuals eventually become more violent and less interested in things they once enjoyed.

Obsessive-Compulsive Disorder

Obsessive-compulsive disorder is characterized by recurrent obsessions and compulsions that are time consuming and cause noticeable distress in the person. **Obsessions** are thoughts, images, or ideas that repeatedly go through a person's mind. **Compulsions** are acts that correspond with these obsessions. An example of an obsession would be fear of germs and the compulsion would be repetitive handwashing or cleaning one's home. Other common obsessions are the need for perfection and exactness or fear of harming someone close. Common compulsions are the need to rearrange items in a certain way, such as newspapers or dishes, and saving things that no longer have any need. The home health aide may walk into a home full of old newspapers and magazines with little space for the client to move around. The first thought might be to toss them away and make space for the client. This would be the logical thing to do, but a client with this disorder will not allow this to happen. The client would be extremely upset and distressed if this were to happen.

Delirium

Delirium is a sudden disturbance of consciousness, making it difficult for a person to focus or shift his or her attention. A person who is delirious often looks confused or intoxicated. Delirium is not a disease, but a set of symptoms that result from an underlying disease. Signs are change in alertness, feelings, and perception; change in level of consciousness; movement; confusion; and incoherent speech. In the final stages of cancer, the pain the client is having is so strong that the client receives a strong dose of painkiller, which may cause the client to exhibit delirium.

Mood Disorders or Bipolar Disorders

Mood disorders are the most common mental disorders for people of all ages. Mood disorders include depression, and its opposite, mania (extreme happiness and hyperactivity). **Depression** is a term that is used to describe a range of emotions, from blue feelings to a severe clinical condition.

The new term given to mood disorder is **bipolar disorder**. A person with bipolar disorder can alternate from being extremely sad to overly joyful and back again, with little reason for these mood swings.

Depression is a mental illness that causes a persistent sadness that makes it difficult to do day-to-day tasks. Often a person with depression is not concerned about personal appearance and neglects hair, teeth, and skin care. A person with depression may look sad without complaining about being sad. Depressed individuals may also stay in bed more than usual.

Common signs of depression include the following:

- persistent sadness
- feeling guilty
- "empty" mood
- feelings of hopelessness and pessimism
- feelings of worthlessness and helplessness

- loss of interest or pleasure in hobbies and activities that the client once enjoyed, including sex
- decreased energy and fatigue
- difficulty in making decisions
- either decreased or increased appetite
- thoughts of death or suicide, and may even attempt suicide

People suffering from clinical depression are unable to enjoy any aspect of their lives and have great difficulty focusing and paying attention. Although a person may not complain about feeling depressed, he or she might frequently complain about things that can add up to depression. For example, many older adults have physical problems, but people who are preoccupied with their physical illnesses may be depressed. They may say things like "I don't know what's the matter with me. I just don't feel right." These complaints may be covering up their depression.

Depression can also affect the way a person thinks. Depressed people can have false beliefs about themselves. Depressed people can be irritable, disagreeable, and at odds with everything.

Many home health agencies can provide mental health services by a licensed professional, so be sure to alert your case manager if you believe that your client is depressed or suicidal.

An aide must take all suicidal threats expressed by the client seriously and report these immediately to the case manager.

Suicide

A few warning signs and symptoms that the depressed client may be planning suicide are when a client does the following:

- makes a will
- gets his or her affairs in order
- suddenly visits friends and family members
- buys a gun, hose, rope, or pills or other forms of medications
- displays significant mood changes, either a decline or improvement.
- writes a suicide note

Psychotic Disorders

Psychosis is a serious condition in which the thinking process is distorted by hallucinations, delusions, or both. The most common form of psychotic disorder is schizophrenia.

Schizophrenia is a serious mental disorder producing various degrees of chronic mental dysfunction and varying degrees of mental impairment. There are different forms of this disease, and each form has its own specific signs and symptoms. Common symptoms of this disorder are disorganized thoughts, bizarre behaviors, attention deficits, and withdrawal. When talking, the person with schizophrenia will switch from one topic to another with no correlation; if asked a question, the person will give an irrelevant answer. These individuals often carry on a conversation with themselves and often suffer from delusions (false beliefs) and hallucinations (hearing voices or seeing objects that are not really there). Common delusions with this disorder involve themes of grandeur, persecution, or religion. The client might tell a home health aide that he or she is the pope or the president. The client may also tell you that "the CIA or the FBI is out to get them." This person may also display bizarre posture and movements. She or he may sit in one position for hours and then suddenly get up and start pacing for hours using the same path over and over again. Individuals with schizophrenia do not realize they are not acting normally and have no control over their actions. If you are caring for a client with schizophrenia, be sure the client takes his or her medications as ordered. Do not try to reason with the client, as this will make the client more upset and more difficult to manage.

Generally, people with severe psychotic episodes will be treated in a hospital to ensure their safety. In less severe cases, antipsychotic medications are prescribed to decrease excitement and agitation and to improve the thought processes.

Effects of Emotions on Health

Sometimes a physical illness can aggravate a mental illness, but a person's emotional health may also affect his or her physical health. Wellness means different things to different people; people feel better on some days than on others. Temporary discomforts are not necessarily a health hazard or danger. A tension headache caused by an emotional crisis can make a person feel ill for a short time. When the upset is resolved, the person forgets the pain and feels well again. Persons who are acutely or chronically ill also have good and bad days. To a great extent these changes are related to their emotional outlooks. When routines have gone smoothly or when a special friend has called or visited, a person may feel very well despite physical problems. On a day when the home health aide comes late and is in a bad mood, the client may complain of feeling much worse than the physical condition warrants.

No two people react the same to external stimuli. The stress situation causing one person to feel unwell may have no effect on another person. People react to personal crises in their own ways. It has been proven that an emotionally depressed person is more likely to catch a cold or develop a physical disorder. Wellness may be described as freedom from discomfort—both physical and mental. Emotional health may strongly influence a person's state of wellness.

The home health aide can help the client by being aware of the client's mental health status and responding to the client in a supportive and nonjudgmental way. The aide should be aware of the signs of depression, and report any changes in behavior to the case manager.

In addition, the home health aide must pay close attention to his or her own stress level and find constructive ways to cope with stressful situations on the job.

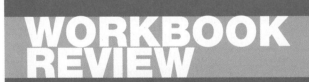

WORKBOOK REVIEW

Go to the workbook and complete the review exercises and activities for Unit 11.

REVIEW

1. List four common emotional reactions.

   _____

   _____

   _____

   _____

2. What is the difference between an internal stimulus and an external stimulus?

3. Explain how a physical response can result from an emotional reaction.

   _____

   _____

4. Define mental health and adjustment.

   _____

   _____

5. Characteristics of a mentally healthy person include which of the following?
   a. Sees reality as it is
   b. Responds to change
   c. Sets reasonable strategies for living
   d. All of the above

6. List four behavioral changes seen in a depressed client.

   _____

   _____

   _____

   _____

7. List two common types of delusions.

   _____

   _____

8. Fill in the blank: If a person states that he or she is hungry, this is a(n) _____ stimulus.

9. List three constructive ways to manage stress.

   _____

   _____

   _____

10. Fill in the blank: A person is said to have a(n) _____ _____ if he or she is having difficulty functioning in society as a result of changes in thoughts, behavior, personality, or emotions.

11. A compulsion is a(n)
     a. act.
     b. desire to perform an act.
     c. lie.
     d. none of the above.

12. A client sees things on the wall, such as bugs, that are not really there. This is an example of a
     a. delusion.
     b. hallucination.
     c. compulsion.
     d. all of the above.

13. Emotions can cause physical reactions such as which of the following?
     a. Heart beats faster
     b. Respirations increase
     c. Mouth becomes dry
     d. All of the above

14. Characteristics of a mentally ill person include which of the following?
     a. Can tolerate mild stress and has a good self-image
     b. Has compassion or feelings for others
     c. Can accept limitations and possibility of death
     d. None of the above

Case Studies

15. You arrive at Mrs. Smith's home in the middle of the afternoon. She is still wearing her pajamas. She tells you she hasn't eaten much the last several days; she appears lethargic and uncommunicative. What steps could you take to determine if she is depressed? What should you do to help Mrs. Smith?

16. One of your clients, an elderly man with multiple health problems, also has a history of depression. During one of your visits, he seems particularly depressed and irritated about his chronic health problems, which cause him a great deal of pain and restrict his independence. He tells you "I've had it!" and "Sometimes I think it just would be easier if I weren't around anymore." What steps should you take to help your client? Should you call your case manager?

SECTION 5
Body Systems and Common Disorders

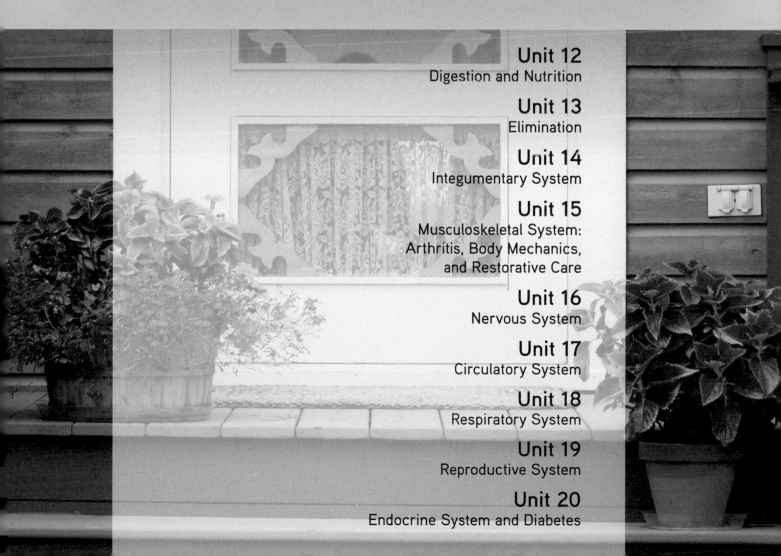

UNIT 12
Digestion and Nutrition

KEY TERMS

aspirating
bariatric
bland diet
clear-liquid diet
diabetic diet
diuretic
emesis
empty calories
enzymes

fiber
food allergy
full-liquid diet
gastrostomy
gluten-free diet
hiatal hernia
high-calorie diet
high-fiber diet
lactose

low-calorie diet
low-sodium diet
malnutrition
Meals on Wheels
metabolism
MyPlate
nutrition
peristalsis
pureed diet

reflux
renal diet
total parenteral nutrition
  (TPN)
ulcers
vegetarian

LEARNING OBJECTIVES

After studying this unit, you should be able to:

- List the organs of the digestive system and their function

- Discuss common disorders of the digestive system

- Explain the nutritional guide MyPlate

- List four guidelines for planning menus for the client

- Name six guidelines for purchasing food

- Describe five guidelines for preparing food

- Identify common food allergies

- List at least seven special diets and foods allowed on each diet

- List medical conditions that special diets would be used for

- Explain care for clients with various types of feeding tubes

- Demonstrate the following:

  PROCEDURE 17   Feeding the Client

Nutrition is the sum of a combination of processes by which the body receives and uses food and nutrients. The body needs food for energy, cell growth, and comfort and satiety. The single most important use of food is to provide proper nutrition to the body. The digestive system changes food into a form that can be used by all the cells of the body. Those parts of food that cannot be used by the body are expelled as waste products, called feces or stool.

Digestive System

Food is the fuel burned by the digestive system to provide energy for the entire body. This use of food can be compared to gasoline in a car that burns to give power to the car or oil in a furnace that produces heat. In the body, the fuel is food; the process of burning this fuel is called metabolism.

Metabolism depends on the proper functioning of each organ of digestion (Figure 12-1). The digestive process begins the moment food is taken into the mouth. The teeth and tongue tear the food into small pieces and mix it with saliva so that it can be swallowed easily. In the saliva, chemical substances called enzymes start to break down the starchy foods into products that can be used by the rest of the body. From the mouth, the partially processed food is swallowed, moving into the esophagus. An involuntary wavelike muscle action called peristalsis moves food through the esophagus and then into the stomach. Sometimes the body rejects or refuses food during the digestive process. When this occurs, the voluntary and involuntary muscles work together to force the food backward. This is called vomiting or emesis.

The stomach is an elastic, muscular organ that holds the food and secretes and mixes in gastric juices. The stomach passes the food into the small intestine. Enzymes

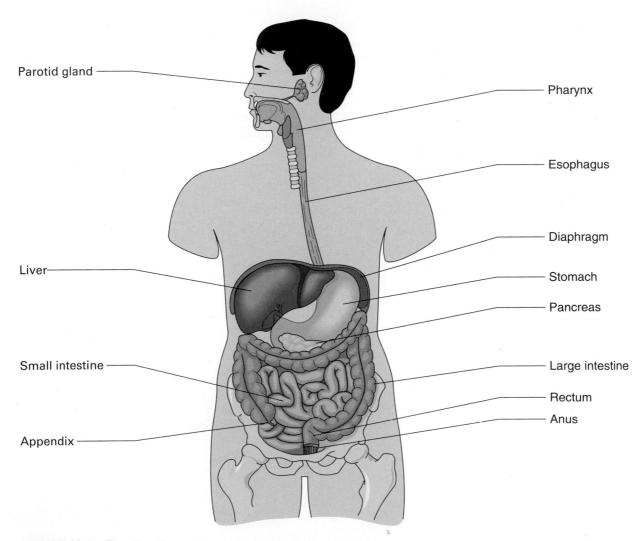

Parotid gland

Liver

Small intestine

Appendix

Pharynx

Esophagus

Diaphragm

Stomach

Pancreas

Large intestine

Rectum

Anus

FIGURE 12-1 The digestive system.

in the intestinal juice are especially important in the digestive process. The liver produces bile, which is necessary to absorb fat. Bile is produced in the liver but is stored in the gallbladder. Bile enters the small intestine and breaks up fats in the duodenum so they can be digested and absorbed. The duodenum is the first 10 inches of the 19- to 20-foot small intestine. The jejunum is the second portion of the small intestine. It is about 9 feet long. The ileum is the third portion and is about 9 feet in length. The pancreas also releases digestive enzymes into the duodenum. Insulin, which controls sugar metabolism, is released into the bloodstream from a specific area within the pancreas.

The digestive juices work together to break down food into a simpler form. The usable products of this breakdown are called nutrients. The nutrients are absorbed through the walls of the small intestine. The nutrients are then carried by the bloodstream to all parts of the body. Some portion of food remains in the small intestine because it cannot be broken down or absorbed. This remaining material moves into the large intestine in a semiliquid state. The large intestine, also called the colon, is about 5 feet long. In this area, much of the liquid from the food is absorbed into the body. This helps maintain the balance of fluids in the body. Peristalsis moves the remaining solid material into the lower part of the colon. When enough waste has collected, the voluntary muscles expel it through the anus. This is a normal bowel movement.

Common Disorders of the Digestive System

Ulcers, hiatal hernia, and heartburn are common disorders of the digestive tract.

Ulcers

Ulcers occur when there is a break in the protective mucous membrane of the stomach or the duodenum. The client may complain of heartburn or a feeling of fullness after eating. If left untreated, ulcers can start to bleed. Treatment consists of medications, change in diet, and adjustment in lifestyle.

Hiatal Hernia

Hiatal hernia occurs when the upper part of the stomach protrudes through the esophageal opening of the diaphragm into the lung cavity. It is very common in older adults. It is treated primarily by eating small amounts of food at a time and sleeping with the head of the bed elevated with blocks. Sleeping with the head of the bed slightly elevated will prevent backflow of stomach juices.

Heartburn/Acid Reflux

So-called heartburn results from a backflow of the digestive juices into the lower portion of the esophagus, which is called **reflux**. These juices, because of their high acid content, cause irritation of the lining of the esophagus. Those affected experience a burning sensation, frequently occurring at night. The client will experience belching that can cause vomitus to go into the mouth. Other symptoms might be a burning sensation in the chest and mouth. A coughing spell often follows one of these attacks.

Tips to prevent reflux are:

- Avoid fatty and spicy foods
- Limit chocolates
- Limit alcohol, caffeine intake, and fizzy beverages
- Do not lie down after eating
- Do not eat at bedtime
- Eat food in small amounts

Nutrition

One of the most rapidly growing fields in health care is nutrition, which may be in part due to an epidemic of overweight and obesity in the United States. Home health care agencies have nutritionists on staff, as do other health care facilities such as nursing homes. It is becoming a common practice for hospitals and nursing homes to provide a nutritionally sound plan to clients as part of their discharge instructions. The dietitian considers the age, weight, sex, mobility, and medical condition of the client when setting up a food plan. It is the responsibility of the home health aide to follow this plan.

Protein is needed to rebuild body tissues. Each gram of protein in a client's diet will produce four calories. Carbohydrates are used for energy in the body. Each gram of carbohydrates produces four calories. Fat produces energy in the body and produces nine calories per gram, which is almost twice as much as that produced by carbohydrates and protein (www.health.gov).

Some dietitians further suggest that the amount of **fiber**, found in whole grains, leafy vegetables, fruits, beans, and peas, be increased in the daily diet. Fiber flushes out food wastes and may help to prevent constipation and cancer of the colon.

In addition, dietitians believe that the average individual should have a regular exercise program. A half-hour walk 5 or 6 days a week is beneficial to keep the body active.

Dietitians know that individual diets must consider a person's ethnic background and food likes and dislikes. Also to be considered is any physical condition that prevents a client from eating certain foods. **MyPlate** is the current nutrition guide recommended by the U.S. Department of Agriculture (USDA). MyPlate uses a place setting with a plate divided into five groups: fruits (20%), grains (30%), vegetables (30%), protein (20%), and a smaller circle representing dairy, such as a glass of low-fat milk or a serving of yogurt. MyPlate adds additional information such as "make half your place fruits and vegetables," drink low-fat milk, and vary your protein food choices. The guidelines recommend portion control of food, while still enjoying various foods; drinking water instead of sugary drinks; and comparing the sodium content of foods like soup and frozen meals and choosing the foods with lower amounts of sodium. MyPlate is a simple way to visualize how to eat at mealtime (Figure 12-2). See Figure 12-3 for a sample 1,800-calorie diet with all the dietary requirements.

Dietary Guidelines for Americans

The following are among the recommendations of the USDA's Dietary Guidelines for Americans:

- Balance calorie intake with physical activity to manage weight.

- Consume more of certain foods and nutrients, such as fruits, vegetables, whole grains, fat-free and low-fat dairy products, and seafood.

- Consume fewer foods with sodium (salt), saturated fats, *trans* fats, cholesterol, added sugars, and refined grains. Enjoy your food, but eat less. When eating out, choose lower-calorie menu options. If you drink alcoholic beverages, do so sensibly.

These guidelines call for moderation, balance, and variety—avoiding extremes in diet. Both eating too much and eating too little can be harmful. Also, be cautious of diets based on the belief that a food or supplement alone can cure or prevent disease.

Food Labels

The Nutritional Labeling and Education Act of 1990 requires that all packaged and processed foods carry labels

Breakfast	2 cups multigrain cereal
	½ cup blueberries
	1½ cups skim milk
Snack	1 cup orange juice or a banana
Lunch	3 slices whole-wheat bread
	4 ounces low-fat deli meat
	2 tsp mustard
	1½ tbs light mayonnaise
	1 bowl lettuce
	1 apple
Snack	6 saltine crackers
	2 ounces reduced-fat cheese
	½ cup milk
Dinner	3–4 ounces baked fish
	1 medium baked potato
	2 tbs reduced-fat sour cream
	1 cup broccoli
	1 cup skim milk

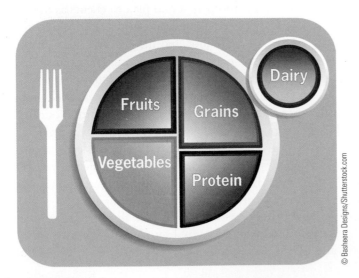

© Basheera Designs/Shutterstock.com

FIGURE 12-2 Steps to a Healthier You: MyPlate.

FIGURE 12-3 Sample 1,800-calorie meal plus all the dietary requirements.

with nutritional information. These labels can help you plan your client's diet. A nutrition label lists the amount of fat, carbohydrates, cholesterol, and sodium per serving of the labeled food. It will also list the Daily Value needed for each nutrient. Review the labels in Figure 12-4A, B, and C. Which food contains the highest amount of sodium? Fat? Calories?

If a food is labeled low fat or low salt, it needs to meet federal requirements. Because so many people are on salt-restricted diets, the food industry is required to list the amount of sodium in food using the following description:

Very low sodium	35 mg or less per serving
Low sodium	140 mg
Light sodium	50% less than average
Lightly salted	at least 50% less sodium than a regular package

(A)

(C)

(B)

FIGURE 12-4 Food labels—all food labels are required to list the calories and other nutrients per serving. (A) Label from sliced pineapple, (B) label from soup, (C) label from a can of peas.

Eat a Variety of Foods

You need more than 40 different nutrients for good health. Essential nutrients include vitamins, minerals, amino acids from protein, certain fatty acids from fat, and sources of calories (protein, carbohydrates, and fat). These nutrients should come from a variety of foods, not from a few highly fortified foods or supplements.

No single food can supply all nutrients in the amounts needed. For example, milk supplies calcium but little iron; meat supplies iron but little calcium. To have a nutritious diet, people must eat a variety of foods.

One way to ensure variety—and with it, an enjoyable and nutritious diet—is to choose foods each day from the five food groups described in MyPlate (see Figure 12-2).

Vitamins and minerals taken regularly in large amounts can be harmful. If you use MyPlate as a guide and eat a variety of food that is well balanced and taken in moderation, vitamin, mineral, and other supplements are not necessary. Exceptions in which your health care provider may recommend a supplement are:

- Pregnant women often need an iron supplement.
- Certain women who are pregnant or breast-feeding may need a folic acid supplement to meet their increased requirements for some nutrients.
- People who are inactive and do not eat properly may need supplements of nutritional drinks (e.g., Ensure) that are enriched with vitamins and minerals.
- People who are going through chemotherapy or radiation therapy may need supplements.

Smart Eating Choices

Most health authorities recommend a diet with less fat, saturated fat, and cholesterol to prevent heart problems (Figure 12-5).

A diet low in *trans* fat and saturated fat and cholesterol can help maintain a desirable level of blood cholesterol. For adults, this level is below 200 mg. As blood cholesterol increases above this level, greater risk for heart disease occurs.

A healthy diet should include two cups of vegetables and fruits each day that are rich in fiber, which helps lower cholesterol. Fiber contains substances that may help prevent heart and blood vessel diseases.

Also important are grains, make sure a minimum of three servings a day come from whole grains sources. Nutrients in whole-grain bread may help regulate blood pressure and maintain heart health.

Choose fat-free or low-fat products, such as low-fat milk, low-fat cottage cheese, or low-fat yogurt. Butter and margarine clog arteries. Use small amounts of olive oil

Fats and Oils
- Use fats and oils sparingly in cooking.
- Use small amounts of salad dressings and spreads, such as butter, margarine, and mayonnaise. One tablespoon of most of these spreads provides 10 to 11 grams of fat.
- Choose liquid vegetable oils most often because they are lower in saturated fat.
- Check labels on foods to see how much fat and saturated fat are in a serving.

Meat, Poultry, Fish, Dry Beans, and Eggs
- Limit your portion of meat, poultry, and seafood to 6 ounces, 2–3 servings per day. A 3-oz portion is a piece of meat the size of a deck of cards, or 3/4 cup of flaked fish.
- Trim fat from meat; take skin off poultry.
- Occasionally, eat cooked dry beans and peas instead of meat.
- Select luncheon meats with fewer than 3 grams of fat per ounce, such as lean roast beef, turkey breast, lean ham, or turkey pastrami.

Milk and Milk Products
- Consume at least 2 or 3 servings daily. (Count as a serving: 1 cup of milk or yogurt or about 1½ oz of cheese.)
- Select skim or low-fat dairy products, nonfat or low-fat yogurt, and nonfat or low-fat cheese most of the time. One cup of skim milk has only a trace of fat, 1 cup of 2% milk has 5 grams of fat, and 1 cup of whole milk has 8 grams of fat.

FIGURE 12-5 Plan for a diet low in fat, saturated fat, and cholesterol.

and canola oils instead. Eat fatty fish (like salmon, tuna, sardines) twice a week to provide omega 3 fatty acids. Eat less meat and cheese to make room for more plant-based food. Add flax seeds to yogurt, cereal, soup, and salads for potential cancer protective fiber. Eat a small handful of nuts daily, as they are full of fiber and healthy fats. Don't drink your calories. The simple sugars they contain provide many nutrient-free calories without filling you up and may even make you crave high-calorie foods.

The Importance of Water

One item that many people overlook in their daily diet is water. It is generally recommended that each individual drink 6 to 10 glasses of water daily. This is necessary for proper digestion; it also helps to maintain proper elimination. Wastes are eliminated from the body by the kidneys. This flushing process is helped by the amount of water taken into the body. Water keeps feces from becoming hardened and decreases chances of constipation. Water also prevents dehydration. A home health aide should encourage the client to drink water throughout the day. Fresh water should be provided often and be readily available for the client's use.

Recently, more and more individuals are drinking bottled water. There has been quite a promotion to purchase bottled water in place of soft drinks. In some areas of our country, tap water may not taste good, and with bottled water being reasonably priced, people are drinking more water.

Developing Good Eating Habits

Is it possible to look at a person and tell whether that person's body is well nourished? A well-nourished person usually has shiny hair, clear skin, good posture, and firm flesh. The person also appears alert and energetic. To be well nourished, people must select the correct foods and follow smart eating choices. Lower forms of animals seem to have natural body wisdom. They eat only those foods that are good for them and they do not overeat. People, however, have so many foods to choose from that they often make mistakes and overconsume.

Often people living alone do not get the proper nourishment. They may not have the desire to eat, or they may not have the knowledge or energy to purchase and prepare nutritious meals. Instead, they feed themselves by snacking or eating out, which can lead to excessive intake of fat and cholesterol.

Another dilemma is seen with clients on low-salt diets who will insist on having a salt shaker on the table. Even though they have been told not to use salt by the dietitian, they continue to use it. As a home health aide, you cannot tell the client that salt is off limits or take the salt shaker away. This is a client's right. This is also true with clients who are overweight and are on a low-calorie diet, but do not follow it. The home health aide should report these situations to the case manager.

Empty-Calorie Foods

Favorite foods are often oversalted, oversweetened, or high in fat content. Examples of such favorite foods are potato chips, candy, soda, and french fries. Teenagers especially have a tendency to eat these foods. In everyday language, these foods are called junk foods, but the proper descriptive name for them is empty-calorie foods. Empty-calorie foods are high in sugars and fats; they are very low in proteins, minerals, and vitamins. Overindulgence in these empty-calorie foods leads to poor nutrition and overweight.

Refer to Figures 12-6 and 12-7. Figure 12-6 provides definitions of important nutritional terms. Knowing these terms will help you understand the value of meal planning for a balanced diet. Figure 12-7 lists vitamins, their important food sources, and their functions.

Obesity

Another dietary problem is overeating. Normally, the body can only burn or use a certain number of calories every day. Calories not used are turned into fat tissue.

In the United States, it has been estimated that 60% of the population is 10 pounds or more overweight. Excess weight forces the heart to work harder and is a major cause of hypertension, heart and lung problems, hip and knee problems, certain cancers, and diabetes. Obesity is a national problem today in all age groups. Bariatric refers to the causes, prevention, and treatment of obesity. Bariatric surgery alters the digestive system to help people with severe weight-related health problems lose weight (Figure 12-8).

Malnutrition

Malnutrition is poor nourishment, which most often occurs when the body does not get a full, balanced diet. Early signs of malnutrition include muscle weakness and a constant feeling of tiredness or fatigue. Later symptoms include a distended or swollen abdomen, a dull film over the eyes, hair that is dry and brittle, and bones that become deformed. This condition is often seen in a client who loses a large amount of weight as a result of chemotherapy or radiation. A feeding tube may be inserted into the client's stomach to treat this condition.

Word	Definition	Examples
Carbohydrates	Sugars or starches that deliver quick energy to the body, 4 cal per 1 gm	Found in grains, potatoes, corn, fruits, and sweets
Proteins	Compounds composed of amino acids needed for growth and tissue repair, 4 cal per 1 gm	Found in meats, fish, milk, eggs, nuts, dried beans
Fats	Made up of glycerin and fatty acids, which provide stored energy to the body, and protect vital organs, 9 cal per 1 gm	Present in meats, butter, milk, peanuts
Minerals	Inorganic elements essential in tissue building and in regulation of body fluids	Iron, calcium, sodium, and zinc
Vitamins	Organic substances vital to certain metabolic functions and needed to prevent deficiency disease. Vitamins are needed only in small amounts but must be obtained from food sources because they are not produced in the body.	Vitamins A, C, B_{12}
Water	A tasteless, odorless liquid compound of hydrogen and oxygen necessary in the digestive process and to regulate body processes	
Calorie	A measure of heat produced by the body when using a specific portion of food	
Metabolism	Sum total of processes needed for the breakdown of food and absorption of nutrients	

FIGURE 12-6   Knowing terms used in nutrition helps us to understand how the body uses food.

Vitamins	Best Sources	Functions
Fat-Soluble Vitamins		

Vitamin A	Leafy vegetables
	Fish liver oils
	Liver
	Egg
	Fruits
	Milk
		Essential for:
		  Growth of bones and teeth
		  Health of eyes
		  Keeping skin healthy

Vitamin D	Sunshine
	Fish liver oil
	Milk
	Egg yolk
	Oatmeal
		Essential for:
		  Growth of bones
		  Regulating calcium and phosphorus
		  metabolism
		  Building and maintaining normal bones
		  and teeth

Vitamin E	Whole grains
	Vegetable oils
	Milk
	Legumes
	Nuts
	Dark-green, leafy vegetables
		Not conclusively defined in humans; may
		  affect the red blood cells
		Recommended for middle-aged women,
		  as it helps in the metabolism of calcium

Vitamin K	Dark-green, leafy vegetables Egg yolks Cabbage Oatmeal	Essential for: Normal clotting of blood
Water-Soluble Vitamins		

Vitamin C
(Ascorbic acid)
	Citrus fruits, pineapple
	Melons and berries
	Tomatoes
	Broccoli
	Green peppers
		Essential for:
		  Maintaining strength of
		  blood vessels
		Health of the teeth and gums
		Aids in wound healing

Thiamine (B_1)	Wheat germ
	Lean pork
	Yeast
	Legumes
	Whole-grain and enriched cereal
	  products
	Liver, other organ meats
		Essential for:
		  Carbohydrate
		  Metabolism
		  Healthy appetite
		  Functioning of nerves

Riboflavin (B_2)	Milk, cheese
	Enriched bread and cereals
	Meat
	Green, leafy vegetables
	Eggs
	Yogurt
		Essential for:
		  Health of skin, eyes, and mouth
		  Carbohydrate, fat, and protein metabolism

Niacin
(Nicotinic acid)
	Meats (especially organ meats)
	Poultry and fish
	Cheese
	Enriched breads and cereals
	Peanuts
		Essential for:
		  Prevention of pellagra
		  Carbohydrate, fat, and
		  protein metabolism

FIGURE 12-7 Fat-soluble vitamins are stored in the fatty tissues of the body, whereas water-soluble vitamins are excreted through body wastes (urine and stool) if not used.

Vitamins	Best Sources	Functions
Water-Soluble Vitamins		
Vitamin B$_6$ (Pyridoxine)	Wheat germ Fish Meats Whole-grain cereals	Essential for: Metabolism of proteins
Pantothenic Acid	Meats Eggs Whole-grain cereals	Aids various steps in metabolism
Biotin	Organ meats Milk Mushrooms Peanuts	Aids various steps in metabolism

Vitamin B$_{12}$ (Cobalamin)	Liver, kidney
	Fish
	Milk, cheese
	Eggs
		Essential for:
		  Metabolism of protein
		  Healthy red blood cells
		  Treatment of pernicious anemia

Folacin (Folic acid)	Dark-green, leafy vegetables
	Liver, kidney
	Green leafy vegetables
		Essential for:
		  Formation of red blood
		  Cells
		  Metabolism

FIGURE 12-7   *(Continued)*

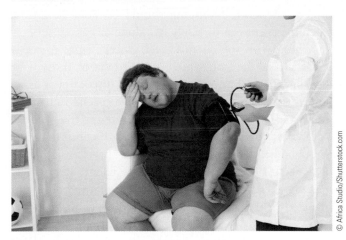

FIGURE 12-8   A bariatric client may need to be on a low-calorie diet.

© Africa Studio/Shutterstock.com

General Guidelines for Meal Planning

There are some general rules to follow when planning nutritious meals for clients. The home health aide should consider the ethnic and regional preferences of the client when planning a menu.

If the client is on a special diet, the dietitian will prescribe a sample diet to follow. There will also be a list of foods allowed on this special diet. The sample diet and list of foods are a great resource in planning menus for a week.

Additional guidelines for preparing food include:

1. Wash your hands before preparing food.

2. Check to see that you have all the ingredients needed to prepare the meal.

3. Prepare an amount of food that will be eaten in one or two meals.

4. Use leftovers in creative ways.

5. Wash fresh fruits or vegetables before using.

6. Clean as you go and be sure to clean up after the meal. Do not leave a mess for others to clean up.

7. Sugar and salt substitutes should be used for clients with sugar and salt restrictions.

8. Make food as appealing as possible.

9. When opening cans, wash the top of the can before piercing with a can opener. This will prevent germs from entering the food.

10. Check food for spoilage and if in doubt discard the food. Be sure to check the expiration dates on dairy, canned goods, cold cuts, and meat products.

11. Serve hot foods hot, and cold foods cold.

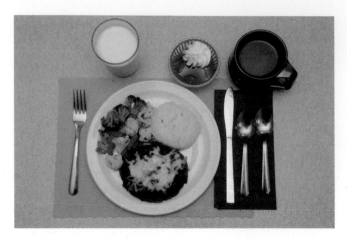

FIGURE 12-9 An attractive, well-balanced meal.

Eating Patterns

Generally, people expect to have three meals a day—breakfast, lunch (dinner), and dinner (supper; Figure 12-9). The midday and evening meals are a cultural choice. For example, farmers who work hard during planting and harvesting often expect and need a hot, full meal at noon. They expend so much effort in the morning that they need to replace energy at noon so they can go back to work. Office workers usually do not need or want more than a light lunch. They usually prefer to have their main meal in the evening in the comfort of their homes. This gives them a chance to be with their families as they all enjoy a hot meal.

Some older adults find that eating the main meal in the evening makes them uncomfortable. They find that they feel better having their main meal at midday and then eating a light meal in the evening. This relieves the feeling of heaviness and discomfort when they go to bed.

Shopping and Meal Preparation

Shopping and meal preparation require time and use of special skills. Planning nutritious meals and buying foods the family can afford require knowledge and use of good judgment. Storing foods properly is also important.

Menus and Shopping Lists

Most meal planning is done for an entire week. Weekly planning saves the home health aide from making frequent trips to the market. Food shopping is not a common duty for a home health aide, due to the cost of paying the aide to shop and the car expense to do the shopping. The following steps are helpful planning guides:

- Sit down with the client and/or the client's family and ask what foods and menus they want. This could be an important activity for the client because it may foster the client's feelings of being useful and in charge of the care.
- Plan menus for a full week. Make sure that the menu follows any specific guidelines provided by the dietitian.
- Make a shopping list and include all items needed in the household. Shopping time can be reduced by organizing the shopping list so that all items of one type are under one heading.
- Look in the newspaper and check the prices of products advertised. Cut out any coupons of items on the shopping list.
- Plan to use only the amount of money budgeted for food and supplies. Always save the receipts for the client for repayment.

Purchasing Food

Planning done in the home saves the home health aide time at the store. Shopping should be done at a time when the client can be safely left alone or has a visitor.

Check with the client's local grocery store to see if it has special days on which older adults or those with disabilities can shop and receive extra discounts or assistance. Many large grocery stores have special individual motorized carts to ride while shopping at their stores. Volunteers might be available in your community or through the client's church to assist the client to shop or actually do the shopping for the client. If possible, it is beneficial to get your client out of the house and involved in the actual grocery shopping. This gives the client a chance to see other people and also make choices in the grocery shopping. Another benefit is for the client to actually see the "real" cost of food and how expensive certain items are.

Meal Preparation

Frozen meals are an excellent option for clients who live alone. Today there is a huge variety of meals to choose from at a variety of prices. The meals can be readily prepared and give the client a variety of choices of food. The meals are easily stored and can be made quickly in a microwave.

Meals on Wheels (a service that brings hot meals to shut-ins and the elderly) usually provides the food at

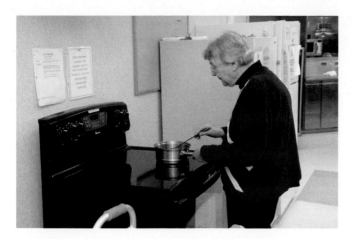

FIGURE 12-10   Client cooking her own meal.

midday. A sandwich for the evening meal is often included. In some areas, the meals are delivered once a week with seven meals to be put in the freezer. Contributions for the meals are based on income.

Some older adults who can ambulate prefer the companionship of a meal shared with friends at a local senior citizen center.

Some people prefer to have five or six smaller meals that can be divided into a light breakfast, an early light lunch, a mid-afternoon snack, a small dinner, and a late-night snack (Figure 12-10). Cancer clients are often encouraged to follow this practice. If the cancer client has difficulty swallowing, the food can be liquefied in a food processor. The aide should also remember that persons who are weak may lose their appetites as a result of their condition and may need to eat more often with smaller portions.

Food Allergies

The incidence of food allergies varies widely, from as little as 0.2% of the population to up to 50%. Food reactions are most common in infancy, diminishing in childhood and adulthood.

A true **food allergy** is any negative reaction to a food, or a food component, that involves the immune system. The reaction can be immediate (within minutes to hours of eating the food), or delayed (symptoms do not appear for 6 to 24 hours after eating the food). Symptoms from a food allergy can be mild to life-threatening, depending on a person's tolerance and the amount of the food or food component ingested. Food allergies can produce a range of symptoms, including skin rashes, digestive tract problems, and respiratory disorders.

Any food item can cause an allergic reaction; however, some of the food categories associated with an allergic response include chocolate, cow's milk, corn, eggs, fish, nuts, strawberries, tomatoes, and wheat.

Sometimes a person is allergic to a raw food, but has no difficulties with the same food if it is cooked. Those with a food allergy may also have an allergic reaction to foods in the same food family (Figure 12-11).

Some people, although not allergic to food per se, are allergic to the molds that grow on some foods. Mold allergies produce milder symptoms, such as headaches, fatigue, or nasal congestion. Beer, wine, canned tomato products, cheese, dried fruits, and certain types of breads are potential mold accumulators.

Food Preparation and Appeal

Foods may be prepared in a number of ways. They may be eaten raw. Some can be broiled, baked, fried, boiled, or steamed. Overcooking causes the loss of minerals, vitamins, and other nutrients. Some meats, particularly pork, ground beef, and chicken, must be thoroughly cooked to kill any bacteria that may be present in the meat.

When planning and preparing meals, a home health aide should keep the following in mind:

- Variety
- Appearance
- Flavor and aroma
- Satiety (hunger satisfaction)
- Individual preferences (Figure 12-12)
- Special diet ordered

Variety.   Variety is necessary to avoid dulling the appetite. People become bored with the same menu day after day. This can cause a loss of interest in food. Variety in the menu helps improve the client's interest in eating.

Appearance.   Appearance is the way food looks when it is served. Nicely arranged food adds to the pleasure and enjoyment of eating. Foods that appeal to the eye perk up the appetite. Properly cooked vegetables, for example, retain their natural color. The color enhances the appearance of the vegetables on the plate. The attractiveness of the meal can be illustrated by two examples. Imagine a plate of food consisting of a chicken breast, mashed potatoes, white bread, and cauliflower. This meal would be nutritious but it would look dull and colorless. If the potatoes or cauliflower were replaced by a garden salad and string beans, the meal would look much brighter and more appealing.

Plant Families					
Apple	**Citrus**	**Cola nut**	**Goose foot**	**Gourd**	**Grass**
apple	quince	coffee	beet	cantaloupe	barley
crab apple	grapefruit	chocolate	spinach	cucumber	corn
loquat	lemon	cola drinks	Swiss chard	melon	oats
pear	orange	tea		pumpkin	rice
quince	tangerine			winter squash	rye
					wheat
Heath	**Laurel**	**Lily**	**Mint**	**Cruciferous**	**Pea**
blueberry	avocado	asparagus	basil	broccoli	bean
cranberry	bay leaf	garlic	bergamot	cabbage	soybean
huckleberry	cinnamon	leek	marjoram	cauliflower	lentil
loganberry		onion	peppermint	mustard	pea
		sarsaparilla	oregano	Brussel sprouts	peanut
			sage	turnip	alfalfa
			savory		tamarind
			thyme		
Plum	**Rose**	**Sunflower**	**Walnut**		
almond	blackberry	artichoke	walnut		
apricot	raspberry	chamomile	hickory nut		
blackberry	strawberry	chicory	pecan		
cherry		endive			
peach		lettuce			
plum		sunflower			
Animal Families					
Birds	**Crustaceans**	**Fish**	**Mammals**	**Mollusks**	
chicken	crab	catfish	cow (milk)	abalone	
egg	crayfish	cod	goat	clam	
duck	lobster	flounder	lamb	cockle	
goose	prawn	halibut	pork	oyster	
pheasant	shrimp	mackerel	rabbit	scallop	
turkey		salmon	sheep	mussel	
		sardine			
		snapper			
		sole			
		trout			
		tuna			

Source: FOOD and MOOD by Elizabeth Somer. Henry Holt and Company, LLC.

FIGURE 12-11 If you are intolerant of or allergic to a food, you also may react to other foods in the same food family.

Flavor and Aroma. Flavor and aroma set the digestive juices into action. Seasonings most often used are salt, pepper, and garlic. However, many herbs, such as thyme, rosemary, parsley, sage, and basil, can be added to bring out the aroma and sharpen the flavor. Often these herbs and spices can be used when a client is on a salt-free diet. Also, fresh lemon juice can be squeezed over meat and vegetables.

Satiety. Satisfying the pangs of hunger is another reason people eat. Some foods make the stomach feel full but not uncomfortable. This feeling is called satiety. If daily

Ethnic Group	Bread and Cereal	Eggs, Meat, Fish, Poultry	Dairy Products	Fruits and Vegetables	Seasonings, Etc.
Chinese	Rice, wheat, millet, corn, noodles	Little meat and no beef, fish, including raw fish, eggs of hen, duck, pigeon	Water, buffalo milk occasionally, soybean milk, cheese	Soybeans, soybean sprouts, bamboo sprouts, soy curd cooked in lime water, radish leaves, vegetables, fruits	Sesame seeds, ginger, almonds, soy sauce, sesame oil, soybean oil, peanut oil
African American	Hot breads, cookies, pastries, cakes, cereals, white rice, cornbreads	Chicken, salt pork, ham, bacon, sausage, salted salmon, salt herring, fish	Milk and milk products, little cheese	Kale, mustard greens, Turnip greens, cabbage, hominy, grits	Molasses, deep frying
Jewish	Noodles, crusty white seeded rolls, rye bread, pumpernickel bread, challah, bagels	Kosher meat (from forequarters and organs from beef, lamb, veal), milk not eaten at same meal (not a rule for all Jewish people), fish, chicken	Milk and milk products, cheese	Vegetables (sometimes cooked with meat), fruits, cooked fruits (compote)	Salt, garlic, dill, parsley
Italian	Crusty white bread, cornmeal and rice (northern Italy), pasta (southern Italy)	Beef, veal, chicken, eggs, fish	Milk in coffee, cheese (many different kinds)	Broccoli, zucchini, other squash, eggplant, artichokes, string beans, tomatoes, peppers, asparagus, fresh fruit	Olive oil, vinegar, salt, pepper, garlic, basil, wine
Puerto Rican	Rice, beans, noodles, spaghetti, oatmeal, cornmeal	Dry salted codfish, meat, salt pork, sausage, chicken, beef	Coffee with hot milk	Starchy root vegetables, green bananas	Lard, herbs, oil, vinegar, hot peppers
Near Eastern	Bulgur (wheat)	Lamb, mutton, chicken, fish, eggs	Fermented milk, sour cream, yogurt	Nuts, grape Leaves	Sheep's butter, olive oil

FIGURE 12-12 Traditional ethnic, regional, and racial food patterns.

Ethnic Group	Bread and Cereal	Eggs, Meat, Fish, Poultry	Dairy Products	Fruits and Vegetables	Seasonings, Etc.
Greek	Plain wheat bread	Lamb, pork, poultry, eggs, organ meats	Yogurt, cheeses, butter	Onions, tomatoes, legumes, fresh fruit	Olive oil, parsley, lemon, vinegar,
Mexican	Lime-treated corn, rice	Little meat (ground beef or pork), poultry, fish	Cheese, evaporated milk as beverage for infants	Pinto beans, tomatoes, potatoes, onions, lettuce	Chili pepper, salt, garlic, herbs

FIGURE 12-12   (*Continued*)

menus are well planned, the satiety value will be provided. Bulk foods such as bread, macaroni, beans, and spaghetti are good fillers.

Individual Preferences.   An important factor in meal planning is providing foods the client likes to eat. There is no logic to explain why some people like certain foods and dislike others. Some individuals want steak served rare; others will only eat it well done. Some people dislike spinach, cabbage, beets, or mushrooms. The home health aide must try to prepare foods the client likes.

Special Diets

Special diets may be ordered by the dietitian to meet a client's specific health needs. If a client is on a low-salt (low-sodium) diet, foods that contain salt (sodium) need to be limited; if the client is diabetic, foods containing high amounts of sugar are limited.

A description of some special diets follows. Figure 12-13 lists recommended foods and foods to avoid for these special diets and why these diets are ordered.

Cardiac Diet.   Individuals with heart problems are prescribed a diet low in salt, low in cholesterol, low in caffeine, and high in potassium. Persons with high blood pressure are treated with a drug called a **diuretic**. A diuretic helps to lower blood pressure by removing extra fluid from the body. However, this drug may cause the mineral potassium to be flushed from the body. The loss of potassium may cause muscle cramps and muscular weakness. Persons taking diuretics may need extra foods containing potassium in their diets. Examples of foods that are high in potassium are bananas, oranges, raw vegetables, and raisins.

Vegetarian Diet.   A **vegetarian** diet is one that generally does not contain red meat. Some include eggs, some fish, some milk, and some even poultry. A lacto-ovo-vegetarian will eat eggs and dairy products, but no meat, poultry, or fish. A vegan is a vegetarian who omits all animal products. Vegetarian diets can be very healthy.

Lactose-Intolerance Diet.   Many people have a difficult time digesting dairy products and are considered **lactose** intolerant. There are milk and dairy substitutes such as lactaid, soymilk, soy yogurt, and soy cheeses available today. Those foods should be eaten to ensure adequate calcium intake. Also, lactose-intolerant individuals can take lactose tablets to help them digest dairy products.

Gluten-Free Diet.   A **gluten-free diet** excludes the protein gluten. Gluten is found in grains such as wheat, barley, rye, and tricale (a cross between wheat and rye) This diet is used for clients with celiac disease.

Renal Diet.   A **renal diet** restricts sodium, potassium, phosphorus, and/or fluids. Foods allowed are canned fruit, rice, pasta, sugar, and candy. No more than 1 serving of milk a day is allowed. Foods not allowed are excessive servings of fruit and vegetables high in potassium, dairy products, and processed meats. This diet is ordered for clients with kidney disease.

Diabetic Diet.   A **diabetic diet** is a diet that recommends eating healthy foods in moderate amounts and sticking to a regular meal plan. It is a healthy eating plan rich in nutrients and low in calories and fats, with emphasis on fruits, vegetables, and whole grains. This diet is ordered for clients with diabetes.

Diet	General Use	Foods Allowed	Foods to Limit/or Avoid
Low-calorie diet	Overweight	Skim milk, fresh fruits, lean meat or fish, vegetables, sugarless jello	Fried foods, rich gravies and sauces, jams, jellies, rich desserts
High-calorie diet	Underweight	Peanut butter, eggnog, jellies, ice cream, desserts, frequent snacks, milk shakes	None
Bland diet	Stomach or intestinal precaution; ulcers	All food groups	Highly seasoned, fried foods, raw vegetables and fruit, whole grains and cereals, spices such as chili peppers or powder, black pepper, red pepper, caffeinated and alcoholic beverages
Diabetic carbohydrate-control diet	Diabetes	Canned fruits in natural juices, fresh fruits, meat, vegetables, bread, diet gelatin, and diet soda; use MyPlate recommendations for diabetics	Foods containing sugar, alcoholic beverages, gravy, sauces, chocolate, regular soda
Low-sodium diet (2 grams or 2,000 milligrams)	Fluid retention; heart problems; high blood pressure	Foods cooked without salt, regular meat, vegetables, fruits, salt substitute	Smoked, cured, and canned fish and meats; cold cuts; cheese; potato chips; pretzels; pickles; bouillon; mustard; catsup; salad dressings; soy sauce
Low-fat, low-cholesterol diet	Heart disease and certain gastrointestinal disorders	Veal, poultry, fish, skim milk, buttermilk, yogurt, low-fat cottage cheese, fat-free soup broth, fresh fruits and vegetables, cereals, gelatin, angel cake, ices, carbonated beverages, coffee, tea, jams, jellies	Fatty meats, bacon, butter, whole milk, cheese, kidney, liver, heart, fried foods, rich desserts, sauces, eggs, sour cream
Clear-liquid diet	Preoperative/ postoperative or digestive disturbances	Tea or black coffee with sugar, apple juice, plain gelatin (no fruit), clear broth, popsicles	Solid foods
Full-liquid diet	Gastrointestinal problems; chewing problems; cancer	All foods in clear-liquid diet, strained cream soups, strained cereals, milk, ice cream, pudding	Solid foods
Soft diet	Gastrointestinal conditions; chewing problems; when clients are weak or have no teeth to chew	All food groups but needs to be chopped up finely	Fresh fruit/raw vegetables, nuts, fried and highly seasoned foods
Pureed diet	Difficulty in swallowing or chewing	Pureed meats, vegetables, and fruits; cereals; ice cream	Solid or whole foods
High-fiber diet	Constipation	Whole-grain breads and cereals, raw and cooked vegetables, fruit juices, dried beans, bran or bran flakes, nuts, seeds, and dried fruits	

NOTE: This chart is a general guide to special diets. Always follow the dietitian's prescribed diet plan.

FIGURE 12-13   Special diets that are ordered for clients with specific medical conditions.

Feeding the Client

On occasion, it may be necessary for the aide to assist with feeding the client who is unable to feed himself or herself, or who needs assistance with feeding (Figure 12-14). The following guidelines are helpful:

- The best position for eating is sitting up in a chair. If this is not feasible, you can position the client up in bed with the use of a few pillows. The food will be digested better if the client is in a sitting position.

- The aide should sit by the side of the client while feeding and be at the eye level of the client. If the client has one-sided weakness, sit on the client's strong side.

- Check to see if dentures are in or have the client brush his or her teeth.

- Wash the client's hands and face—refresh the client.

- If possible, have the client eat in a pleasant environment and preferably not in the bedroom.

- Feed small amounts of food at a time. Feed slowly; let the client set the pace. Thermal bowls and cups will assist in keeping the food at the right temperature.

- Make sure the consistency of the food is appropriate.

- Do not mix foods together. Feed each food item separately, identifying the food to the client.

- Offer liquids between solid foods.

- Most clients will prefer to feed themselves if possible. Many different feeding devices available today make this possible (Figures 12-15, 12-16A, B). The feeding device will need to be chosen according to the client's disability.

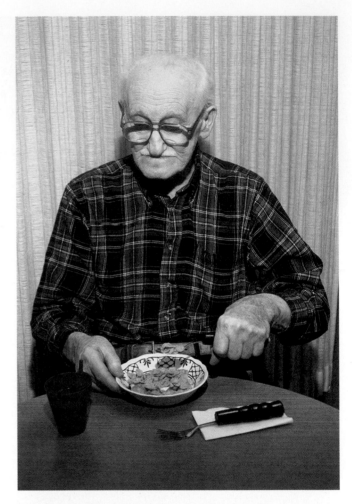

FIGURE 12-15   A client using a feeding device.

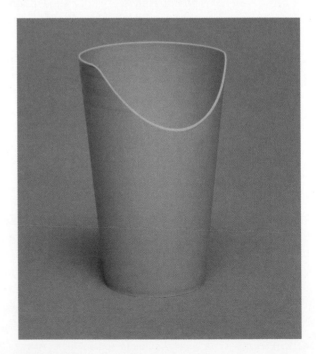

FIGURE 12-16A   Special feeding cup.

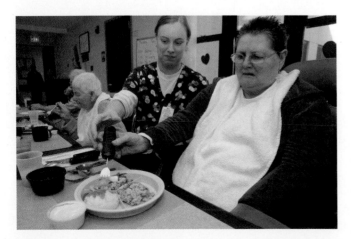

FIGURE 12-14   Feeding a client in an assistive living facility.

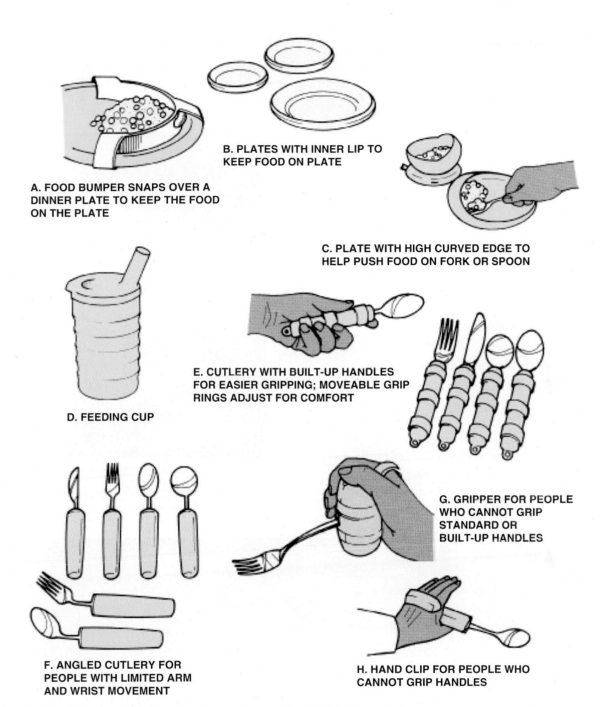

B. PLATES WITH INNER LIP TO KEEP FOOD ON PLATE

A. FOOD BUMPER SNAPS OVER A DINNER PLATE TO KEEP THE FOOD ON THE PLATE

C. PLATE WITH HIGH CURVED EDGE TO HELP PUSH FOOD ON FORK OR SPOON

E. CUTLERY WITH BUILT-UP HANDLES FOR EASIER GRIPPING; MOVEABLE GRIP RINGS ADJUST FOR COMFORT

D. FEEDING CUP

G. GRIPPER FOR PEOPLE WHO CANNOT GRIP STANDARD OR BUILT-UP HANDLES

F. ANGLED CUTLERY FOR PEOPLE WITH LIMITED ARM AND WRIST MOVEMENT

H. HAND CLIP FOR PEOPLE WHO CANNOT GRIP HANDLES

FIGURE 12-16B Eating and drinking aids for the client with disabilities.

- A child's feeder cup or plastic glass may be used if the client cannot drink from a regular cup. Do not use a syringe to feed the client.

- If the client has use of only one hand, a suction plate or plate guard may be used.

- If a regular spoon is too hard in the mouth, use a plastic spoon in this situation.

- If your client chokes easily, mix a commercial thickener into liquid foods. Many liquid drinks are available pre-thickened; the aide will not need to add the commercial thickener to such products. This may prevent the client from **aspirating** (drawing by suction) liquids into the lungs. Clients choke more readily on thinner liquids than thick liquids.

- 32 ounces of whole milk
- 1 cup of nonfat dry milk
- Mix and chill
- 275 calories per 8-ounce serving
- 19 g of protein

Optional: Can add 1 packet of Carnation Instant Breakfast or similar product to the fortified milk mixture.

FIGURE 12-17   An easy extra nourishment drink to prepare for a client who needs extra calories.

- Do not eat the client's food. Bring your own food to the client's home.

- If you need to record food intake, do it in percentages, such as 20% or 90%.

- If the client is blind, you need to tell the client where each food is on the plate in relation to a clock.

- If the client has a poor appetite and is becoming malnourished, it is advisable to offer high-calorie and high-protein drinks often throughout the day (Figure 12-17). Commercially prepared nourishments come in a variety of preparations and flavors. If using commercially prepared drinks, serve them cold and try not to waste them, as they are expensive. See Procedure 17, Feeding the Client.

Alternative Nutrition

Some clients are fed through a feeding tube inserted through an opening in the abdominal wall (Figure 12-18). This tube is called a **gastrostomy**. The client can also be

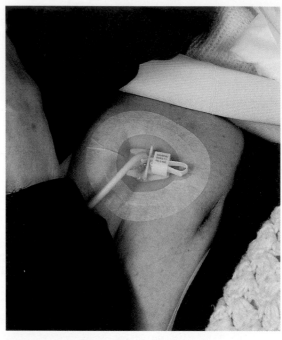

FIGURE 12-18   If the client is unable to eat, a feeding tube may be inserted into the client's abdomen to the stomach to maintain proper nutrition. The nurse inserts the feeding tube.

PROCEDURE 17   FEEDING THE CLIENT

Purpose
- To provide proper nutrition for clients who are unable to feed themselves or who need assistance in feeding
- To provide a pleasurable experience for the client
- To encourage the client to use adaptive devices for feeding

Procedure
1. Wash your hands.
2. Prepare the client to eat. Place the client in an upright position. Place a large napkin over the client's chest.
3. Bring the food to the client. Tell the client what foods you have prepared.

4. Ask the client which food is desired first. (Getting the client's cooperation and participation is important.)
5. If possible, have the client hold finger foods or bread.
6. Feed the client at the pace the client is able to chew and swallow the food.
7. Rotate different foods on the tray. Offer liquids frequently.
8. When the client is done eating, remove the food and chart the amount the client ate and drank. Amount of food eaten is recorded in percentages.
9. Wash your hands.

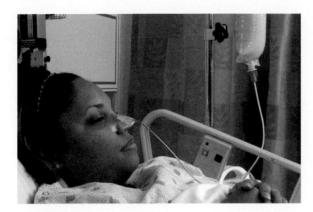

FIGURE 12-19 A young female fed through a nasogastric tube.

fed through a nasogastric tube, which is inserted through the nose and into the stomach (Figure 12-19). Administration of these feedings is done by a case manager or family member.

Clients who cannot be nourished by being fed through the mouth/nose or through a gastrostomy may receive nutrition intravenously. The client would have a small catheter (tube) inserted into the blood vessel by a health care provider. Through this line or catheter, the client may receive **total parenteral nutrition (TPN)**. The fluid that goes through this line contains a high-dextrose (sugar) solution that contains all the necessary nutrients. It is administered via a special pump (see Figure 12-20) to make sure the rate is consistent and to prevent fluid overload. A special control apparatus monitors the rate at which fluid nourishment is supplied to the client. The solution is hung by the case manager or family member. The home health aide will be given instructions on how to manage the client while the feeding is in progress, and how to troubleshoot the pump.

In providing nursing care for clients with tube feedings, the aide will need to:

* Check the tubing for kinks and do not allow the client to lie on the tubing.
* Check the taping of the tubes.

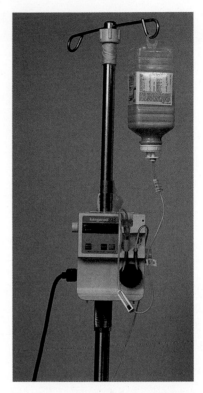

FIGURE 12-20 The feeding tube or TPN feeding is regulated with a special monitor placed on a pole. It is the case manager's responsibility to teach the family how to administer and monitor a tube feeding.

* Give the client frequent oral care.
* Follow the client's care plan for proper positioning during and after feedings.

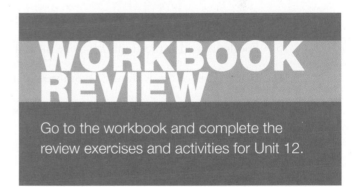

WORKBOOK REVIEW

Go to the workbook and complete the review exercises and activities for Unit 12.

REVIEW

1. List the five food groups according to MyPlate.

   _____

   _____

   _____

   _____

   _____

2. Name four considerations for making the client's meals appealing.

   _____

   _____

   _____

   _____

3. Name six special diets that may be ordered to meet a client's specific health needs.

   _____

   _____

   _____

   _____

   _____

   _____

   _____

4. A client with a chewing problem may be placed on what type of special diet?

5. Foods cooked without salt are to be included in what type of special diet?

6. What types of foods should be omitted in a diet for a client with hypertension?

7. A client's appetite may be increased when she or he is
   a. served food she or he likes.
   b. eating alone.
   c. smelling bad odors.
   d. inactive.

8. The digestion process begins in the
   a. stomach.
   b. mouth.
   c. esophagus.
   d. small intestine.

9. Identify, by circling, the two items on each tray that should *not* be on the listed special diet:

   Low Cholesterol

   batter-fried fish fillets

   baked potatoes with sour cream

   steamed green beans

   angel food cake with fresh
   raspberries

   Clear Liquid

   apricot nectar

   beef broth

   cherry gelatin cubes

   apple juice

   coffee with cream and sugar

10. Clients with heart problems are usually placed on which of the following?
    a. Low-sugar diet
    b. High-salt diet
    c. Low-protein diet
    d. None of the above

11. Place the letter that best represents the nutrient function in Column II next to the appropriate nutrient name
    in Column I.

    Column I

    1. ____ vitamin B_{12}
    2. ____ vitamin K
    3. ____ vitamin C
    4. ____ vitamin D
    5. ____ vitamin B_1

    Column II

    a. essential for normal blood clotting
    b. regulates calcium and phosphorus metabolism
    c. used in treatment of pernicious anemia
    d. essential to maintain strength of blood vessels
    e. essential for carbohydrate metabolism

12. Clients who are malnourished need to be on a diet that is ____ and ____.

13. List five guidelines for preparing meals.

    _____

    _____

    _____

    _____

    _____

14. T   F   It is not uncommon for clients to have food allergies to chocolates and strawberries.

15. T   F   Good sources of vitamin C include melons and berries.

16. T   F   A gastrostomy tube is a special tube for feeding that is placed in the esophagus.

17. The drawing of foreign material into the lungs is called
    a. dyspnea.
    b. aspirating.
    c. reflux action.
    d. anorexia.

Case Studies

18. A client with severe hypertension asks you to prepare soup and a salami sandwich for lunch. Is this a good idea? What steps could you take to encourage your client to make healthy food choices?

19. You are making a visit to a new client who appears to be quite thin. You notice that there is not much food in her cupboard or in the refrigerator. In her freezer are several packages of frozen dinners. Is this client at risk for malnutrition? What steps could you take to ensure that your client receives adequate nutrition?

UNIT 13
Elimination

KEY TERMS

bladder	fluid balance	kidneys	renal failure
clean-catch specimen	frequency	kidney dialysis	restricted fluids
colonoscopy	functional incontinence	kidney stones	stoma
colostomy	hematuria	lithotripsy	stress incontinence
condom catheter	hemodialysis	meatus	suppository
constipation	hernia	millimeter	total incontinence
cystitis	hesitancy	oliguria	umbilical
defecation	hiatal	ostomy	ureters
diarrhea	ileostomy	ostomy bag	urethra
dysuria	impaction	overflow incontinence	urge incontinence
edema	incontinent	perineum	urgency
enema	inguinal	peritoneal dialysis	urinary catheter
flatus	Kegel exercises	pyuria	vomitus

LEARNING OBJECTIVES

After studying this unit, you should be able to:

- Describe organs and functions of the urinary tract system

- Discuss four urinary tract disorders

- Define the terms used to describe signs and symptoms of urinary disorders

- Describe four types of urinary incontinence

- Describe three characteristics of normal bowel movements

- Discuss three disorders of the gastrointestinal tract

- List the components of fluid balance

- Identify fluids that are recorded for intake and output

- List the reasons for recording fluid intake and output

- Discuss bowel and ostomy care

- Demonstrate the following:

  PROCEDURE 18 Measuring and Recording Fluid Intake and Output

  PROCEDURE 19 Giving and Emptying the Bedpan

  PROCEDURE 20 Giving and Emptying the Urinal

  PROCEDURE 21 Assisting Client to Use the Portable Commode

  PROCEDURE 22 Collecting a Clean-Catch Urine Specimen

  PROCEDURE 23 Caring for a Urinary Catheter

  PROCEDURE 24 Connecting the Leg Bag

  PROCEDURE 25 Emptying a Urinary Drainage Unit

  PROCEDURE 26 Applying a Condom (External Catheter)

  PROCEDURE 27 Retraining the Bladder

  PROCEDURE 28 Giving a Commercial Enema

  PROCEDURE 29 Giving a Rectal Suppository

  PROCEDURE 30 Regulating the Bowels

  PROCEDURE 31 Applying Adult Briefs

  PROCEDURE 32 Collecting a Stool Specimen

  PROCEDURE 33 Changing an Ostomy Bag

Urinary System

The urinary system consists of the kidneys, ureters, bladder, and urethra (Figure 13-1). The kidneys are the primary organs of this system. Their function is to filter waste material from the bloodstream. As the blood passes through the kidneys, it undergoes a purifying and recycling process; waste material and excess water are filtered from it. As the blood continues through the kidneys, much of the filtered water and some minerals are reabsorbed into the bloodstream. This reabsorption is necessary to maintain the body's liquid balance. The waste material and excess water (now called urine) pass from the kidneys into the bladder through tubes called ureters. The bladder is a muscular organ for storing urine. When the bladder has accumulated about a pint of urine, nerves sense discomfort. Involuntary muscle contractions of the bladder then empty the urine into the urethra, a tube that empties urine from the bladder. These muscular contractions can be controlled and become voluntary to a large extent. The normal daily output of urine is 1500 to 2000 mL (millimeters; 1 1/2 to 2 quarts). When the normal bladder contains about 200 to 330 mL of urine, a person has an urge to urinate or void. Each time the person voids, the urine cleans the urethra of any pathogenic organisms that may have entered through the meatus. Normal urine color is clear, light yellow with a mild ammonia odor.

Signs and symptoms of urinary problems may include:

- Dysuria—painful urination
- Hematuria—finding traces of blood in the urine
- Oliguria—voiding in small amounts
- Pyuria—having pus in urine
- Flank pain—pain in the area between the ribs and the hip bone in the person's back
- Change in stream of urine—urine is expelled slower or at different rates
- Color of urine—change to deep red, brown, or yellowish green
- Frequency—going to the bathroom more often than usual and only voiding a small amount of urine
- Hesitancy—delay in starting to void
- Retention—inability to void
- Urgency—having to void immediately

If you notice any of these signs or symptoms when caring for a client, you need to report them. If a urinary tract disorder is treated early, the results of the treatment are better. It is also a good idea to be aware of the preceding terms and what they mean so that if these words are used on a client's care plan, you will better understand the client's problems.

Prevention of Urinary Tract Infections

A goal of good health maintenance in caring for your client is to prevent urinary tract infections. Guidelines to follow are:

- Wipe the perineal area from front to back after voiding or defecating (having a bowel movement).
- Increase the fluid intake of the client throughout the day.

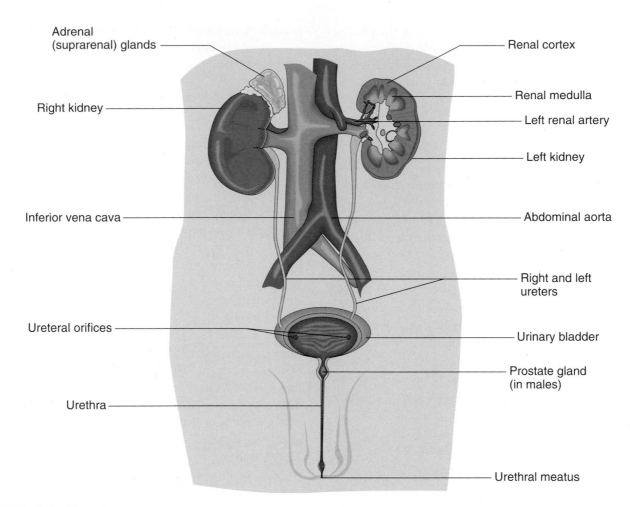

Adrenal (suprarenal) glands

Right kidney

Inferior vena cava

Ureteral orifices

Urethra

Renal cortex

Renal medulla

Left renal artery

Left kidney

Abdominal aorta

Right and left ureters

Urinary bladder

Prostate gland (in males)

Urethral meatus

FIGURE 13-1   The urinary system.

- Avoid bath salts, oils, and vaginal sprays.
- Drink cranberry juice, which will make the urine less odorous and helps to prevent urinary tract infections.
- Empty the bladder completely when voiding.
- Wear cotton underwear.

Common Disorders of the Urinary System

Incontinence, cystitis, renal failure, and kidney stones are four common disorders of the urinary system.

Incontinence

Some individuals have no voluntary control of their bladder muscles. This causes them to be incontinent, or to expel urine unexpectedly. Incontinence occurs in babies before toilet training because they have not yet developed control over the muscles in the urethra. The severity of urinary incontinence ranges from occasional leaking of urine while sneezing to the inability to control urination at all.

Types of Urinary Incontinence

Stress incontinence refers to the involuntary loss of small amounts of urine during activities that increase intra-abdominal pressure, such as coughing, running, laughing, or lifting heavy objects. Typically caused by weakened pelvic floor muscles or a weakened or damaged urethral sphincter, stress incontinence is most common in women but may affect men following prostate surgery. A client with stress incontinence can be taught to do Kegel exercises (pelvic floor strengthener). The client is told to tighten the pelvic muscles, as though to stop the urine stream when voiding, and then release. The client should try to do this about 10 times at each voiding and do it three or four times a day. Eventually, this will tighten the muscles around the meatus (opening where urine is expelled).

Urge incontinence is the involuntary loss of urine because of the inability to reach the bathroom in time.

The bladder muscle contracts and may give the client a few seconds only to reach the toilet. Most common in older adults, this type of incontinence usually is caused by weakened pelvic floor muscles, urinary tract infections, bladder irritants, Parkinson's disease, Alzheimer's disease, stroke, or nervous system damage. This condition can also be called overactive bladder.

Overflow incontinence refers to the continuous or periodic dribbling of urine because of an atonic bladder (bladder that has lost tone), or an anatomic obstruction, such as an enlarged prostate or a urethral stricture. The client tries to urinate, but only produces a weak stream of urine and is unable to empty his or her bladder. The drug Tamsulosin® can be used to treat this condition.

Functional incontinence is seen in the older adult. The client has involuntary urination because of the inability to reach a bathroom due to a specific disability, such as a physical or cognitive impairment, an inaccessible toilet, inattentive or inaccessible caregivers, or an unwillingness to move.

Total incontinence refers to a continuous leaking of urine, day and night, or the periodic uncontrollable leaking of large amount of urine.

Cystitis

Cystitis occurs when the membrane lining of the urinary bladder becomes inflamed. It can be caused by bacterial infection or a kidney inflammation that has spread to the bladder. Signs and symptoms of cystitis are urinary frequency and urgency, dysuria, nausea, anorexia (loss of appetite), and fever. The health care provider may order a urine specimen to be collected on the client to find out what organism is causing the infection. If an organism is found in the urine, the common treatment consists of medication, avoiding sodas with caffeine, and increasing fluid intake.

Kidney Stones

Kidney stones are usually caused by an excess of calcium. The urine becomes crystallized (hardened) and stones may block the ureters and cause painful urination. The stones can be of various sizes: some large, some very small. Signs and symptoms of renal colic are sudden severe pain in the flank area, hematuria (due to the stones trying to pass through the ureters), nausea, and fever. If the health care provider suspects that a client may have kidney stones, the client's urine will need to be strained through a strainer every time the client voids. The reason for this is that if a client passes a stone, no more treatment is needed. If the stones are not passed, a special procedure to dissolve the stones through laser therapy may be

needed. A technique is available now for some clients, whereby the stones can be destroyed by sound waves (lithotripsy) rather than by surgery.

Renal (Kidney) Failure

When a client's kidneys no longer produce urine in the body, waste materials build up in the body, and if nothing is done, the client can die. Early signs of renal failure are weakness, fatigue, and lethargy. Eventually, signs like hypertension, edema, and fluid retention appear throughout the body. This condition can be treated by kidney dialysis or kidney transplant. There are two types of kidney dialysis. One is called hemodialysis, which is done with the use of a machine that takes wastes out of the body. A surgical opening is created in the client's arm in which the health care provider will insert two tubes into the client's blood vessels, one in an artery and one in a vein. The machine is connected to the client through these tubes, which then start cleaning the blood of waste products. This procedure can be done several times a week, and the process usually takes 3 to 4 hours. This type of dialysis is done at a kidney dialysis center. The procedure will cause the client to be tired, and he or she may need to rest for a few hours after the dialysis. The second form of kidney dialysis is called peritoneal dialysis. In this method, a tube is placed in the client's abdomen and a large bag of fluid is connected to this tube and then drained out. The advantage of this method is that it can be done in a client's home. This procedure may need to be done at different intervals throughout the day. This method may take as little as 2 hours or as long as 10 hours depending on the weight of the solution. If you have a client receiving this type of treatment, the case manager will instruct you on your specific duties. You may just need to bring the solution to the client, and then the client will follow through with the procedure. The client on dialysis will need to follow a renal diet and may be on fluid restriction.

Common Disorders of the Gastrointestinal Tract

Hernias

A hernia is a protrusion or projection of an organ or part of an organ through the wall of the cavity that normally contains it. Causes of hernias are many, such as age, injury, and abdominal pressure from lifting heavy loads or coughing. Treatment is by surgery (herniorrhaphy) or mechanical reduction. Common types of hernias are: **hiatal**, the protrusion of the upper part of the stomach through the diaphragm and into the chest; **inguinal**, protrusion near the groin area; and **umbilical**, protrusion near the navel.

Gall Bladder Disorders

The function of the gall bladder is to store and concentrate bile between meals. The gall bladder is located next to the liver. Gallstones form when the bile contains more cholesterol than can be kept in storage. Signs and symptoms of gall bladder disorders are pain radiating to the back and right shoulder, occurring several hours after eating, and flatulence. Cholecystitis is inflammation of the gall bladder. Cholelithiasis is formation of stones in the gall bladder. Clients with gall bladder problems are treated by a low-fat diet and if necessary a surgery called a cholecystectomy, which is removal of the gall bladder.

Diverticulitis

This condition occurs when the tiny sacs inside of the intestines become inflamed and irritate the intestines. Research shows that more than 50% of individuals over the age of 50 have some form of this disease. It is usually discovered when a client has a **colonoscopy** (exam of the colon). A colonoscopy is done by using a long flexible tube attached to a video camera to view the inside of the colon. The client will need to have a bowel prep prior to this test to clean out the colon. Signs and symptoms of diverticulitis are constipation or diarrhea, cramping pain in the abdomen, and increased rectal gas. Diverticulitis is

treated with diet and medication, and if it becomes too severe, surgery may be indicated.

Hemorrhoids

Hemorrhoids are varicose veins that occur inside the rectum or around the outside of the rectum. They are caused by a weakness in this area, which can occur with straining on defecation or pregnancy. They can be very painful, itch, and can bleed if irritated. Treatment consists of the application of special cream, cold packs, and avoidance of constipation.

Measuring and Recording Fluids

Intake is a measure of all the fluids that a person drinks. Output is all the fluid that passes out of the body. The abbreviation for measuring fluid intake and output is I&O. This may be done for a client who has heart or kidney disease. If there is too little fluid in a client's system, the client is said to be dehydrated. If there is too much fluid in a client's system, the client is said to have fluid overload or **edema** (swelling of body tissues with water retained by the body). If there is edema or other fluid retention in a client's body, the health care provider may order **restricted fluids**. This means that the client's total intake of fluids is restricted to a specific amount. The amount varies and can be as little as 600 mL a day. A reverse of this condition involves too little fluids in the body, for which the health care provider may order to force fluids, which means to encourage the client to drink above normal amounts of fluid. Vomiting and diarrhea are frequent causes of dehydration. When the body fluid is in normal range, **fluid balance** exists. See Procedure 18, Measuring and Recording Fluid Intake and Output.

PROCEDURE 18   MEASURING AND RECORDING FLUID INTAKE AND OUTPUT

Purpose

- To identify food items that need to be measured for fluid intake
- To measure and record fluid intake and output accurately

Fluids that should be included in the measurement of intake include:

Measure for Intake

ice	water
juices	pop
coffee	ice cream

yogurt	soup
jello	pudding

any other food that is liquid at room temperature

Measurement for Intake

NOTE: You may need to remind family members to keep tract of the intake, when an aide is not attending the client.

1. A measuring device like a measuring cup used for cooking is usually used to measure fluid intake. Measurements are done using the metric scale, which is milliliters or mL. Remember that 30 mL equals 1 ounce (Figure 13-2).

(continued)

PROCEDURE 18 MEASURING AND RECORDING FLUID INTAKE AND OUTPUT (*continued*)

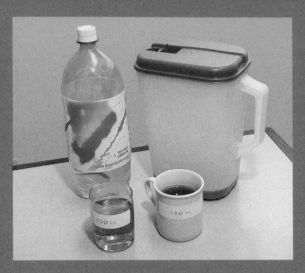

FIGURE 13-2 It is a good idea to measure the capacity in millimeters (mL) of commonly used glasses and cups. This will be helpful in recording the intake of a client.

2. After the client has drunk the liquid, record the amount. If the client drank an 8-oz bottle of soda, record 240 mL = 30 × 8 = 240. If the client drank only 6 oz = 6 × 30 = 180 mL. If the client drank a cup of coffee, you will need to measure the amount of liquid the cup holds, by pouring water into the cup and measuring it using the measuring device (Figure 13-3).

3. After a 24-hour period, the amount of fluids is added and recorded on the client's record. In acute care facilities, the intake is totaled and recorded every shift.

Measure for Output

vomitus (emesis) liquid stools
urine
blood or drainage from wounds

Procedure

1. Assemble supplies:
   large measuring container for output
   disposable gloves

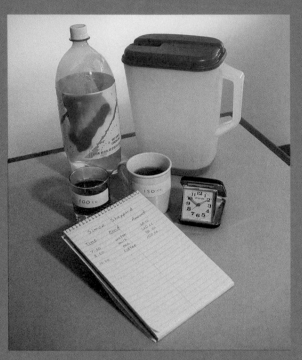

FIGURE 13-3 Intake is recorded in millimeters (mL) after the client has drunk the liquid.

2. Wash hands and apply gloves.
3. Measure all liquids eliminated by the client.
4. Ask the client to use a urinal or bedpan for all voiding. If the client can use the toilet, a special plastic hat (potty hat) can be placed in the toilet to collect the urine (Figure 13-4).
5. Pour urine from the bedpan or urinal into a measuring device (Figure 13-5). Measure the amount of urine at eye level on a flat surface. Record the amount. Always record output in mL.
6. Be sure to explain to the client how to keep exact records. The client or family will need to record the output at times when the aide is off duty.
7. Clean and disinfect equipment after each use.
8. Remove gloves and wash hands.

(*continued*)

PROCEDURE **18**   MEASURING AND RECORDING FLUID INTAKE AND OUTPUT *(continued)*

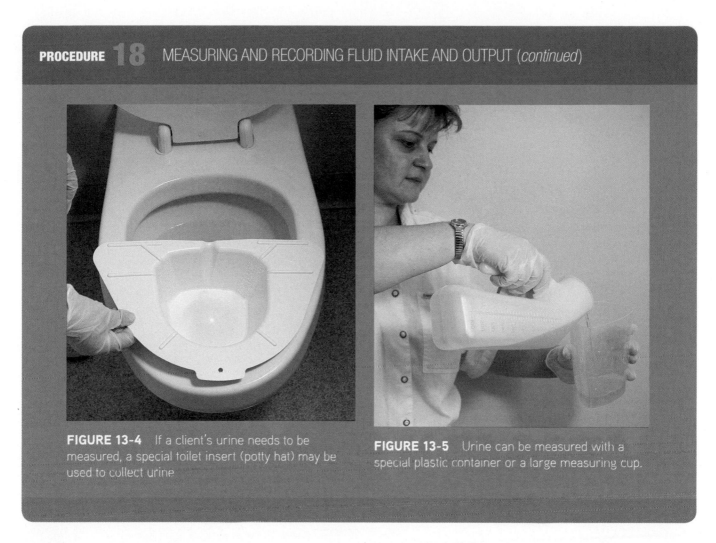

FIGURE 13-4   If a client's urine needs to be measured, a special toilet insert (potty hat) may be used to collect urine

FIGURE 13-5   Urine can be measured with a special plastic container or a large measuring cup.

Giving and Emptying the Bedpan or Urinal

The bedpan is used for clients who are confined to bed. The bedpan should be given whenever the client requests it. The aide should follow a regular schedule of offering the bedpan or urinal. If the client does not remember to ask, the home health aide should offer to bring the bedpan or urinal. The aide can politely remind the client by asking, "Do you need to use the bedpan or urinal?"

A female client will use the bedpan for both urinating and defecating (Figure 13-6). A male client will need a urinal (Figure 13-7) if he needs to urinate. If the client is very small or has a body cast, a smaller bedpan or fracture pan can be used.

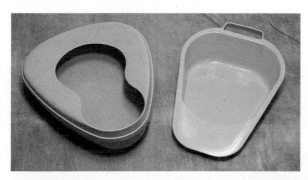

FIGURE 13-6   Regular bedpan (*left*) and fracture bedpan (*right*).

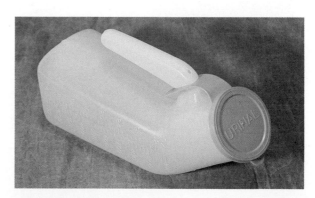

FIGURE 13-7   Male urinal.

PROCEDURE 19   GIVING AND EMPTYING THE BEDPAN

Purpose

- To provide for routine elimination of bladder and bowels
- To observe or measure urinary or fecal output

Procedure

1. Assemble equipment and supplies needed:
   disposable gloves
   bedpan and bedpan cover
   toilet tissue
   moistened washcloth or disposal wipes
2. Wash hands and apply gloves.
3. Tell the client what you plan to do and provide for privacy.
4. Place the bedpan near the bed. Place toilet tissue near the client's hand.
5. Fold the top covers at an angle. Remove the client's bottom clothing.
6. To raise the buttocks, have the client bend the knees and push on the heels. As the client lifts, place your hand under the small of the client's back.
7. Lift gently and slowly with one hand. Slide the bedpan under the hips with the other hand. The client's buttocks should rest on the rounded shelf of the bedpan. The narrow end should face the foot of the bed. If the client cannot assist, turn the client to one side and position the bedpan over the buttocks (Figure 13-8). Roll the client onto the bedpan. The aide holds the bedpan in place when the client is lying on his or her backside and then turns the client and removes his or her gloves. Elevate the client's head with pillows or raise the head of the bed if it is electric.
8. Pull a sheet over the client for added privacy. Make sure the client is as comfortable as possible.
9. Remove the bedpan with gloved hands when the client is finished using it. Remove the bedpan by having the client bend the knees and push on the heels. Place one hand under the small of the client's back and lift. Remove the bedpan with the other hand. If the client cannot lift, have the client turn to the side while holding on to the bedpan so it does not spill.
10. If possible, have the client wipe him- or herself. If client is not able to do this, the aide must wipe the client. Remember to wipe from front to back on a female client. Discard tissues in the bedpan.
11. Replace the client's clothing. Give client a wet washcloth or disposable wipe to clean his or her hands.
12. Take the bedpan to the toilet, observe contents, and measure if necessary. Empty contents into toilet. Flush. Fill bedpan with cold water and empty. Clean bedpan by using warm soapy water or disinfectant and a toilet brush. Empty the water into the toilet and rinse the bedpan. Dry well.
13. Return the bedpan to the proper storage area.
14. Remove gloves and wash hands.
15. Record color and amount of urine; record color, amount, and consistency of stool.

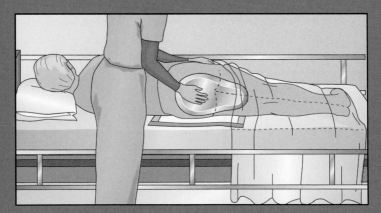

FIGURE 13-8   Roll the client away from you while supporting the client with one hand on the client's hip and arm. Place the bedpan with the other hand. Then roll the client back onto the bedpan.

PROCEDURE 20 GIVING AND EMPTYING THE URINAL

Purpose

- To provide for routine elimination of urine for a male client

Procedure

1. Wash your hands and apply gloves.
2. Lift the top bedcovers and place the urinal under the covers so that the client can grasp the handle. If he cannot do this, you must place the urinal in position and ensure that the penis is placed in the opening of the urinal (Figure 13-9). If possible, assist the client to stand when using the urinal.
3. Remove gloves and dispose of them properly. Leave client alone if possible. You may give the client a bell to ring when he is done.
4. Put on gloves and remove the urinal once the client is done using it.
5. Take the urinal to the bathroom and observe the contents. Measure if required. Empty the urinal. Rinse with cold water. Rinse with disinfectant or water; dry and store properly. The client may want the urinal at his side; if so, give the urinal back to him. Many older male adults have problems with urinary frequency and want the urinal handy.
6. Remove gloves and wash hands.
7. Record amount and color of urine, if required.

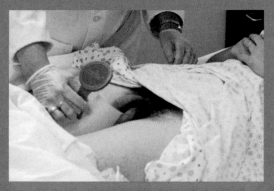

FIGURE 13-9 If the client is unable to place the urinal, the aide will place the penis into the opening of the urinal.

PROCEDURE 21 ASSISTING CLIENT TO USE THE PORTABLE COMMODE

Purpose

- To assist client to use a portable toilet who, because of mobility problems, cannot use a regular toilet

Procedure

1. Assemble equipment:
   commode and bucket
   toilet paper
   moistened washcloth with soap applied or disposal wipes
   disposable gloves
2. Wash hands and apply gloves.
3. Bring commode to area closest to client. Detach bucket from commode, if you need to wipe the client. If you place water in the bucket, it will make it easier to clean and empty.
4. Transfer the client to the commode and pull down the client's underwear. Give the client toilet paper.
5. If the client is stable, leave the room to provide privacy.
6. After the client is done, check to see if you need to wipe the client.
7. Remove gloves and assist the client to the chair or bed.
8. Return to the commode and apply gloves. Empty the bucket in the toilet. Rinse with disinfectant and cold water. Return the bucket to the commode. Store the commode in the designated area.
9. Remove gloves and wash hands.
10. Record amount of urine or stool.

Collecting a Urine Specimen

A **clean-catch specimen** is requested to obtain a urine sample that is as free of contamination as possible. This is required to provide a urine sample for a diagnostic test and to ensure that the test results are as accurate as possible. See Procedure 22, Collecting a Clean-Catch Urine Specimen.

PROCEDURE 22 COLLECTING A CLEAN-CATCH URINE SPECIMEN

Purpose

- To obtain and send specimen to laboratory for analysis

Procedure

1. Assemble supplies:
   disposable gloves
   sterile urine specimen container with completed label
   biohazard transportation bag
   clean bedpan or urinal
   antiseptic wipes
2. Wash hands and apply gloves.
3. Explain the procedure to the client. Provide for privacy.
4. Wash the client's genital area or have the client do so, with antiseptic wipes. It is especially important for the urinary opening (meatus) to be cleansed.
5. Give the client a specimen container.
6. Have the client begin to void into the bedpan, urinal, or toilet. After a small amount of urine has been voided, have the client catch some of the urine in midstream in the sterile specimen container. You will only need 2 ounces, or 60 mL. After the specimen has been collected, the client can resume voiding into the bedpan, urinal, or toilet.
7. Immediately place the sterile cap on the specimen container so the specimen will not become contaminated. Apply label.
8. Place labeled specimen container inside a biohazard transportation bag.
9. Remove gloves and wash hands.
10. Store the specimen bag according to the instructions until its transportation to the local laboratory. You may need to put it into a cold storage place temporarily.
11. Document time of collection and type of specimen.

Caring for Urinary Catheters

A **urinary catheter** is a tube inserted into the bladder to drain urine. Germs can easily enter the bladder while the catheter is in place. Therefore, cleaning around the urinary opening is important. The catheter is inserted by the nurse. The catheter is replaced weekly or once a month. The collection bag, tubing, and catheter are referred to as the *closed drainage system* (Figure 13-10). The system should never be disconnected except to reconnect it to a leg bag. The reason the system should not be disconnected is to prevent germs from entering the system (Figure 13-11). Always check to see if the tubing is lying in correct position, not kinked (Figure 13-12). You should never raise the collection bag higher than the level of the client's bladder (Figure 13-13). This is to assist the gravity drainage and prevent backflow of urine into the bladder. Never pull on a catheter. If possible, cover the bag with a cloth to prevent the embarrassment of your client. Newer closed drainage systems have a stop valve in the tubing and in the bag, which will prevent backflow of urine.

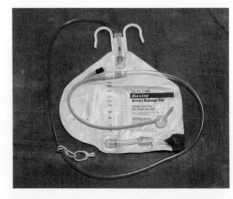

FIGURE 13-10 Closed urinary drainage system. Note tubing, urinary drainage bag, and indwelling catheter with bulb inflated.

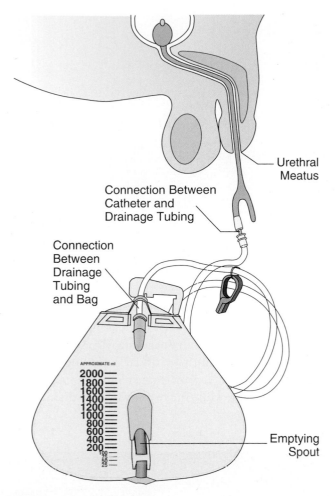

Urethral Meatus

Connection Between Catheter and Drainage Tubing

Connection Between Drainage Tubing and Bag

APPROXIMATE ml
2000
1800
1600
1400
1200
1000
800
600
400
200

Emptying Spout

FIGURE 13-11 Special care must be taken to protect the possible sites of contamination in the closed urinary drainage system.

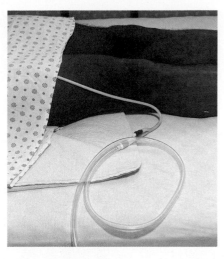

FIGURE 13-12 Tubing should be placed on top of the leg. The excess tubing should be coiled on the bed.

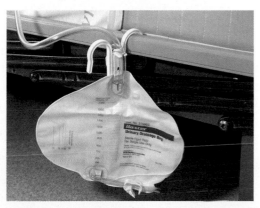

FIGURE 13-13 The urinary drainage bag should be attached to the bed frame. Check to see that the tubing does not fall below the level of the drainage bag.

PROCEDURE 23   CARING FOR A URINARY CATHETER

Purpose

- To clean the area around where the catheter enters the body
- To prevent infection of the urinary tract
- To decrease odors and make the client comfortable
- To maintain closed drainage system

Procedure

1. Assemble supplies:
   disposable gloves
   towel and bed protector
   washcloth and basin of warm water with soap or disposal wipes
   plastic bag for waste
2. Wash your hands and apply gloves.
3. Tell the client what you plan to do. Provide for privacy.
4. Position the client on his or her back. Place towel or bed protector under the client's buttocks. Expose only the small area where the catheter enters the body.

For the male, gently grasp the penis and draw the foreskin back. Clean around the catheter first and then around the meatus. Wash using a circular

(continued)

PROCEDURE 23 CARING FOR A URINARY CATHETER *(continued)*

motion. Rinse and dry in the same manner. Clean catheter at least 4 inches down from the meatus. *For the female*, separate the labia, cleanse from front to back; begin at the center, then cleanse each side, moving in only one direction away from the meatus, using a clean area of the cloth for each stroke. Rinse the washcloth or use new wipes and clean the catheter at least 4 inches down from the meatus. Dry carefully. Observe

for any skin breakdown, signs of infection, crusting, leakage, or bleeding.

5. Remove towel or bed protector.
6. Remove gloves and discard into plastic bag.
7. Cover client and discard equipment and wastes properly.
8. Wash hands.
9. Document procedure, your observations, and the client's reaction.

The leg urinary collection bag is smaller than the bedside urinary collection bag to provide a smaller collection bag for the client when out of bed. The leg bag is attached to the outside of the client's thigh (upper leg). Another option is to have an extension tube put on the leg bag and have it attached to the lower leg. The leg bag allows for greater mobility for the client, but must be emptied more frequently, as it is smaller. A client may use the leg bag while in the wheelchair or ambulating, and it can be connected to the closed drainage bag when in bed for the night. The leg bag must be rinsed according to agency directions. A clean cap or stopper must be used at the end of the tubing while the bedside urinary drainage bag is not in use.

PROCEDURE 24 CONNECTING THE LEG BAG

Purpose

- To connect a leg urinary drainage bag

Procedure

1. Assemble equipment:
   disposable gloves
   urinary leg bag with straps
   alcohol wipes
   paper towels
2. Wash your hands and apply gloves.
3. Tell the client what you plan to do. Provide for privacy.
4. Place a paper towel underneath the catheter connection area.
5. Disconnect the catheter from the tubing. Wipe the end of the catheter with an alcohol wipe (Figure 13-14). Remove the cap from the end of the leg bag and connect the leg bag to the catheter. Wipe the end of the closed drainage bag tubing with an alcohol wipe. Place the cap on the end of a closed drainage system.

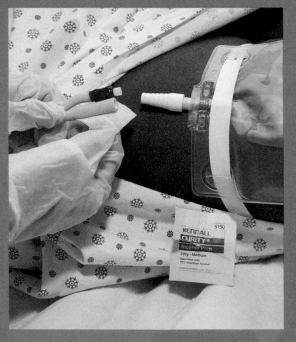

FIGURE 13-14 Wipe the end of the catheter with an alcohol wipe before connecting the leg bag.

(continued)

PROCEDURE 24   CONNECTING THE LEG BAG (*continued*)

6. Attach the leg straps and bag to the leg of the client. Check to see if the part marked "top of bag" is in the correct position.
7. Empty and measure urine from the closed drainage bag.
8. Clean and disinfect the bag and store in designated area.
9. Remove gloves and wash hands.
10. Document procedure completed.

PROCEDURE 25   EMPTYING AN URINARY DRAINAGE UNIT

Purpose

• To empty urinary drainage bag

Procedure

1. Assemble equipment:
   disposable gloves
   alcohol wipes
   measuring device
   paper towel
2. Wash hands and apply gloves.
3. Tell client what you plan to do.
4. Place a paper towel underneath the measuring device on the floor below the drainage bag.
5. Open the drain or spout and allow the urine to drain into the measuring device (Figure 13-15A). Do not allow the tip of tubing to touch the sides of the measuring device.
6. Close the drain and wipe it with an alcohol wipe. Replace it in the holder on the bag (Figure 13-15B).
7. Note the amount and color of urine. Empty the urine into the toilet. Wash and rinse the measuring device.
8. Remove gloves and wash hands.
9. Record amount.

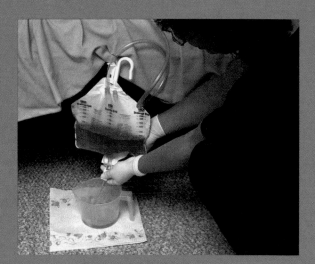

FIGURE 13-15A   Open the drain on the bottom of the urinary drainage bag, and be sure to place a paper towel underneath the container.

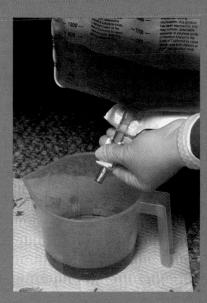

FIGURE 13-15B   Allow the urine to drain into the container. Note that the end of the drain is not touching the sides of the container. Wipe the drain off with an alcohol wipe before replacing.

PROCEDURE **26**   APPLYING A CONDOM (EXTERNAL CATHETER)

Purpose

- To drain urine from the urethra through a tube to a drainage bag

Procedure

1. Assemble equipment:
   disposable gloves
   condom catheter (Figure 13-16A and B)
   disposal wipes
   washcloth or small towel
   special adhesive (optional)
   drainage bag
2. Wash hands and apply gloves.
3. Tell the client what you plan on doing and provide for privacy.
4. Place the client on his back and expose only the perineal area.
5. Clean and dry the penis.
6. Place the tip of the penis into the condom.
7. Roll the condom over the penis.
8. If using a self-adhesive condom, it needs to be gently squeezed on top to seal it.
9. Special adhesive may come with the condom to apply after it is rolled to the top.
10. Connect to the urinary leg bag or closed drainage bag.
11. Remove gloves and wash hands.

NOTE: The condom catheter is used primarily on younger men who have no control over their urination. A downside of this type of catheter is that the urine is in constant contact with the skin, which can cause the tip of the penis to become reddened and sore; also, leakage can occur because sometimes the fit is not the best. If leakage does occur, another brand of catheter may be indicated.

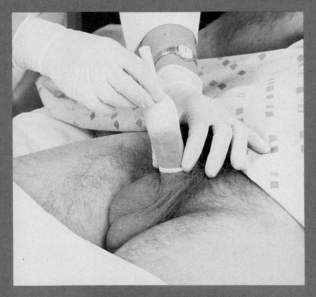

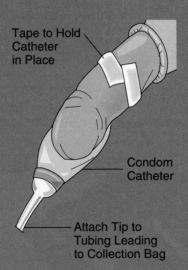

Tape to Hold Catheter in Place

Condom Catheter

Attach Tip to Tubing Leading to Collection Bag

FIGURE 13-16   A. Condom (external) catheter being placed on penis. B. Correctly applied and secured condom.

Retraining the Bladder

A home health aide may need to keep a record for a few days of how often and how much the client voids throughout the day and night. Once the client's voiding pattern is known, the case manager can analyze the client's voiding record and formulate a schedule for the aide to follow. The schedule developed by the case manager will include regularly scheduled times for the aide to have the client drink a measured amount of fluids, and then to toilet the client at regular intervals. This is done for clients who are incontinent and can be retrained to control their urination and bowel movements.

PROCEDURE 27 RETRAINING THE BLADDER

Purpose

• To regain bladder control

Procedure

The schedule developed by the case manager will include regularly scheduled times for the aide to have the client drink a measured amount of fluid. After the client has drunk the liquid, the aide notes the time; 30 minutes later the aide will toilet the client.

The aide will need to encourage the client to void each time the client is positioned on the commode or toilet. It is helpful at times to run water from the faucet to give the client an urge to void. Other methods of encouraging the client to void are to have the client apply light pressure to the bladder area to stimulate the urge to empty the bladder, pour warm water over the genital area, or lean forward on the toilet to stimulate emptying the bladder.

Remember that the client needs to be toileted at regular intervals to prevent accidents. The client will need consistent positive reinforcement to remain dry. At first it may be necessary to take the client to the bathroom every 2 hours; intervals may be lengthened as control is gained. A common cause of incontinence is delay in getting the client to the bathroom. It is of utmost importance to take the client to the bathroom on a *regular* time schedule.

The plan will also call for the aide to maintain the client's fluid intake at about 2500 mL/day, except for persons with fluid restriction (i.e., congestive heart failure or renal failure). The aide should encourage the client to wear regular underwear to enhance the client's self-esteem and to help the client from reverting back to the previous incontinence habit.

Bowel Movements

When a person has a bowel movement, this rids the body of waste products that have accumulated after food has been digested. Everyone has a different pattern in frequency of bowel movements. For some individuals having three bowel movements a day may be normal, whereas another individual may have a bowel movement every 3 days. The medical term for having a bowel movement is **defecation**. When a client has a defecation, the stool or feces should be observed for: *color*—black, tarry, brown, tan; *consistency*—hard, formed, liquid, pasty; *amount*—large, medium, or small. If a client has frequent bowel movements and the stool is very runny and loose, the client has **diarrhea**. When a person passes gas through the colon, the medical term for rectal gas is **flatus**. **Constipation** is difficulty in having a bowel movement. If a client does not have a bowel movement for 3 days, the client may develop a fecal impaction. An **impaction** is a large amount of hard stool in the lower colon or rectum that cannot be expelled normally. Signs of an impaction are pain in the lower abdomen and continuous liquid stools, which are caused by leaking around the hard stool. If a client does

develop an impaction, the nurse will need to remove the stool manually.

Constipation is the most common bowel problem that occurs in the client. Causes are due to lack of activity, medications, diet, and disease. The care plan should indicate measures to alleviate or prevent constipation. Measures often used to prevent this problem are: increase in fluid intake; increase in mobility; increase in fiber in the diet; use of laxatives or stool softeners. Documentation of bowel movements in the home is often done to prevent constipation and impactions.

Enemas and Rectal Suppositories

An **enema** is the technique of introducing fluid into the rectum to remove feces and flatus (gas) from the rectum and colon. The two common prepared enemas are the chemical (often referred to as Fleets) and oil-retention enemas. A chemical enema contains a small amount of solution, just enough to stimulate the client to have a bowel movement. Oil-retention enemas are given to soften hard feces in the rectum and are usually followed by a soap solution enema. A rectal **suppository** is a cone-shaped, easily melted, medicated mass that can readily be inserted into a client's rectum. The suppository contains ingredients that, once absorbed by the lining of the colon, will give a stimulus to the colon to evacuate stool. Either of these techniques may be necessary to relieve the client of constipation, to make the client more comfortable, or to prepare the client for diagnostic tests.

PROCEDURE **28** GIVING A COMMERCIAL ENEMA

Purpose

• To help cleanse the bowel

Procedure

1. Assemble supplies (Figure 13-17):
   disposable gloves
   commercial prepackaged enema
   protective pad
   bedpan or commode
   toilet paper
   lubrication jelly
   water, washcloth, soap, towel
2. Wash hands and put on gloves.
3. Tell the client what you plan to do.
4. Provide for the client's comfort and privacy.

5. Place a protective pad underneath the client's buttocks.
6. Have the client turn to the left side. Turn the covers back to expose only the buttocks.
7. Remove the cover on the tip of enema. Apply extra lubricant to the tip to ensure easy insertion.
8. Separate the buttocks and insert the tip into the rectum at least 3 inches. Slowly squeeze the plastic container (Figure 13-18). This forces the solution to flow evenly into the rectum.
9. Remove the enema tip while holding the client's buttocks together.
10. Instruct the client to hold the enema for at least a few minutes.
11. Position the client on a bedpan, commode, or toilet.
12. Remove gloves and wash hands.
13. Apply clean gloves and assist the client in cleaning the area around the anus and buttocks after the client has finished defecating.
14. Return the client to a comfortable position.
15. Remove gloves and wash hands.
16. Record results of enema—color, amount, consistency; for example: 10:00 AM, Fleets enema given, good results—large, brown, formed stool.

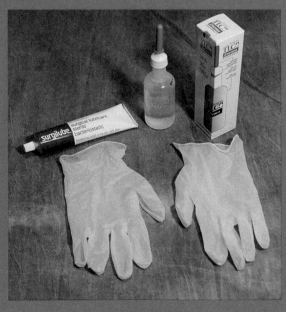

FIGURE 13-17 Equipment needed to give a commercial enema.

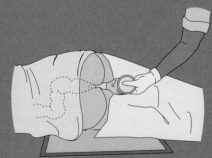

FIGURE 13-18 Administering a commercial enema.

PROCEDURE 29   GIVING A RECTAL SUPPOSITORY

Purpose

- To stimulate a bowel movement

NOTE: Suppositories are usually stored in the client's refrigerator and are wrapped in foil. The suppository will melt once inserted into the warm environment of the rectum and colon. It will take the suppository at least 5 to 10 minutes to melt. It is important that the aide inform the client to wait a few minutes after the suppository is inserted before trying to have a bowel movement.

Procedure

1. Assemble supplies:
   disposable gloves
   rectal suppository
   lubricant
   protective pad or paper towels
2. Wash hands and apply gloves.
3. Tell the client what you plan to do and provide privacy.
4. Open foil-wrapped suppository.
5. Turn the client to one side and place a protective pad under the buttocks.
6. Lubricate your gloved finger well, then insert the gloved finger with suppository, tip end first, into the rectum (Figure 13-19). Push the suppository along the lining of the rectum with your index finger as far as your finger allows. Be careful not to insert the suppository into the feces. The suppository needs to be next to the lining of the rectum for it to be effective.
7. Remove gloves and wash hands.
8. After 10 to 20 minutes have passed, assist the client to the toilet or commode.
9. After the client has had a bowel movement, assist the client back to bed or a chair. If you need to wipe the client, apply gloves.
10. Remove gloves and/or wash hands.
11. Record results. Note color, consistency, and amount of stool.

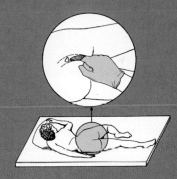

FIGURE 13-19   Carefully place the rectal suppository into the rectum, about 3 inches for adults.

Bowel Regulating Programs

Among the elderly, constipation is often encountered. If a client is unable to exercise and move about regularly, bowel action becomes sluggish. Sometimes medications, especially painkillers, can cause constipation. If a client has hemorrhoids, there may be a fear of pain and so the client avoids trying to have a bowel movement. There are several methods that can assist clients to evacuate. Each method is designed according to the client's specific need. For instance, if any medication is to be administered, or a digital exam is to be performed (a lubricated finger is inserted into the rectum and irritates the rectum area for a minute), it needs to be part of the daily routine. A bowel regulating program is developed with the client to set up a designated time for a bowel movement. Consuming dietary foods that are high in fiber and bulk, drinking eight glasses of water a day, and exercising will help the client to achieve this goal. Medications such as Metamucil, stool softeners, suppositories, or enemas may be needed to supplement the program.

PROCEDURE 30   REGULATING THE BOWELS

Purpose

- To retrain a client to be continent of bowel movement
- To regulate a client to have regular bowel movement

Procedure

1. The health care provider assesses the prior habits of the client. If the client always had a bowel movement early in the morning, this would be important to know in planning the client's bowel regulating program.
2. A plan is designed and implemented. Important elements of the plan are:
   - Intake of high-fiber foods
   - Adequate intake of liquids
   - Regular exercise
   - Toileting client at regular intervals
   - Praise by aide of slightest progress
   - Privacy for client for bowel movements
3. Follow the bowel regulating program developed by the health care provider. If the plan appears to be working, note the success of the program. If the plan does not work, revise the plan. It is also important to give some suggestions to the health care provider of possible solutions for regulating the bowels.

Adult Briefs

The adult disposal brief is used to keep the incontinent client dry and to minimize embarrassment to the client in the event of accidents. The adult brief will also reduce odor, save on bed linens, and reduce urinary infections and pressure sores. The adult brief comes in various styles and sizes. One design may be an insert to go inside a specially designed brief. Another popular type is a "wraparound brief" fastened with Velcro-like tabs (Figure 13-20 A, B). It is important to have the correct size for your client to ensure effectiveness. If an adult brief is too large, it will be ineffective and leakage will occur; if the brief is too small, the brief will also be ineffective and leak. It is a good idea to place a maximum-absorbency brief on the client at night. It is also important to read the instructions on the package on how to apply each particular style of brief. Many briefs have a strip on them that changes color when the brief needs to be changed. The brief should be checked at regular intervals and changed as needed. Do not apply powder to the client's perineal area when

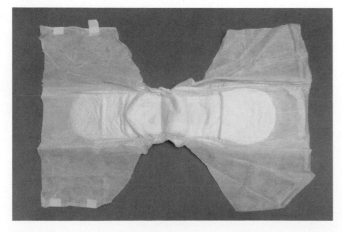

FIGURE 13-20A   Adult brief with side tabs.

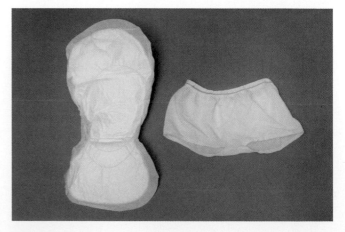

FIGURE 13-20B   Adult disposal pant with insert.

adult briefs are used. Many of the briefs have specially treated wipes to use to clean the client's perineal area (**perineum**) when changing the briefs. They are very reasonable in cost and are recommended over soap and water. If a certain brief does not appear to be working, report this to the case manager. There are many different types on the market, and some work better on some clients than others.

PROCEDURE 31   APPLYING ADULT BRIEFS

Purpose

- To confine urine or feces to one area when the client is incontinent
- To reduce odor and skin breakdown
- To reduce laundering of linens and clothes

Procedure

1. Assemble supplies:
   adult brief
   cleansing wipe
   disposable gloves
   plastic bag
2. Wash hands and apply gloves.
3. Tell the client what you plan to do and provide privacy.
4. Remove the soiled brief and place it in a plastic bag.
5. Cleanse the genital area with a cleansing wipe and place in a plastic bag.
6. Apply a new brief underneath the client's buttocks. Be sure to position the brief correctly under the buttocks. Bring the lower end of the brief through the client's perineal area. Fasten the tabs on the brief. Adjust the brief to fit closely by pulling it snugly into the groin.
7. Remove gloves and wash hands.
8. Dispose of soiled brief outside of the client's room to prevent odors.
9. Record output—urine or stool and approximate amount—if required.

Collecting a Stool Specimen

On occasion it may be necessary to collect a stool sample for a diagnostic test. Stool samplings for guaiac blood or occult blood are usually done three times on three different bowel movements.

PROCEDURE 32   COLLECTING A STOOL SPECIMEN

Purpose

- To collect a stool sample for a diagnostic test

Procedure

1. Assemble supplies:
   disposable gloves
   bedpan or other collecting container
   specimen container or Hema-screen packet with label completed
2. Inform the client of the need for a specimen.
3. After the client has had a bowel movement in the bedpan or a toilet, apply gloves and, using a wood applicator, remove stool (Figure 13-21A). Place a small amount (approximately 1 tablespoon) of stool in a labeled container (Figure 13-21B) if the stool is going to be sent to the laboratory. Notify the agency that you have the specimen, as

(*continued*)

PROCEDURE 32 COLLECTING A STOOL SPECIMEN *(continued)*

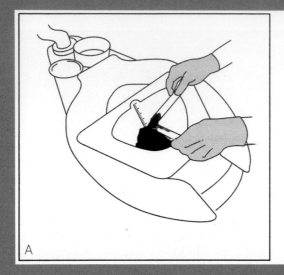 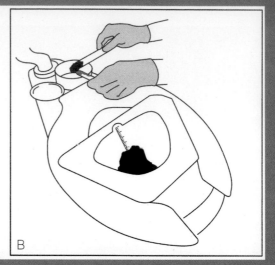

FIGURE 13-21 Using tongue blades to transfer the stool specimen from the collection container (A) to the specimen container (B).

some samples need to go to the laboratory right away.

4. If the test is for occult blood or guaiac, place a small amount of stool on Hema-screen packet with the applicator stick included in the test. Close the tab and turn the packet over. Pull the tab back slowly. Read the results 30 to 60 seconds later.

A blue discoloration around the perimeter indicates that blood is present.

5. Dispose of soiled equipment, remove gloves, and wash hands.

6. If need be, send the stool specimen to the laboratory in a biohazardous bag.

7. Document stool specimen collection and results.

Caring for an Ostomy Bag

An **ostomy bag** is sometimes called a stoma bag. It is used for clients who have had a surgical operation called a colostomy or an ileostomy. In these operations, the intestine is cut and brought to the outside of the body (Figure 13-22). Body wastes (feces) are expelled through an opening in the abdomen instead of the rectum. This opening in the abdomen is called a **stoma** (Figure 13-23). The ostomy bag is placed over the opening to collect the wastes (Figure 13-24). A **colostomy** is an artificial opening into the large intestines in which the stool coming into the bag will usually be formed like regular stool. An **ileostomy** is an artificial opening into the small intestines in which the stool will be more liquid and odorous. A client with an

ileostomy will need to wear an ostomy bag at all times. These two openings can be either permanent or temporary, depending on the initial reason for the **ostomy**. An ostomy bag should be changed or emptied when it becomes one-third or one-half full. Once regulated, the client can change or empty it at about the same time each day. The best time of the day to schedule a pouch change is first thing in the morning when the stoma is less active. In addition to changing the bag, the client may need to irrigate the intestines. If the client needs to do this, the client would have been taught at the hospital by the enterostomal therapist nurse or WOCN how to irrigate (wash out) the intestine. An aide may assist the client with this procedure.

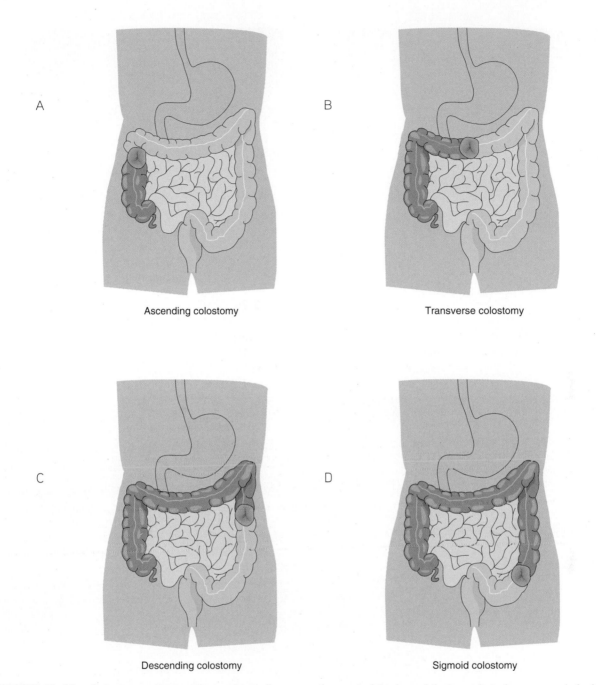

A. Ascending colostomy

B. Transverse colostomy

C. Descending colostomy

D. Sigmoid colostomy

FIGURE 13-22   Colostomy sites may vary depending upon the part of the bowel that needs to be removed. A. Ascending colostomy. B. Transverse colostomy. C. Descending colostomy. D. Sigmoid colostomy.

Until a client has adjusted to using the ostomy bag, there may be strong feelings of embarrassment. The home health aide can help the client accept the inconvenience by being understanding. The aide should not show displeasure in assisting the client.

The bags and attachments come in many styles today. They are lighter, odor proof, and fit more tightly. Many types of bags and appliances are available; a few require a belt to attach the appliance; others do not require a belt. Colostomy bags can be one-piece disposable pouches or two-piece disposable pouches. A popular method of attachment is with a skin barrier to the area around the stoma (Figure 13-25A). This skin barrier protects the real skin from irritation and contamination with the client's feces and also serves as a place where the colostomy bag can be put on and taken off. Another popular method for attaching a colostomy bag is with a wafer, which is changed once a week. The WOCN or enterostomal therapist will give you special instructions on the type of skin attachment and bag the client is using (Figure 13-25B and Figure 13-26).

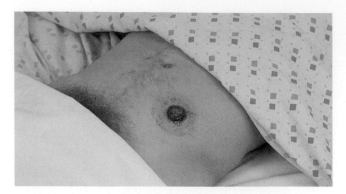

FIGURE 13-23   A stoma on the outside of the client's abdomen.

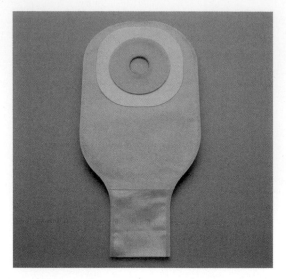

FIGURE 13-24   Stoma protector and drainage bag. (*Permission to use this copyrighted material has been granted by the owner, Hollister Incorporated.*)

PROCEDURE 33   CHANGING AN OSTOMY BAG

Purpose

- To keep the client clean
- To prevent skin breakdown around the stoma
- To regulate and establish a daily routine for removing fecal wastes

Procedure

1. Assemble supplies:
   disposable gloves
   washcloth
   basin of warm water and soap
   clean ostomy bag
   plastic bag
   skin ointment (if ordered)
   toilet tissue
2. Wash your hands and apply gloves.
3. Tell the client what you plan to do and provide privacy.
4. Gently remove the soiled colostomy bag from the stoma. Place it in a plastic bag. Colostomy bags are often reused. If the bag is to be reused, take the bag to bathroom and empty the contents and rinse the bag out.
5. If there is stool on the skin, remove it with toilet tissue. Wash the area around the stoma with mild soap and water. Pat the area dry.
6. Apply ointment if ordered. Observe the area around the stoma for redness or open areas.
7. Apply the client's pouch.
   - If a one-piece pouch or bag is being used, remove the self-stick backing from the new ostomy appliance. Press the new bag to the area around the stoma, being sure to seal tightly.
   - If a two-piece pouch is being used, be sure to cut the opening to the correct size. (A few bags are premeasured and this step is not necessary.) Remove the adhesive backing on the face plate. Firmly apply the face plate to the client's skin around the stoma, working from the stoma outward. Then apply the bag to this face plate. Let your client assist you as much as possible. Be sure to follow any special manufacturer's instruction in application of the appliance.

(*continued*)

PROCEDURE 33   CHANGING AN OSTOMY BAG (*continued*)

8. Assist the client to connect the belt to the appliance, if the client is using this type of appliance.
9. Remove wastes. Observe stool for color, amount, and consistency. If necessary, spray the room with deodorizer.

10. Remove gloves and wash hands.
11. Document procedure and time, your observations, and the client's reaction.

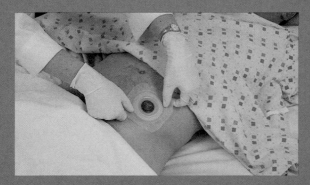

FIGURE 13-25A   Applying the skin barrier to the stoma.

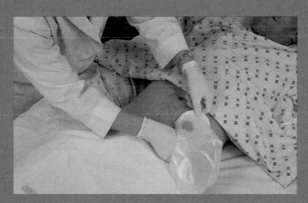

FIGURE 13-25B   Press the pouch into place.

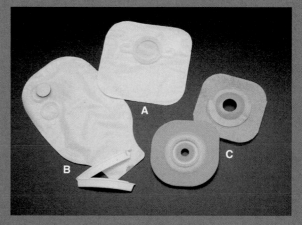

FIGURE 13-26   A. Closed stoma bag used for stool collection; notice the plastic seal around the bag. B. Larger stoma bag, which could be used for irrigation. C. Sample of artificial skin and Karaya ring skin attachments. (*Permission to use this copyrighted material has been granted by the owner, Hollister Incorporated.*)

WORKBOOK REVIEW

Go to the workbook and complete the review exercises and activities for Unit 13.

REVIEW

1. What is the medical term for inflammation of the bladder?

2. When measuring intake and output, 1 ounce is equal to how many mL?

3. Fill in the blank: _____ incontinence refers to the involuntary loss of small amounts of urine during activities such as coughing, running, laughing, or lifting heavy objects.

4. Fill in the blank: _____ incontinence refers to an involuntary loss of urine because of the inability to reach the bathroom in time.

5. When collecting a clean-catch midstream urine specimen, always
   a. do it in the morning.
   b. take the first few drops of urine.
   c. maintain a sterile collection container.
   d. none of the above.

6. A surgically placed opening in the abdomen, such as a colostomy, is called a
   a. scar.
   b. stoma.
   c. wound.
   d. hernia.

7. Using the following terms, match each term with the correct definition.

   edema   millimeters   dehydration
   restricted   fluid balance   forcing fluids
   intake   output   meatus

   _____ a. A decrease in the amount of water in the body tissues due to intake of insufficient fluids or excretion of excess fluids
   _____ b. The fluid eliminated from the body and recorded
   _____ c. The measurement of fluid taken in by the body
   _____ d. Swelling of body tissues with water retained by the body
   _____ e. Output is measured in this unit of measurement
   _____ f. Opening where urine comes out
   _____ g. Encourage client to consume adequate amounts of liquids
   _____ h. Client eliminates about the same amount of fluid that is taken in
   _____ i. Client needs intake of fluids limited

8. Using the following terms, match each term with the correct definition.

   dysuria   oliguria   hematuria
   condom catheter   frequency   stoma
   commode   potty hat   impaction

   _____ a. Painful or difficult voiding
   _____ b. Large amount of hardened stool at end of rectum
   _____ c. In-toilet specimen collector
   _____ d. Blood in urine
   _____ e. Portable toilet
   _____ f. External catheter
   _____ g. Voiding in very small amounts
   _____ h. Having to urinate often
   _____ i. Outside opening on the abdomen for a colostomy

9. When is the intake of fluids recorded?
   a. After the client drinks the fluid
   b. After each swallow
   c. When the client says she or he will drink it
   d. At the end of the shift

10. Describe normal characteristics of urine in regard to the following:
    a. Amount in 24 hours: _____
    b. Color: _____
    c. Clearness: _____
    d. Odor: _____

11. List four organs of the urinary system.

    _____

    _____

    _____

    _____

12. Care of the client with an indwelling catheter is aimed at preventing
    a. urinary incontinence.
    b. bleeding.
    c. infection.
    d. voiding.

Case Studies

13. Mr. Jones is on a bladder retraining program, and the nurse has developed a schedule that requires you to toilet him every 2 hours. When it is time for Mr. Jones to be toileted, he tells you that he does not need to go. What steps could you take to encourage him to cooperate with this procedure? What methods could you suggest that may stimulate his bladder to release urine?

14. You have been assigned to change Mrs. Smith's ostomy bag. In doing so, you notice that the color of the stoma has changed significantly since the last time. What should you do?

UNIT 14
Integumentary System

KEY TERMS

bony prominences   epidermis   podiatrist   shearing

dermis   friction   pressure sore

LEARNING OBJECTIVES

After studying this unit, you should be able to:

- Identify parts and functions of the integumentary system

- Describe common skin disorders

- Describe the appearance of pressure sores

- Locate the pressure points on the body where pressure sores usually occur

- Describe nursing care measures to prevent pressure sores from developing

- List guidelines for application of ointment to the skin

- Demonstrate the following:

  PROCEDURE 34 Applying Clean Dressing and Ointment to Unbroken Skin

  PROCEDURE 35 Assisting with Tub Bath or Shower

PROCEDURE 36 Giving a Bed Bath

PROCEDURE 37 Giving a Back Rub

PROCEDURE 38 Giving Female Perineal Care

PROCEDURE 39 Giving Male Perineal Care

PROCEDURE 40 Assisting with Routine Oral Hygiene

PROCEDURE 41 Caring for Dentures

PROCEDURE 42 Shaving the Male Client

PROCEDURE 43 Giving a Warm Foot Soak

PROCEDURE 44 Giving Nail Care

PROCEDURE 45 Shampooing Hair in Bed

Integumentary System

The skin, hair, and nails make up the integumentary system. The skin is the largest organ of the body. It covers the entire outer surface of the body. Skin is made up of two layers of tissue. The outer layer is the epidermis and the inner layer is the dermis (Figure 14-1). Other parts of the integumentary system are the nails, hair, oil and sweat glands, and mucous membranes.

The integumentary system protects the body but also has other functions. It regulates body temperature and works with the nervous system to sense touch, pressure, pain, heat, and cold.

The pores or natural openings in the skin surface are protected by oil glands and sweat glands. As the body perspires (sweats) through the skin pores, the air evaporates the perspiration and the body feels cooler. Secretions from these glands are helpful in keeping germs from entering the pores. When the skin is cut or there is an open sore, germs can enter the body easily. Once germs get beyond the skin, the other body defenses start to work. White blood cells surround the germs and try to stop them from going deeper into the body. The pus that forms on a skin wound is made up of dead white blood cells that have fought off the germs.

Hair protects the body in several ways. The eyebrows keep sweat from falling into the eyes. The tiny hairs inside the nose and ears stop small particles from entering and causing damage. The eyelashes keep small objects from getting into the eyes. These hairs all act very much like a screen door on a house in keeping out unwanted organisms. The skin itself is a protective covering that helps to maintain body temperature and excretes waste products through perspiration.

Common Disorders of the Integumentary System

Pressure Areas

Clients who spend most of their time in a bed or chair because of weakness or injury can develop pressure sores. Other names for pressure sores are bedsores, pressure ulcers, or decubitus ulcers. Pressure sores can cause serious health problems. The care given to the skin of a person confined to bed or a wheelchair is extremely important. Breakdown most often occurs where the skin covers the bones. These places are called bony prominences (Figure 14-2). A pressure sore is an injury to tissues, such as skin and muscle, usually caused by

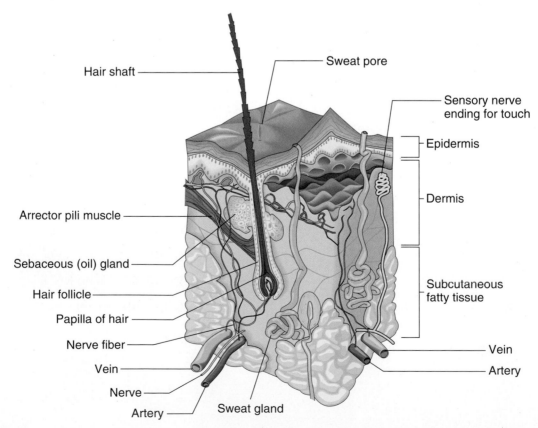

Hair shaft

Sweat pore

Sensory nerve ending for touch

Epidermis

Dermis

Arrector pili muscle

Sebaceous (oil) gland

Hair follicle

Papilla of hair

Nerve fiber

Vein

Nerve

Artery

Sweat gland

Subcutaneous fatty tissue

Vein

Artery

FIGURE 14-1 Cross section of the skin.

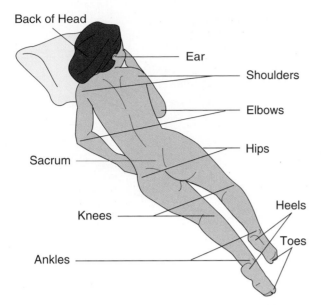

FIGURE 14-2   Areas of the body where pressure sores most often appear.

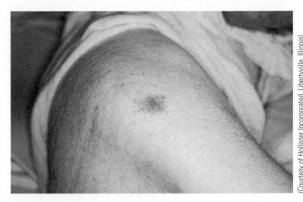

(Courtesy of Hollister Incorporated, Libertyville, Illinois)

FIGURE 14-3A   Stage 1—warm-looking reddened area.

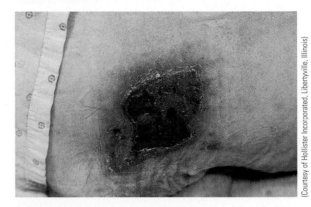

(Courtesy of Hollister Incorporated, Libertyville, Illinois)

FIGURE 14-3B   Stage 2—blister forms.

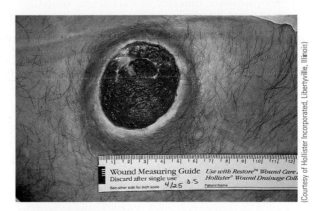

(Courtesy of Hollister Incorporated, Libertyville, Illinois)

FIGURE 14-3C   Stage 3—blister breaks open.

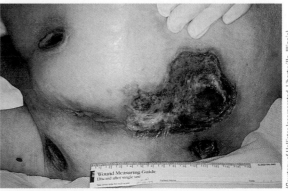

(Courtesy of Hollister Incorporated, Libertyville, Illinois)

FIGURE 14-3D   Stage 4—open sore with underlying structure exposed.

constant pressure. This constant pressure decreases the amount of blood flow to tissues. Because of decreased blood flow, the affected area becomes starved for nutrients and oxygen.

The back of the head, buttocks, coccyx, elbow, knees, and heels are common places to watch for signs of skin breakdown. A **pressure sore** is a breakdown in the skin that covers a bony area. Some common causes of pressure sore development are injury to the skin due to leaving a client in one position too long, **friction** (sliding from side to side or from one surface to another) and **shearing** (when the skin of the client moves in one direction, and the underlying bone moves in another), poor skin cleansing, poor nutrition, and incontinence.

Signs of Pressure Sores

Pressure sores are characterized by stages, depending on the degree of severity.

Stage 1: A warm-looking reddened area. Within 18 to 24 hours the reddened area can become an open sore. If not treated it will soon develop into Stage 2 (Figure 14-3A).

Stage 2: A blister will form and there will be small breaks visible on the client's skin. If not treated it will soon progress to Stage 3 (Figure 14-3B).

Stage 3: The blister breaks open and there is a well-defined sore visible (Figure 14-3C).

Stage 4: The open area extends to the muscle, bones, and underlying structures (Figure 14-3D). These sores can vary in size and are places where infections can easily and quickly set in.

Preventing Pressure Sores. Certain medical conditions such as diabetes, stroke, and paralysis make the client more susceptible to skin breakdown. Clients with circulatory problems or clients who are obese or very thin are also more susceptible. Nursing care is aimed at prevention, as once a pressure sore occurs, more skilled nursing care is required. The home health aide must pay particular attention to the bony prominence areas on the client. Skin should be cleansed when necessary at routine intervals and the skin should be kept clean and dry. The aide should avoid hot water and use a mild cleansing agent that minimizes irritation and dryness of the skin. If soap is used on the skin it must be completely rinsed off, as soap has a drying effect on the skin. Care must be exerted to minimize the force or friction used on the skin as it is cleaned. If the skin gets dry, it is more vulnerable to the development of pressure sores. Environmental factors that may increase the incidence of pressure sores are low humidity in the home and exposure to cold. Dry skin should be treated with good moisturizing lotions applied at frequent intervals around the clock. If the client is incontinent or has wound drainage that cannot be controlled, chux or briefs that absorb moisture and present a quick-drying surface to the skin can be used. Topical ointments that act as barriers to moisture can be used with the briefs. A nutritious high-protein diet should be offered and, if need be, a nutritional protein supplement can be given to the client. Nutrition plays a big part in the development of pressure sores. Once an individual becomes malnourished, pressure sores can develop quickly if the client is bedridden. The client also needs to be kept as mobile as possible. It is important that the client's position be changed often and passive range-of-motion exercises be provided as part of a daily routine.

Many special devices are available to place on the bed or on the specific part of the body to aid in the prevention of pressure sores. Examples are alternating air pressure mattress (Figure 14-4A), egg-crate mattress (Figure 14-4B), gel foam cushion for wheelchairs, lamb's wool or sheepskin pad (Figure 14-4C), bed cradle (Figure 14-4D), elbow pad (Figure 14-4E), heel pad (Figure 14-4F), and ankle elevator (Figure 14-4G).

An alternating air pressure mattress is a mattress filled with air (Figure 14-4A). This works by continuously changing the pressure areas on the client's back. One can improvise an air mattress designed for camping instead of

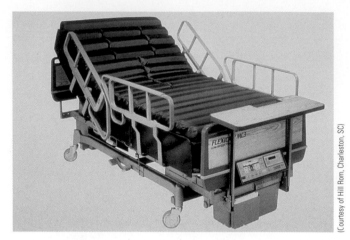

(Courtesy of Hill Rom, Charleston, SC)

FIGURE 14-4A Alternating air pressure mattress.

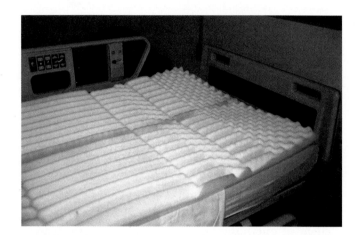

FIGURE 14-4B Egg-crate mattress.

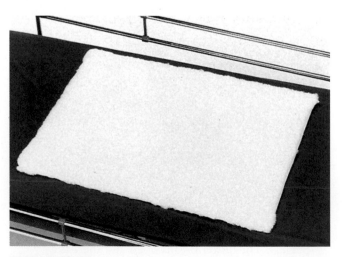

FIGURE 14-4C Lamb's wool or sheepskin pad.

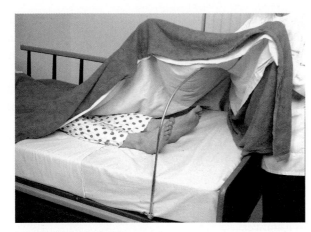

FIGURE 14-4D Bed cradle.

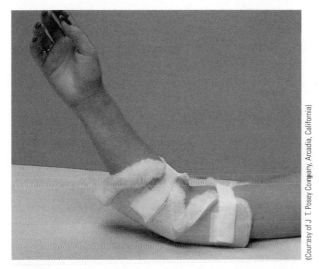

FIGURE 14-4E Elbow pad.

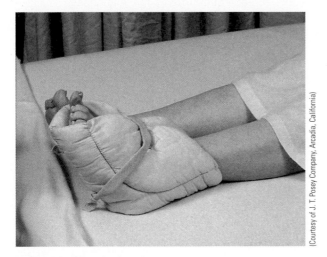

FIGURE 14-4F Heel pad.

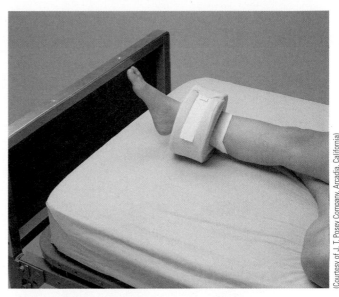

FIGURE 14-4G Ankle elevator.

buying a medical air mattress. A water mattress is also effective in reducing pressure on the skin, but causes problems when transferring clients in and out of bed, because it is not as firm as a regular mattress.

An egg-crate mattress is a mattress made of foam rubber that is molded like an egg crate (see Figure 14-4B). They are inexpensive but effective in reducing pressure on the skin. You can also purchase one the size of a seat for the client to sit on during the day when in a chair. A gel foam cushion is a special cushion filled with a solution or gel. This style of cushion is effective in the prevention of pressure sores for a client who sits in a wheelchair for long periods of time.

Sheepskin or lamb's wool pads prevent pressure sores by acting as a barrier between the client's skin and the sheets (see Figure 14-4C). A bed cradle is another device to keep linens off the client's legs and feet (see Figure 14-4D). In the home a client may substitute a box or other device to keep linens off the legs and feet. Elbow pads that have a sheepskin lining will protect the elbow from irritation due to the bed linens (see Figure 14-4E and H). Elbow and arm pads can protect the client's arm (see Figure 14-4H). Sheepskin will also help moisturize the skin. Heel pads made of either foam or sheepskin will protect the heel from breaking down in a bedridden client (see Figure 14-4F). If the ankle needs to be elevated off the bed to protect it from

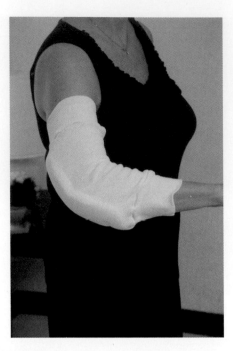

FIGURE 14-4H Elbow and arm pad.

irritation and skin breakdown, an ankle elevator can be used (see Figure 14-4G). These special devices can prevent the skin from rubbing against the bed linens, but do not take the place of good skin care.

Another treatment for pressure sores is the application of dressings such as Duoderm or Hydrocol. A nurse applies this product to the skin and it is left on for 3 to 7 days. These products are special dressings that can protect an area, dry it out, and help it heal. The dressings contains special ingredients that assist in healing the pressure sore, which are very effective in most cases. This product can be left on the skin when bathing in the tub or in a shower.

The home health aide should watch for skin irritation when applying braces and splints, and report the first sign of a reddened area to the case manager. Some other common skin disorders and their treatments are described in Figure 14-5.

Disorder	Description	Treatment
Acne	Chronic inflammatory disease of the sebaceous (oil) glands and hair follicles. Characterized by eruptions, cysts, nodules, or pustules that may lead to scarring and pitting of the skin. Often appears at puberty when major body changes commence. Usually appears on the face, neck, and shoulders.	Diet modification Topical medication Cleansing of the skin Surgical skin peeling and removal
Psoriasis	Scaly, itchy skin eruptions that appear at any age.	Topical ointments for mild cases Ultraviolet light and tar preparations for moderate cases Vitamin D_3 can be given orally
Dermatitis	Skin inflammation that causes itching, redness, and skin lesions (sores). May be caused by skin irritants such as poison ivy, allergies, sunburn, or adverse reaction to heat or cold.	Topical medication and avoidance of causal factors
Scabies	Skin lesions caused by mites that burrow into the skin. Transmitted by direct contact, clothing, and linen. Itching may persist several days after treatment. Noticed around fingers, wrists, axilla, waist, under the breasts, abdomen, buttocks, and genitalia. Infection of the lesions is common.	Topical medication Antibiotics if infection occurs Antihistamines to relieve the itching

FIGURE 14-5 Common skin disorders and their treatments.

Applying Over-the-Counter (OTC) Ointments

There are numerous types of creams, salves, and ointments available today that can be applied to the skin. Some are used for infections, others for rashes, and some for relief of pain or just plain lubrication of the skin. Home health aides are allowed to apply these ointments to unbroken skin areas. Be sure to read the directions on the care plan for each ointment that needs to be applied. A few ointments need to be applied sparingly, which means just a thin layer applied to the skin. Other ointments need a heavy application to be effective. Often clients will have three or four ointments that need to be applied. Double-check to make sure you are applying them to the right area of the body. Always wear gloves when you are applying the ointments so as not to absorb them into your own body.

Applying Skin Dressings

Occasionally it may be necessary to apply a dressing for minor cuts and scrapes. Applying a clean dressing and ointment to broken skin helps to protect the area from contamination and irritation. Although most dressings will be changed by the nurse, occasionally the dressing change is done by the home health aide, with the approval of the nurse. In these cases, the aide should observe and record the color, amount, and consistency of the drainage; the progress of the healing; and the surrounding skin condition. See Procedure 34, Applying Clean Dressing and Ointment to Unbroken Skin.

PROCEDURE 34   APPLYING CLEAN DRESSING AND OINTMENT TO UNBROKEN SKIN

Purpose

- To help skin heal and avoid infection
- For relief of pain

Procedure

1. Assemble supplies:
   disposable gloves
   two or more 4 × 4 gauze pads prepackaged
   over-the-counter ointment (if ordered)
   receptacle for wastes (e.g., plastic bag)
   tape and scissors
2. Wash your hands and apply gloves.
3. Tell the client what you plan to do and provide for privacy.
4. Position the client so the area with the dressing is accessible while maintaining client comfort (Figure 14-6A).
5. Remove the old dressing. If the dressing does not lift off easily, pour warm water over it to loosen it. Discard the used dressing in an open waste receptacle (plastic bag). Note color, amount of drainage, and condition of surrounding skin.

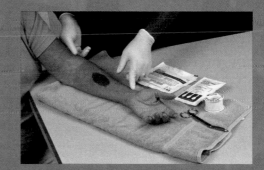

FIGURE 14-6A   Assemble equipment and position the client so that the area with the dressing is accessible.

6. Open the package of gauze pads without touching the pads (Figure 14-6B). Be careful not to have the dressing touch bed linens or the client's clothing. Cut the tape. Apply medication in a thin layer to the affected area. Apply ointment if ordered. Apply dressing. Do not touch the center of the dressing. Hold all dressings on the corners only. Apply the tape correctly (Figures 14-6C and 14-7).

(continued)

PROCEDURE 34 APPLYING CLEAN DRESSING AND OINTMENT TO UNBROKEN SKIN (*continued*)

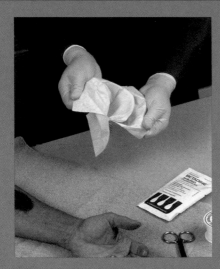

FIGURE 14-6B Correct method of opening dressing.

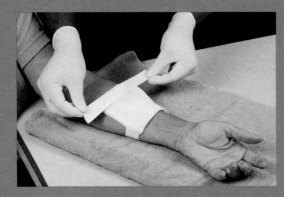

FIGURE 14-6C Applying tape correctly over the dressing.

7. Position the client comfortably.
8. Discard wastes. Remove gloves and wash hands.
9. Return supplies to designated storage area.
10. Document dressing was changed; also any abnormal observations of the wound and skin condition, such as signs of redness, swelling, heat, foul odor, or amount of drainage.

Topical Applications to Unbroken Skin

1. Obtain correct topical medication. Check label of medication with care plan.
2. Wash hands and apply gloves.
3. Position the client so area is accessible, while maintaining client comfort.
4. Apply medication in a thin layer to affected area only. Note color and appearance of skin. Is the affected area large or small? Is there drainage? Is the skin red?
5. Remove gloves and reposition the client.
6. Wash hands.
7. Return medication to correct storage area.
8. Document application of ointment and appearance of skin.

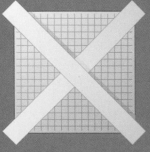
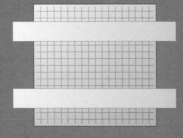
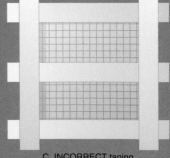

A. Correct taping   B. Correct taping   C. INCORRECT taping

FIGURE 14-7 Correct taping allows for air circulation.

Hygiene

Good hygiene is an important part of the care a home health aide provides to a client. Practicing good hygiene is important to maintain skin integrity and prevent infection, as well as to refresh and clean the client. The home health aide may be responsible for providing bathing, oral care, and personal care to the client. It is important for the aide to be sensitive to cultural reactions of clients with regard to providing this type of care. A client's cultural ideas about health, illness, hygiene, and rules for behavior may be different from your own. It will be helpful for you to understand your client's customs, practices, and beliefs so you can provide the best care and be respectful of individual differences. If you are unsure of your client's cultural patterns with regard to personal hygiene, it is a good idea to talk with your case manager. In the home care setting it is also important to be adaptable. For example, you may have to use a plastic bowl if there is not a basin to bathe the client or a tablecloth if a clean sheet is needed and there are none.

Bathing a Client

A tub bath or shower will clean and refresh the client, as well as stimulate the circulation in the skin. While bathing a client, the aide should check the client's skin for any signs of irritation or any change in the client's condition.

Giving a Bed Bath

If the client is bedridden, the bath will need to be given in bed. A partial bath is given on days a complete bed bath is not given. The bed bath is usually given in the morning or when the home health aide arrives at the home. This procedure is one of a series of procedures performed in the same time period of time, such as oral care. This will require the home health aide to organize and plan ahead. All materials and supplies needed can be gathered and placed conveniently so that each separate procedure can be completed easily. A partial bath is given in the same manner as a bed bath, except that the legs and feet are not washed. If the client is able, this type of bath can be given by the bathroom sink.

If you work in an assistive living facility, the bathing facilities are very user-friendly. The tub will have a door to walk the client into the tub (Figure 14-8). This type of tub is very accessible for the client to get in and out of, and also makes it easier for the aide to assist the client with the bath. The shower will have an upscale bathing

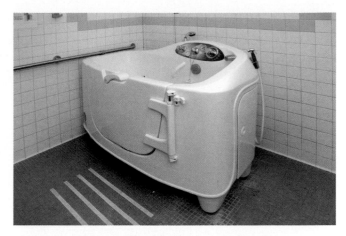

FIGURE 14-8   Tub in an assistive living facility.

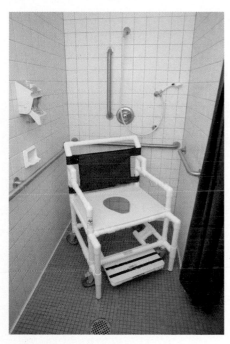

FIGURE 14-9   Shower and shower chair in an assistive living facility.

chair so that the aide can wheel the client in and out of the shower with little difficulty (Figure 14-9). Both the shower chair and tub will need to be cleaned and disinfected after each client use (Figure 14-10A and B). If possible, plan the tub bath or shower for a time convenient for the client. A tub bath or shower should not take more than 15 minutes unless there is a special reason for a longer bath. If client needs to use the bedpan, offer it before the bath. Gather supplies needed for making the bed and put them near at hand. Organize materials needed for oral hygiene, denture care, and nail care to move easily from one procedure to another as needed. See Procedure 35, Assisting with a Tub Bath or Shower, and Procedure 36, Giving a Bed Bath.

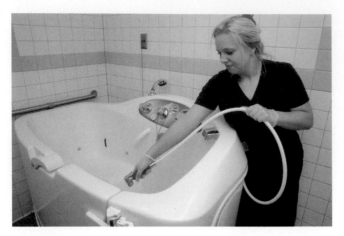

FIGURE 14-10A Cleaning a tub after use.

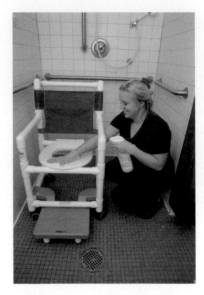

FIGURE 14-10B Cleaning a shower chair.

PROCEDURE 35 ASSISTING WITH TUB BATH OR SHOWER

Purpose

- To clean and refresh the client
- To check client's skin for signs of skin breakdown
- To stimulate circulation in the skin

Procedure

1. Assemble needed supplies and place in bathroom (Figure 14-11):
   clean clothing
   bath seat or stool
   2 washcloths and towels
   shampoo (if needed)
   plastic pitcher (if shampooing client's hair)
   hose attachment (optional)
   comb and brush
   skid-proof bath mat
   liquid soap
2. Wash hands.
3. Tell the client what you plan to do.
4. Fill the tub one-third full with warm water. **NOTE:** Test the temperature on the inside of your wrist to be sure it will not burn the client. The water should be about 115°F (46°C). Place a skid-proof bath mat in the bottom

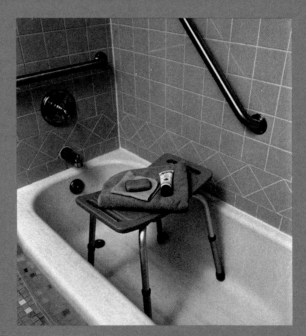

FIGURE 14-11 Gather the equipment needed for a bath.

of the tub. If the client is taking a shower, regulate the flow and be sure the temperature is correct.

(continued)

PROCEDURE 35   ASSISTING WITH TUB BATH OR SHOWER (*continued*)

5. Assist the client to sit on a chair or on the closed toilet seat. Help the client undress. Place soiled clothing in the hamper. Close the bathroom door so the client will not be chilled and to provide for privacy.

6. For a tub bath, help the client to sit on the edge of the tub. If there is a safety bar, have the client hold onto it. When the client has gained balance, help the client to turn and lift both legs into the tub. Give assistance by supporting the client under the arms and helping the client to slowly sit in the tub facing the faucets. If the client cannot sit in the tub, place a bath stool in the water. Help the client to sit on the stool (Figures 14-12 and 14-13). If the bath has a shower head above, the aide needs to turn on the water and adjust the temperature and proceed with bathing the client.

7. If the client needs a shampoo, wet the hair, rub in shampoo, lather, and massage the

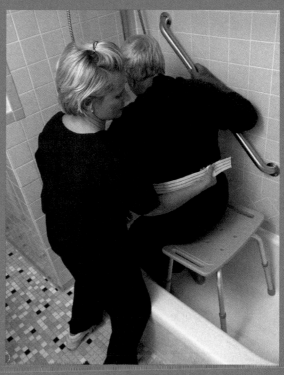

FIGURE 14-13   Have the client sit on tub or shower chair.

head. If possible, have the client tilt the head back. Pour water over the head using a pitcher. Repeat shampoo, massage, and rinse. The client may hold a washcloth over the eyes during the shampoo to prevent soap from entering the eyes.

8. Give the client a washcloth and soap. Allow the client to do as much bathing or washing as possible. Assist as necessary (Figure 14-14). A long-handled sponge can be used by the client to wash his or her back (Figure 14-15). If the shower is running, make sure the flow is not too heavy; check the water temperature often.

9. Remain beside the tub at all times during the bath or shower. **NOTE:** Be ready to help the client at any moment. If the client should feel faint, empty water from the tub, cover the client with a towel to avoid unnecessary chilling, and lower the client's head between the client's knees.

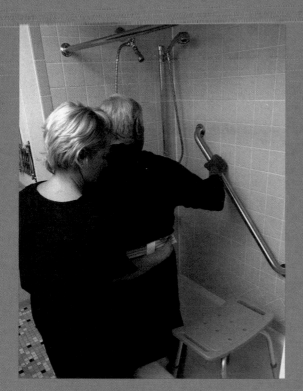

FIGURE 14-12   Instruct the client to hold onto the grab bars.

(*continued*)

PROCEDURE 35 ASSISTING WITH TUB BATH OR SHOWER (*continued*)

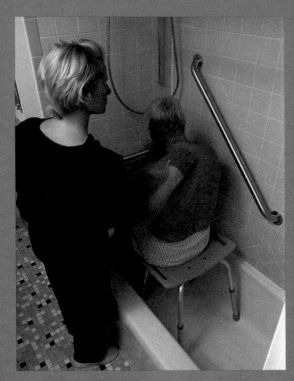

FIGURE 14-14 Assist the client in washing his back.

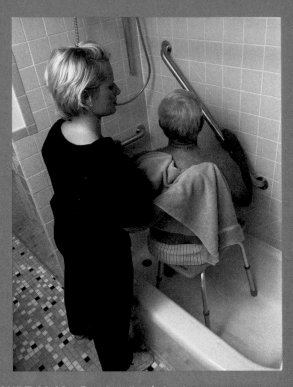

FIGURE 14-16 Dry the client's back.

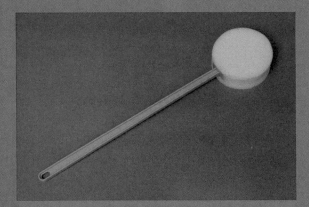

FIGURE 14-15 Long-handled sponge used by the client to wash his back.

10. For a tub bath, help the client raise out of the water. Assist the client out of the water. Assist the client to sit on the edge of the tub. Bring the client's legs over to the outside and assist the client to stand. Allow the client to sit on the closed toilet seat or the chair.

11. Make certain that the client's body is thoroughly dry. Do not dry the client by rubbing with the towel; instead pat the area to be dried. Help dry difficult areas such as the back and shoulders (Figure 14-16). Be sure underarms are completely dry. Protect the skin from unwanted moisture with a moisture barrier lotion. Pay special attention to the feet. Dry the soles of the feet and between the toes. Apply lotion to the client's skin as required (Figures 14-17A and B).

12. For a shower, make sure the client is completely washed and rinsed and then turn off the shower. Towel dry and assist the client out of the shower area.

13. Assist the client to dress in clean clothes.

14. Help the client back to bed, to a wheelchair, or to a chair.

15. Return to the bathroom; apply gloves; and drain, clean, and disinfect the tub or shower stall (Figure 14-18). Place dirty clothes and towels in the hamper. Put supplies away.

(continued)

PROCEDURE 35   ASSISTING WITH TUB BATH OR SHOWER (*continued*)

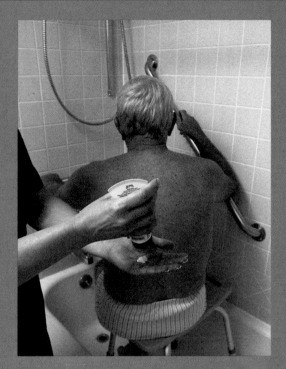

FIGURE 14-17A   Place lotion in your hands to warm.

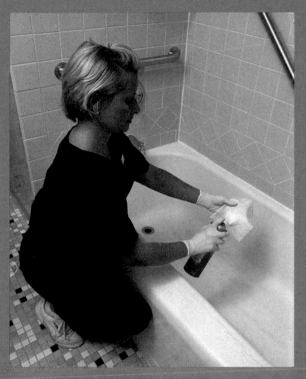

FIGURE 14-18   Be sure to clean the tub with disinfectant after the bath.

16. Remove gloves and wash hands.
17. Document procedure, any observations, and the client's reaction.

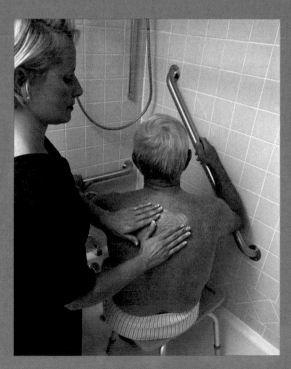

FIGURE 14-17B   Apply lotion to the client's back.

PROCEDURE 36 GIVING A BED BATH

Purpose

- To clean and refresh the client
- To stimulate circulation
- To observe the client's skin for signs of skin breakdown

Procedure

1. Gather supplies for the bed bath, dressing the client, and making the bed:
   body wash and disposable gloves (optional)
   washcloths and towels
   fresh clothes
   body lotion and deodorant
   change of bed linens
   bath basin, two-thirds filled with water
2. Close windows to prevent a draft from blowing on the client. If there are other people in the home, ask not to be disturbed. Provide for privacy.
3. Wash your hands.
4. Tell the client what you plan to do.
5. Remove blankets, leaving the top sheet covering the client. Place one pillow under the client's head.
6. Pull out the bottom part of the top sheet so it covers the client loosely. Remove the client's clothing.
7. Place a basin of water on the chair or dresser at the bedside.
8. Assist the client in moving to the side of bed nearest you. Apply gloves.
9. Moisten washcloth and squeeze out excess water. Form a mitt by folding a washcloth around one hand (Figure 14-19).
10. Using clear water only, wash the client's eyes first. Wipe from the inner corner to the outer corner of the eye, using a different part of the washcloth for each eye (Figure 14-20). Using a mild soap, wash the face, ears, and neck. Pat dry with the face towel.
11. Lift the client's farthest arm and lay a bath towel under the area to keep the bed dry. Wash with soap, rinse, and pat dry, making sure the arm and axilla are clean. Place the client's hand in the basin (Figure 14-21). Dry the client's hand. Repeat for other hand and arm. Apply underarm deodorant or bath powder if client desires.

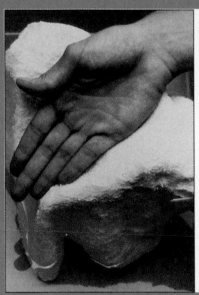
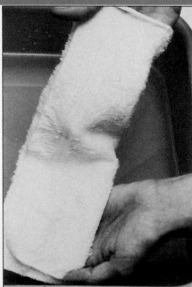
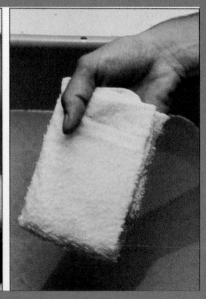

FIGURE 14-19 To make a bath mitt, wrap the washcloth around one hand, bringing the free-hanging end up over the palm and tucking in the end.

(continued)

PROCEDURE 36   GIVING A BED BATH (*continued*)

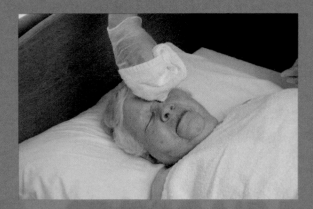

FIGURE 14-20   Cleaning the client's eye.

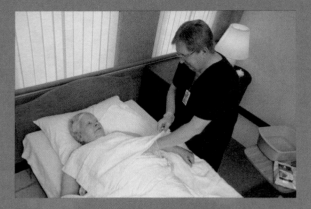

FIGURE 14-22   Washing the client's chest.

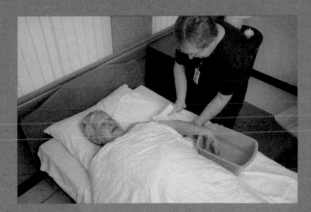

FIGURE 14-21   Place the client's hand into a basin to soak.

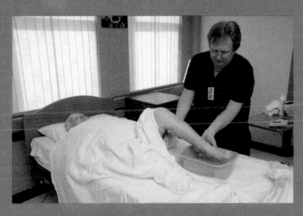

FIGURE 14-23   Place the client's foot into the basin to wash.

12. Give nail care and clean under nails. Trim nails *if allowed*. Refer to Procedure 44 for a description of the proper method to give nail care.

13. Place a towel over the client's chest, then pull the sheet down to the waist. Working under the towel, wash with body wash, rinse, and dry chest (Figure 14-22). Rinse and dry the area under a woman's breasts carefully to prevent skin irritation and redness. The abdomen is washed after the chest is washed. Replace sheet over chest.

14. Have the client bend one knee. Fold the sheet up from the foot of the bed. Expose the thigh, leg, and foot. Place a towel under the area, and put the basin on the towel, placing the client's foot in the basin (Figure 14-23). Wash and rinse the client's foot. Remove the foot from the basin and dry it well.

15. Remove the basin from the bed. Follow the same procedure for the other leg and foot.

16. Lightly apply lotion on the client's legs and feet if skin is dry (never massage the client's legs).

17. Change the water in the basin before proceeding with the bath. If at any time during the bath the water becomes dirty or cool, change it.

18. Place a bath towel lengthwise by the client's back and buttocks. Starting at the hairline, use long, firm strokes while washing the back. Carefully wash the buttocks area (Figure 14-24). Apply lotion to the client's back.

(*continued*)

PROCEDURE 36 GIVING A BED BATH (*continued*)

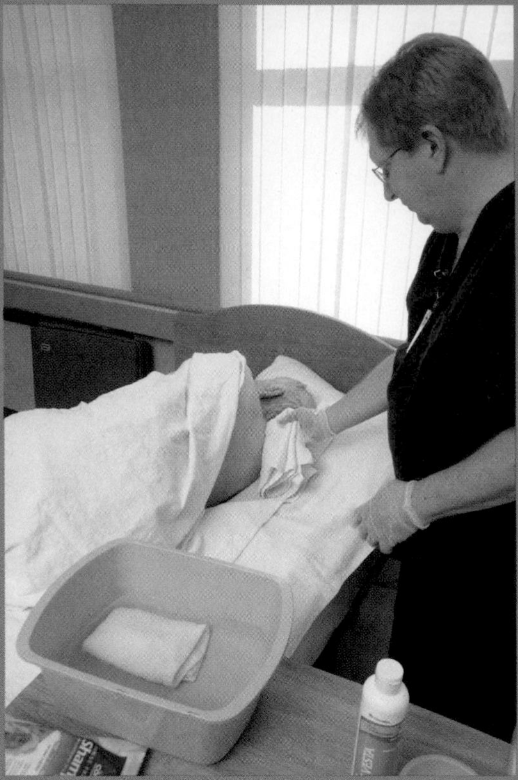

FIGURE 14-24 Washing the client's back and buttocks.

19. Change the water at this point. Remember to wipe a female client from front to back. This method is highly recommended to reduce the spread of germs and prevent infection. Prepare the washcloth with body wash and have the client wash the genital area, if able. Rinse the cloth and have the client wipe and dry the genitals, if capable. Remove gloves and wash hands.
20. Spread a clean towel under the client's head and comb or brush the client's hair.
21. Assist the client into clean clothes.
22. Remove the basin, dirty linens, and other equipment.
23. Change the bed linens using the procedure for making an occupied bed.
24. Leave the client in a comfortable position.
25. Wash your hands.
26. Document procedure and time, observations, and the client's reaction.

A simpler type of bath introduced recently with much success is the bag bath. This type of bath is given often in hospitals and long-term care facilities. A commercial bag bath is available and very easy to use: Just put the package in the microwave for a few minutes and remove. The package usually contains five or six presoaked disposable washcloths. The aide bathes the client using one cloth for the face, one for the arms and upper chest, one for the legs, another for the back, and the last one for the perineal area. The solution on the washcloth not only cleans the skin, but also gives the skin a protective coating so that it is less likely to break down. There is no need to dry the client because the solution is self-drying. If need be, the aide can prepare his or her own bag bath. The special solution needs to be supplied to the client, and the aide will need to prepare it according to directions. After the solution is prepared, place five washcloths in a plastic bag and pour the solution over the washcloths. Place in a microwave oven to warm, then remove and start the bath. This type of bathing has many advantages: it is less drying to the skin, the washcloths are always warm, it needs very little equipment, and it is quite a time saver for the aide.

Back Rub

A back rub is helpful to increase the blood circulation to the back area, and to provide comfort and relaxation to the client. It is also a good opportunity for the aide to observe the skin for signs of skin breakdown. A good back rub or massage is very relaxing for a client with dementia. See Procedure 37, Giving a Back Rub.

PROCEDURE 37 GIVING A BACK RUB

Purpose

- To increase the blood circulation to the back area
- To give comfort to the client and provide relaxation
- To observe the skin for signs of skin breakdown

Procedure

1. Wash your hands.
2. Assemble supplies:
   small towel
   lotion
3. Tell the client what you plan on doing and provide privacy for the client.
4. Position the client on the back or side.
5. Place a small amount of lotion on your hands (Figures 14-25A and B). Rub your hands together to warm the lotion.

6. Begin by starting at the base of the spine; rub toward the neck in the center of the back. Use both hands in one long stroke (Figure 14-26).
7. When reaching the neck, continue down the sides of the back. When reaching the base of the spine, rub up the center again. Repeat several times (Figure 14-27).
8. If necessary, add more lotion and use a spiral motion for several minutes.
9. Remove excess lotion with small towel. Reposition the client.
10. Wash hands and return supplies to proper place.
11. Document backrub and any sign of skin irritation.

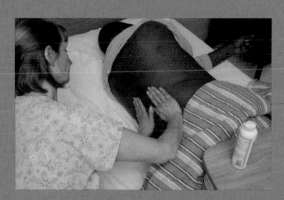

FIGURE 14-26 Use long, smooth strokes as you apply lotion.

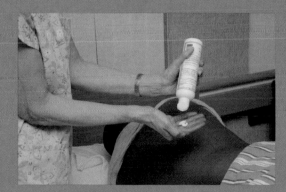

FIGURE 14-25A Place a small amount of lotion on the hands.

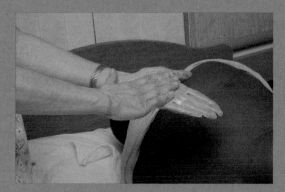

FIGURE 14-25B Rub the hands together to warm the lotion.

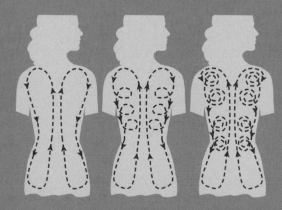

FIGURE 14-27 Give the client a gentle back rub using the strokes as shown.

Perineal Care

Part of good skin care includes keeping the perineum clean, which is the area from the genitals to the anus. Keeping the perineum clean is important to prevent infections and skin breakdown, and to reduce odor, especially if the client has a catheter. Perineal care must be done daily. See Procedure 38, Giving Female Perineal Care, and Procedure 39, Giving Male Perineal Care.

PROCEDURE 38 GIVING FEMALE PERINEAL CARE

Purpose

- To prevent infections and skin breakdown
- To clean the genital and anal area
- To prevent odors

Procedure

1. Assemble supplies:
   disposable gloves
   soap or perineal wash
   basin
   water
   washcloths and towel
2. Wash your hands and apply gloves.
3. Tell client what you plan to do, and provide for privacy.
4. Position the client on her back and place sheet or thin cotton blanket over the client.
5. Position the towel under the client's buttocks.
6. Wet a washcloth with soap and water or perineal wash. Help the client flex her knees and spread her legs if able.
7. Separate the vulva. Clean downward from front to back with one stroke, using a different part the washcloth with each stroke, starting with the inner labia, and then rinse (Figure 14-28). Repeat with the outer labia. Repeat on the other side. Dry with a towel.
8. Help the client lower her legs and turn onto her side away from you.
9. Apply soap or perineal wash to the washcloth.
10. Clean the rectal area by cleaning from the vagina to the anus with one stroke (Figure 14-29). Rinse the washcloth and repeat until the area is clean.
11. Pat the area dry with a towel.
12. Observe the area for any unusual redness, open areas, or abnormal discharge.
13. Cover the client and remove equipment.

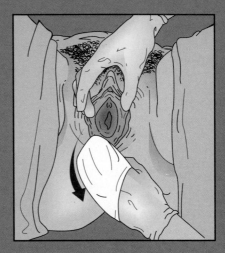

FIGURE 14-28 Separate the vulva. Clean downward from front to back with one stroke.

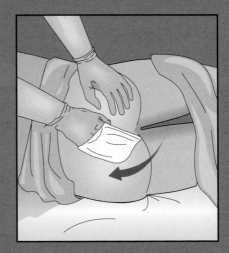

FIGURE 14-29 Clean the rectal area by cleaning from the vagina to the anus with one stroke.

14. Clean equipment and remove gloves.
15. Wash hands.
16. Document procedure completion and any abnormal observations.

PROCEDURE 39 GIVING MALE PERINEAL CARE

Purpose

- To prevent spread of infection
- To promote comfort
- To prevent odors
- To clean the genital and anal area

Procedure

1. Repeat steps 1 through 6 as for female perineal care.
2. Grasp the penis gently with a gloved hand. Clean the tip of the penis using a gentle circular motion (Figure 14-30). You will need to pull back the foreskin if the man is uncircumcised (Figure 14-31). Start at the urinary meatus and work outward. Rinse the area well and then dry. Return the foreskin to its original position.
3. Clean the remaining portion of the penis with firm downward strokes. Rinse well.
4. Wash the scrotum and pat dry.
5. Turn the client to the side and clean the rectal area in the same way as for the female.
6. Follow steps 11 through 16 as for female perineal care.

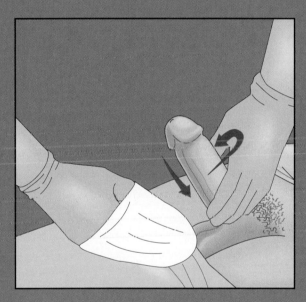

FIGURE 14-30 Grasp the penis gently with a gloved hand. Clean the tip of the penis using gentle circular motion.

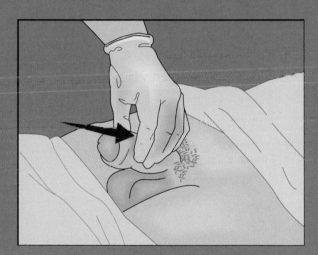

FIGURE 14-31 Pull back the foreskin if the man is uncircumcised.

Oral Care

Some clients will be unable to give themselves oral care. In these instances, the aide must assist the client with oral hygiene, including brushing teeth and caring for dentures. Good oral hygiene is important to keep the client's teeth and gums healthy, to observe the gums for irritation, to refresh the client's mouth, and stimulate the client's appetite. If a client has Down syndrome or is on seizure medication such as Dilantin, special attention to oral care is essential. The medication taken by the client makes the client's gums very tender.

Denture Care

Dentures are very expensive and should be cared for very meticulously. If the client only wants to wears the upper dentures and not the lower dentures, store the lower dentures in a designated area in a container that is clearly marked with the client's name. Occasionally, you will find clients whose dentures do not fit, and they most likely need to be realigned by a dentist because they are very loose. Even though they are loose, please encourage the client to wear the dentures, as this will prevent the client's gums from receding more. The more the clients wear their dentures, the better the dentures will fit. See Procedure 40, Assisting with Routine Oral Hygiene, and Procedure 41, Caring for Dentures.

PROCEDURE 40   ASSISTING WITH ROUTINE ORAL HYGIENE

Purpose

- To keep client's teeth, tongue, and gums healthy
- To refresh client's mouth and improve appetite

Procedure—Using Toothettes and Lemon Glycerine Swabs

1. Assemble equipment:
   disposable gloves
   toothettes or lemon glycerine swabs (Figure 14-32)
   paper towels or small towel
   small container of water
   lip cream
2. Wash your hands and apply gloves. Tell the client what you plan to do and provide for privacy.
3. Place small towels or paper towels under the client's head and turn the head to one side (Figure 14-33).
4. Dip toothettes into water or mouthwash (optional). Lemon glycerine swabs can be placed directly from the package into the client's mouth.

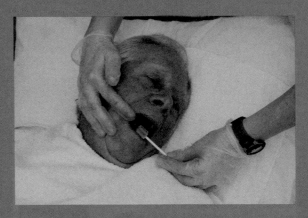

FIGURE 14-33   Cleaning the client's mouth with toothettes.

5. Insert swab into the client's mouth and swab the gums, teeth, and tongue. If need be, repeat with clean swab.
6. Apply pleasant-tasting lip lubricant to lips.
7. Place used swabs in paper towels.
8. Remove your gloves and add to paper towels for disposal.
9. Wash your hands.
10. Document procedure.

Procedure—Routine Oral Care

1. Assemble needed equipment and supplies
   disposable gloves
   toothbrush—manual or electronic
   toothpaste
   cup of water
   towel
   small bowl or basin or emesis basin
   mouthwash (optional)
   tissues or moistened washcloth
2. Wash your hands and apply gloves.
3. Tell the client what you plan to do and position the client in a sitting position (if allowed). Provide for privacy.

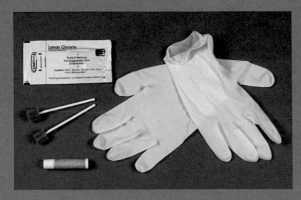

FIGURE 14-32   Toothettes, lemon glycerine swabs, and lip cream.

(continued)

PROCEDURE 40 ASSISTING WITH ROUTINE ORAL HYGIENE (*continued*)

4. Place a towel over the client's chest and under the chin.
5. Moisten the toothbrush and apply toothpaste (Figure 14-34).
6. Let the client brush his or her teeth, if able. If not, carefully brush the client's teeth (Figures 14-35A, B, C, D, and E).

7. The client or the aide should brush the teeth by holding the brush at a right angle to the teeth, starting at the gumline and working upward.
8. Give the client a cup of water; be sure the client rinses the mouth well (Figure 14-36). Hold the basin underneath the client's

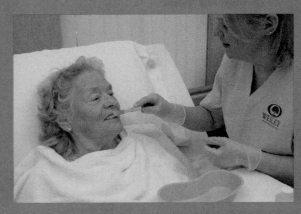
FIGURE 14-34 Brushing the teeth.

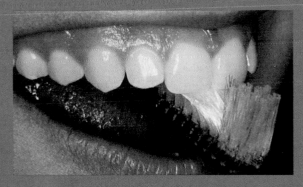
FIGURE 14-35C Brush the top and bottom teeth thoroughly, including the gums.

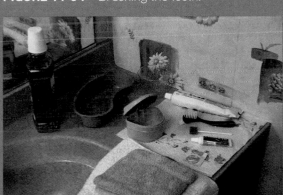
FIGURE 14-35A Supplies for oral hygiene.

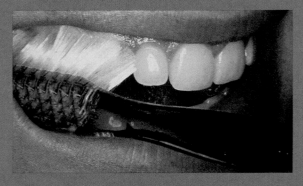
FIGURE 14-35D Be sure to brush behind the front teeth.

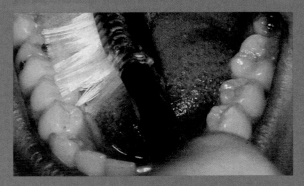
FIGURE 14-35B Hold a soft, wet toothbrush at a 90° angle and brush the back teeth.

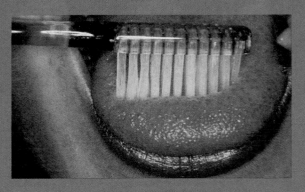
FIGURE 14-35E Brush the tongue.

(*continued*)

PROCEDURE 40 ASSISTING WITH ROUTINE ORAL HYGIENE (*continued*)

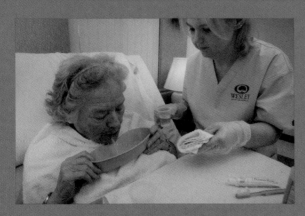

FIGURE 14-36 Client expectorating into emesis basin.

chin and have the client return the fluid. If mouthwash is available, have the client rinse the mouth with the mouthwash. Xylitol® mouthwash or spray may be used by the client to assist in destroying bacteria in the mouth.

9. Offer the client a moistened washcloth to wipe the mouth.
10. Reposition the client.
11. Clean and replace equipment.
12. Remove gloves and wash hands.
13. Document procedure completed and time, any observations, and the client's reaction.

PROCEDURE 41 CARING FOR DENTURES

Purpose

- To clean dentures and refresh the client's mouth
- To provide opportunity to observe the client's gums for irritation or soreness
- To stimulate the client's appetite

Procedure

1. Assemble the needed supplies (Figure 14-37):
   denture brush or toothbrush
   denture cleaner or toothpaste
   denture cleaning tablet (e.g., Efferdent)
   denture cup
   disposable gloves
   mouthwash and small cup
   emesis basin
   washcloth and small towel
2. Wash your hands and apply gloves.
3. Tell the client what you plan to do.
4. Ask the client to remove the dentures (Figure 14-38), helping if needed. Place the

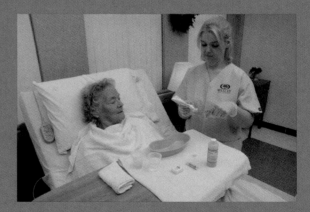

FIGURE 14-37 Supplies for oral care.

dentures in a padded container or denture cup (Figure 14-39A). Be very careful in handling the client's dentures; they may become slippery.

5. Take the dentures to the sink. Place approximately 2 to 3 inches of water and a washcloth in the bottom of the sink (Figure 14-39B). This will protect the

(*continued*)

PROCEDURE 41 CARING FOR DENTURES (*continued*)

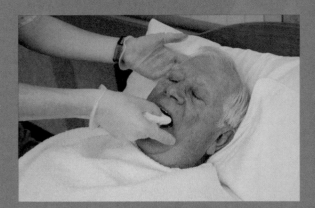

FIGURE 14-38 Removing dentures from the client's mouth.

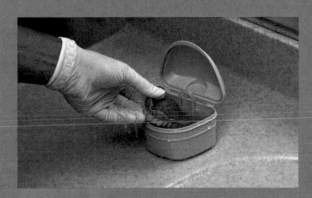

FIGURE 14-39A Place the dentures into a container.

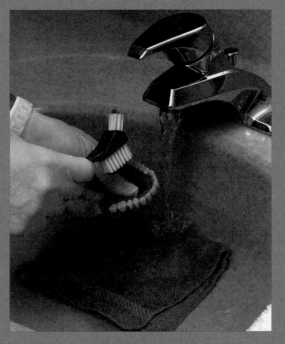

FIGURE 14-39B When cleaning dentures, use cool running water and protect the dentures by placing a washcloth in the bottom of the sink.

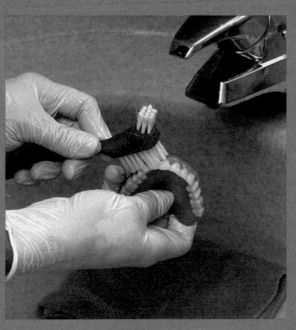

FIGURE 14-39C Be sure to brush all surfaces of the dentures.

dentures in case they are dropped. Turn on the cold water and brush all surfaces of the upper and lower plate (Figure 14-39C). Rinse the denture cup and fill with cold water. If the client is not going to wear the dentures, place denture cleaning tablets in the container. If the client is going to wear the dentures, take the clean dentures in the cup to the client.

6. Assist the client to rinse the mouth with mouthwash. Have the client expel the rinse into the emesis basin.

7. Toothettes can be used to clean the gums and tongue. Observe the client's mouth for signs of irritation or sores.

(*continued*)

PROCEDURE 41 CARING FOR DENTURES (*continued*)

8. Have the client insert the dentures in the mouth, if able. If need be, apply a small amount of dental adhesive to the inside of the dentures (Figure 14-39D).
9. Remove equipment, clean, and return to storage area.
10. Remove gloves and wash your hands.
11. Document procedure completed and any abnormal observations.

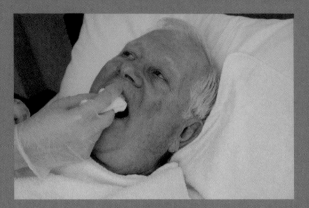

FIGURE 14-39D Replace the dentures in the client's mouth.

Personal Care and Grooming

The home health aide will be responsible for providing personal care to clients to keep clients well groomed so that they look their best and feel good about themselves. Personal care will include bathing, foot soaks, shaving, nail care, and shampooing.

PROCEDURE 42 SHAVING THE MALE CLIENT

Shaving can be planned for the same time that other daily hygiene tasks are done. If the client is taking a blood-thinning medication like warfarin, *always* use an electric razor. An ordinary razor may cause excessive bleeding from a cut in the facial area. For shaving, the electric razor is usually the easiest to use. However, it may be necessary to use a safety razor or disposable razor. If the client is on oxygen, a disposable razor is recommended. If the razor is dull, replace the blade. In some instances, older women also may request to have facial hair shaved to improve cosmetic appearance. Remember standard precautions; wear gloves.

NOTE: You may not shave off a client's mustache or beard without written permission.

Purpose

• To remove unwanted facial hair

Procedure

1. Wash hands and apply gloves.
2. Ask the client if he wants a shave and provide privacy.
3. Assemble needed supplies:
   disposable gloves
   razor and shaving cream
   basin of warm water
   washcloth and towel
   aftershave lotion (optional)

(*continued*)

PROCEDURE 42 SHAVING THE MALE CLIENT (*continued*)

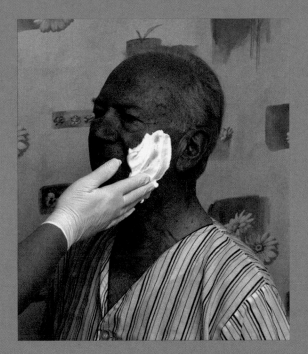

FIGURE 14-40A Apply shaving cream to the face.

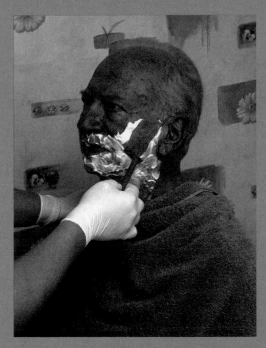

FIGURE 14-40B Shave in the direction of hair growth.

4. Position the client in a sitting position and place a towel under the chin and across his chest.

5. Apply shaving cream (Figure 14-40A). With one hand, pull the skin tight above the area to be shaved. With the razor in your other hand, gently take short, even strokes. Shave in the direction the hair grows (Figures 14-40B–D). If the client is able, let him do as much as possible. If feasible, have the client shave with a mirror in front of him.

6. Rinse the razor frequently. After the shave is completed, rinse the face and pat dry.

7. Apply aftershave lotion (optional).

8. If using an electric razor, apply preelectric lotion before using the razor, as it will make the skin easier to shave. Hold the skin taut as you work the razor around the face. Clean the inside of razor each time you use it. If the cutting blades get dull, ask to have the blades replaced. It is almost impossible to shave an older man's wrinkled face with a dull electric razor.

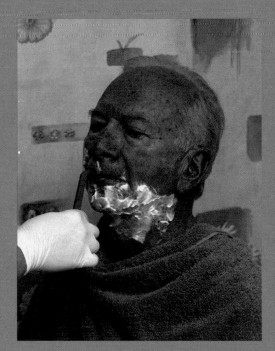

FIGURE 14-40C Be sure to shave the area under the nose and the top of the chin.

(*continued*)

PROCEDURE 42 SHAVING THE MALE CLIENT (*continued*)

9. Clean equipment and return to designated area.
10. Remove gloves and wash hands.
11. Document procedure completed and any abnormal observations.

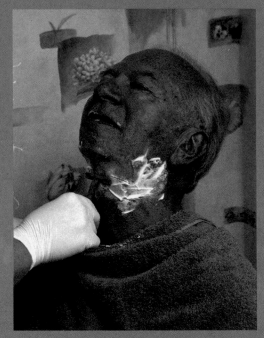

FIGURE 14-40D Shave the area under the client's chin.

PROCEDURE 43 GIVING A WARM FOOT SOAK

Purpose

- To stimulate circulation in a client's feet
- To relieve pain or discomfort
- To soften the toenails to make them easier to cut

Procedure

1. Assemble equipment:
   disposable gloves
   large basin—plastic oblong dishpan
   warm water—100° to 110°F
   large plastic garbage bag or small rug
   small thin blanket
   2 towels

2. Wash hands and apply gloves.
3. Tell the client what you plan to do. Provide for privacy.
4. Have the client sit in a comfortable chair if possible.
5. Place small rug on floor and place basin of water on top of rug.
6. Remove the client's shoes and socks and slowly place client's feet in a basin of warm water (Figure 14-41). Be sure to follow any special instructions for specific soaps or solutions that might be ordered.
7. Place thin blanket over the client's legs and feet.

(continued)

PROCEDURE 43   GIVING A WARM FOOT SOAK *(continued)*

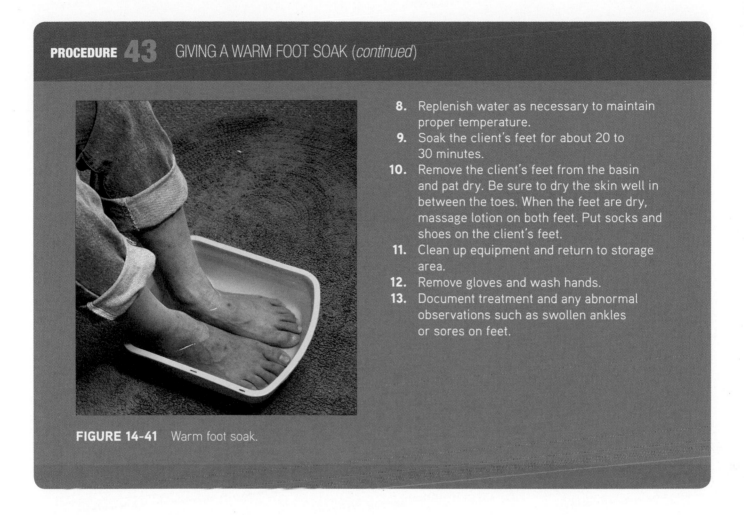

8. Replenish water as necessary to maintain proper temperature.
9. Soak the client's feet for about 20 to 30 minutes.
10. Remove the client's feet from the basin and pat dry. Be sure to dry the skin well in between the toes. When the feet are dry, massage lotion on both feet. Put socks and shoes on the client's feet.
11. Clean up equipment and return to storage area.
12. Remove gloves and wash hands.
13. Document treatment and any abnormal observations such as swollen ankles or sores on feet.

FIGURE 14-41   Warm foot soak.

Nail Care.   The home care aide is not allowed to cut the fingernails or toenails of clients who are diabetic or clients with poor circulation to their legs. Be aware if the client is on a blood thinner medication, as cuts can produce excessive bleeding. Check with your case manager about your agency policy concerning cutting nails. Some agencies will allow a home health aide to cut nails, whereas others will not allow home health aides to cut nails. Nail care is usually given at bath time or when there is a need because of a broken nail or hangnail. A manicure may be done to make the client feel more attractive. In the elderly, you might note very thick toenails, which require special clippers to cut; this usually is done by a **podiatrist** (health care provider who specializes in foot problems). See Procedure 44, Giving Nail Care.

PROCEDURE 44   GIVING NAIL CARE

Purpose

- To keep the client's nails clean and well groomed
- To observe for signs of irritation

Procedure

1. Assemble supplies:
   soap, water, and basin
   nail brush

(continued)

PROCEDURE 44   GIVING NAIL CARE *(continued)*

towel and lotion, preferably lanolin lotion
small scissors or clippers
emery board or nail file

2. Wash your hands.
3. Tell the client what you plan to do and provide for privacy.
4. Soak the toenails or fingernails in soap and water for 10 minutes.
5. Brush the nails with a nail brush. Clean under the nails. Rinse well. Dry the hands and nails.
6. Wear gloves if clipping nails/toenails.
7. If the nails are too long, make a straight cut for toenails and a curved cut for fingernails (Figure 14-42). Check to make sure that you are allowed to cut the client's nails. If you accidentally cut a client's skin while cutting the nails, remember to use standard precautions. Report the cut to the case manager.

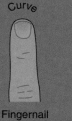 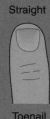

Curve   Straight

Fingernail   Toenail

FIGURE 14-42   Cut fingernails with a curve and toenails straight across.

8. Use a file or emery board to smooth the edges of the nails.
9. Massage lotion on the hands or feet.
10. Clean the basin, brush, and scissors or clippers. Return equipment to proper place.
11. Wash your hands.
12. Document procedure, any observations, and the client's reaction.

PROCEDURE 45   SHAMPOOING HAIR IN BED

Purpose

- To clean the hair and scalp
- To stimulate circulation in the scalp
- To make the client feel and look better
- To prevent accumulation of dandruff or formation of scalp crusts

NOTE: Dry shampoos can also be used if the client is too weak to tolerate a wet shampoo. Follow the directions on the package for the dry shampoo. If you need to shampoo a client's hair and the client is mobile, it is better to do it in the kitchen sink than the bathroom sink. It is easier to bend an older client's head forward rather than backward for the shampoo.

Procedure

1. Assemble equipment:
   shampoo and hair conditioner or rinse
   3 to 4 towels
   inflatable shampoo basin (Figure 14-43)
   2 large empty garbage bags
   large pitcher or empty gallon milk container
   comb and brush
   large empty bucket
   disposable gloves
   hair dryer
2. Wash your hands and apply gloves.
3. Tell the client what you plan to do.
4. Prepare the bed by placing a plastic garbage bag under the head with a large towel on top of it.

(continued)

PROCEDURE 45 SHAMPOOING HAIR IN BED (*continued*)

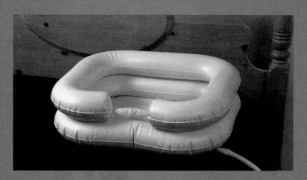

FIGURE 14-43 Inflatable shampoo basin.

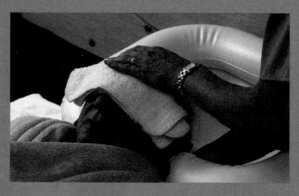

FIGURE 14-44B Place a washcloth or towel under the client's neck and cover the client's eyes with a washcloth.

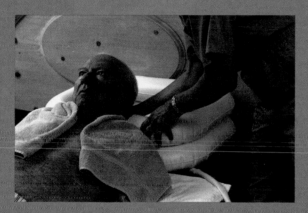

FIGURE 14-44A Placing tray under the client's head for a bed shampoo.

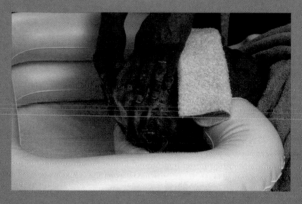

FIGURE 14-44C Wet the hair and apply shampoo, using the fingertips to massage the scalp.

5. Place the bucket on the floor with a plastic bag under the bucket.
6. Place the shampoo basin on top of a large towel on the bed and gently place the client's head in the basin (Figure 14-44A). Be sure to pad the client's neck area with a small towel.
7. Place the end of the tubing into the bucket.
8. Comb your fingers through the hair with a slight fingertip massage of the scalp. Wet the hair with warm water. The client can use a washcloth to cover the eyes for protection (Figure 14-44B).
9. Apply shampoo to the head, lather well, and massage the scalp with your fingertips (Figure 14-44C). If a specific shampoo is ordered, follow any special instructions.

10. Rinse hair with water thoroughly, making sure to remove all traces of shampoo (Figure 14-44D).
11. If necessary, reapply shampoo, lather well, and rinse thoroughly.
12. Apply hair conditioner or rinse. Follow directions on the bottle.
13. Remove the shampoo tray from the bed.
14. Gently and briskly massage the scalp and hair with a dry towel. Repeat with a dry towel as needed. If a hair dryer is available, blow-dry the hair. Gently comb or brush and style hair per the client's preference (Figure 14-44E).
15. Remove and clean equipment. Return equipment to proper place.

(*continued*)

PROCEDURE 45 SHAMPOOING HAIR IN BED (*continued*)

16. Remove gloves and wash hands.
17. Observe scalp for buildup of dandruff or any other substance, sores or any break in the skin, or redness.
18. Document procedure and any abnormal observations.

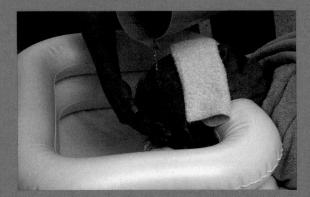

FIGURE 14-44D Rinse the hair, removing all shampoo, and apply hair conditioner.

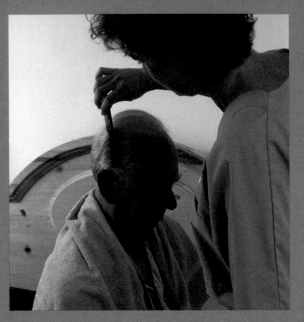

FIGURE 14-44E Comb the hair; place a towel on top of the shoulders to collect any hair.

WORKBOOK REVIEW

Go to the workbook and complete the review exercises and activities for Unit 14.

REVIEW

1. The integumentary system (skin) is composed of:

_____

_____

_____

2. List two functions of the skin.

   _____

   _____

3. Identify the four stages of pressure sore development. Match the stage in Column I with the correct description in Column II.

   Column I

   1. Stage 1
   2. Stage 2
   3. Stage 3
   4. Stage 4

   Column II

   _____ a. skin is gone and underlying tissue is exposed
   _____ b. skin is red in color
   _____ c. blister-like lesion over the area
   _____ d. blister breaks open

4. List five places in the body that pressure sores are most likely to appear.

   _____

   _____

   _____

   _____

   _____

5. You *need* or *don't need* to wear gloves when applying ointments.

6. Over-the-counter ointments *can* or *cannot* be applied by a home health aide.

7. Place in proper sequence the body parts washed in a bed bath.

   ____ a. farthest arm   ____ f. chest
   ____ b. feet   ____ g. abdomen
   ____ c. face   ____ h. perineal area
   ____ d. back   ____ i. nearest leg
   ____ e. nearest arm   ____ j. farthest leg

8. T F   When doing female perineal care, wipe from the urinary opening to the anus.

9. T F   Dermatitis is a skin inflammation that can cause itching and redness that is often caused by allergies.

10. You are assigned a new client, Mr. Jerry Thompson, and the care plan states you are to do all of the following tasks for him in a 3-hour period. In what order would you do the tasks?

    a. Tub bath
    b. Brush dentures
    c. Change linens on bed
    d. Shampoo hair
    e. Apply one ointment to heel and one to reddened area on right lower arm
    f. Change dressing on right lower arm
    g. Nail care
    h. Shave with an electric razor
    i. Soak both feet for 20 minutes

Case Studies

11. You are assigned to care for Mr. Tom Clark, who is terminally ill, and you have 2 hours to give him a bed bath, provide denture care, change the dressing on his right arm, and shampoo his hair using a shampoo basin in bed. How would you plan your time at his home? What supplies will you need?

12. While giving a bath to your client, you notice reddened areas on her coccyx and right ankle. What nursing action(s) would you take?

UNIT 15

Musculoskeletal System: Arthritis, Body Mechanics, and Restorative Care

KEY TERMS

abduction

active range-of-motion exercises

activities

adduction

ambulating

analgesics

anti-inflammatory

arthritis

arthroplasty

atrophy

base of support

body mechanics

bursitis

cartilage

closed fracture

contractures

cyanosis

dangling

dorsiflexion

extension

external rotation

flexion

Fowler's position

fracture

gait belt

gout

internal rotation

joint capsule

ligaments

musculoskeletal disorders (MSD)

open fracture

opposition

osteoarthritis

passive range-of-motion exercises

pivot

pivot disc

plantar flexion

pronation

prone position

prostheses

range-of-motion exercises

rehabilitation

rheumatoid arthritis

rotation

safe patient handling and mobility (SPHM) standards

sprain

stand lift

steroids

supination

synchronize

synovium

tendons

tophi

total hip replacement

total knee replacement

transfer belt

LEARNING OBJECTIVES

After studying this unit, you should be able to:

- Identify components of the musculoskeletal system

- List three functions of the musculoskeletal system

- List four disorders of the musculoskeletal system and their main signs and symptoms

- Differentiate between the following three types of arthritis: rheumatoid, osteoarthritis, and gout

- Describe the nursing care given to clients with arthritis

- Explain nursing care for a client with a recent hip or knee replacement

- Describe safe patient handling and movement standards terms

- Explain the purposes for proper body mechanics

- List 10 rules of good body mechanics

- Identify comfort and safety measures for lifting, turning, and moving clients

- Explain the use of the gait or transfer belt

- Describe the term *dangling* a client

- Describe components of various mechanical lifts

- Identify comfort, alignment, and safety measures for positioning clients in bed

- Describe four different body positions that clients can be placed in

- Describe nursing care for a client with a cast

- Explain the purpose of applying cold to a body part

- Describe how to dress and undress a client with one-sided weakness

- Explain two complications of immobility

- Distinguish between active and passive range-of-motion exercises

- Demonstrate the following:

PROCEDURE 46   Applying a Transfer or Gait Belt

PROCEDURE 47   Dangling a Client

PROCEDURE 48   Turning the Client Toward You

PROCEDURE 49   Moving the Client up in Bed Using a Lift Sheet

PROCEDURE 50   Log Rolling the Client

PROCEDURE 51   Positioning the Client in Supine Position

PROCEDURE 52   Positioning the Client in Lateral/Side-Lying Position

PROCEDURE 53   Positioning the Client in Prone Position

PROCEDURE 54   Positioning the Client in Fowler's Position

PROCEDURE 55   Assisting the Client from Bed to Wheelchair

PROCEDURE 56   Transfer with Pivot Disc

PROCEDURE 57   Assisting the Client from Wheelchair to Bed

PROCEDURE 58   Transferring the Client from Wheelchair to Toilet/Commode

PROCEDURE 59   Transferring the Client Using a Mechanical Lift

PROCEDURE 60   Transferring a Client Using a Stand Lift

PROCEDURE 61   Sliding Board Transfer

PROCEDURE 62   Caring for Casts

PROCEDURE 63   Applying a Cold Application to the Client's Skin

PROCEDURE 64   Dressing and Undressing the Client

PROCEDURE 65   Performing Active Range-of-Motion Exercises

PROCEDURE 66   Performing Passive Range-of-Motion Exercises

PROCEDURE 67   Assisting the Client to Walk with Crutches, Walker, or Cane

Musculoskeletal System

The musculoskeletal system is made up of bones and muscles. It protects the internal body organs and makes body movement possible. The skull, for instance, forms a protective covering for the brain. The spinal column surrounds the spinal nerves leading from the brain.

There are more than 200 bones in the body (Figure 15-1A and B). Bones are joined together by tough elastic fibers called **ligaments**.

Joints allow the bones to be moved in certain ways (Figure 15-2). The elbows and knees have hinge joints, which move in only two directions like hinges on a door. The joints at the shoulder and pelvis are ball-and-socket

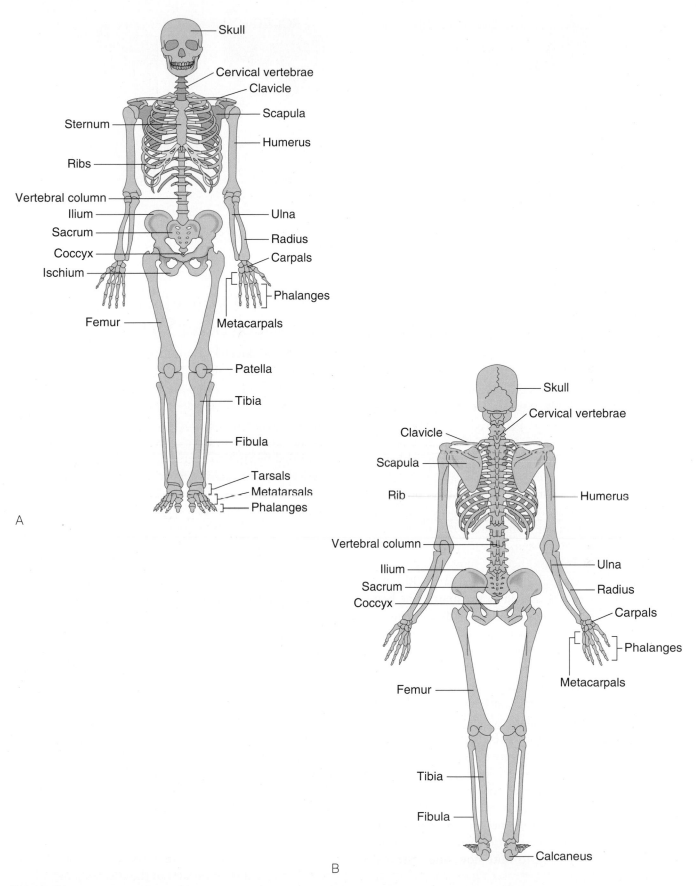

FIGURE 15-1   Bones of the skeleton. A. Anterior view. B. Posterior view.

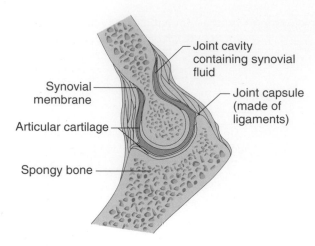
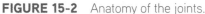
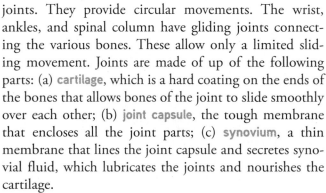
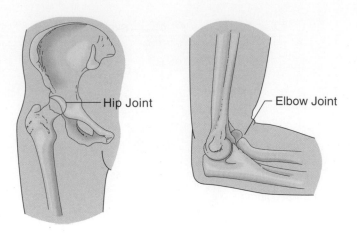

FIGURE 15-2 Anatomy of the joints.

joints. They provide circular movements. The wrist, ankles, and spinal column have gliding joints connecting the various bones. These allow only a limited sliding movement. Joints are made of up of the following parts: (a) cartilage, which is a hard coating on the ends of the bones that allows bones of the joint to slide smoothly over each other; (b) joint capsule, the tough membrane that encloses all the joint parts; (c) synovium, a thin membrane that lines the joint capsule and secretes synovial fluid, which lubricates the joints and nourishes the cartilage.

Skeletal muscles are attached to the bones by tendons and are stretched over joints. Certain muscles produce motion by pulling on the bone when they receive messages from the nervous system. These muscles are called voluntary muscles because their movement is controlled by the brain. For example, the eye sees a $5.00 bill on the floor. The picture is relayed to the brain. The brain, through the nervous system, tells the body to bend over and pick up the bill. This is an example of voluntary muscle action or one that the body chooses to perform.

Other muscles, called involuntary muscles, form the walls of organs. They, too, receive messages through the nervous system but they work automatically, or without any conscious effort by the individual. The heart is an example of an involuntary muscle because it pumps blood throughout the body without any conscious effort.

The musculoskeletal system constantly interacts with other systems. The interior of the bone produces new blood cells for the circulatory system. Muscles move in response to messages from the nervous system. It is not necessary to understand these complex interrelationships. However, it is interesting to note how one system depends on another.

Common Disorders of the Musculoskeletal System

The musculoskeletal system can be invaded by disease-causing microorganisms. However, the most common problems are injuries that are caused by falls or overuse.

Musculoskeletal disorders (MSDs) are injuries or disorders of the muscles, nerves, tendons, joints, or cartilage and disorders of the nerves, tendons, or muscles that are caused by sudden exertion or prolonged exposure to physical factors such as repetition, force, or vibration. This definition excludes conditions such as fractures, contusions, and cuts resulting from sudden physical contact of the body with external objects.

A sprain is a partial tear of a muscle, tendon, or ligament. Sprains usually involve damage to blood vessels and nerves. The site of the sprain may appear swollen and black and blue, with sharp intermittent pain that increases on movement. The cause of a sprain is usually due to trauma to a joint, such as falling down steps when wearing high heels or getting one's foot caught in a door. Treatment consists of immobilizing the joint with an elastic bandage, elevating the extremity, applying ice, and prescribing rest for the client. Depending on the severity of the sprain, it will generally take 3 to 6 weeks or longer to heal.

Bursitis is inflammation of a bursa, which is an enclosed sac containing fluid, which is found between muscles and tendons. The joints most affected with this disorder are the shoulder, elbow (sometimes referred to as tennis elbow), and the knee (sometimes referred to as housemaid's knee). The client may complain of tenderness, swelling, pain, and limitation of movement at the site. Treatment varies but generally consists of rest, painkillers, application of moist heat, and injection of steroids to the affected joint.

A fracture is a break in a bone. A closed fracture is a break in the bone but not in the skin. An open fracture is a break in the skin and the bone is fractured. With this type of break there is a high risk of infection due to the break in the skin where microorganisms can easily enter. Fractures are usually treated with surgery, cast application, and/or traction. Healing of the bones generally takes at least 6 weeks for a younger adult and a little longer for an older adult.

Definition of Arthritis

Arthritis means inflammation of a joint. Many people complain of rheumatism in relation to their many aches and pains. Arthritis affects over 50 million people in the United States and costs more to treat than cancer. There are several types of arthritis. The two main ones are rheumatoid arthritis and osteoarthritis. A comparison of the two types is shown in Figure 15-3. Other types of arthritis are gout and ankylosing spondylitis. The major warning signs of arthritis are:

• Swelling in one or more joints

• Stiffness

• Pain or tenderness in any joint

• Decreased range of motion

• Obvious redness and warmth in a joint

• Unexplained weight loss, fever, or weakness

Risk factors for arthritis are:

• Family history—If parents or siblings have arthritis, you are more likely to develop the disorder.

• Age—Risk increases with age. Incidence of all types of arthritis increases with age.

• Sex—Women are more likely to develop rheumatoid arthritis, whereas gout is more predominant in males.

• Previous joint injury—Individuals who have had previous injury to a joint are more likely to develop arthritis in that joint.

• Obesity—Extra weight puts stress on joints, particularly the knees, hips, and spine.

Rheumatoid Arthritis

Rheumatoid arthritis generally affects people between the ages of 20 and 45, but it is also seen in younger children and older adults. The cause of this condition is that the immune system that normally protects the body works the opposite way and fights the body. The body's immune system attacks joints and inflames the synovium, causing swelling, redness, and pain. It is a disease that affects the entire body; the joints are affected the most, as the disease can eventually destroy cartilage and bone within the joint. There is symmetrical swelling (both hands or both feet are affected, not just one side) of the joints. It can occasionally cause problems with the muscles, skin, blood vessels, nerves, and eyes. The client may have a very mild case, which might cause mild discomfort, or a severe case where widespread joint deformities are present. For clients the morning is usually the most difficult part of the day or after a long period of inactivity, because at these times the pain increases and the stiffness is greater. The characteristic signs and symptoms of this disease are joint pain, stiffness and redness of the joints, and difficulty with range of motion. Other less common signs are mild fever, weight loss, and fatigue. As the disease progresses, joint problems increase in severity. These deformities of the joints are seen in the hips, knees, wrists, fingers, and ankles (Figure 15-4).

Osteoarthritis

Another term for osteoarthritis is "wear-and-tear" arthritis. This type of arthritis affects the weight-bearing joints, such as the spine, hip, and knee. The affected joint or joints become enlarged and painful. There is usually

Rheumatoid Arthritis	Osteoarthritis
Affects the lubricating fluid in the joints	Affects cartilage, connective tissue
Inflammation	Wearing down condition
System disease (total body)	Health not generally affected
Good and bad periods of pain	No particular good periods without pain
Results in deformity	Limits motion only
Affects any joint	Affects weight-bearing joints
Affects all ages—even young people	Affects older age group

FIGURE 15-3   Comparison of rheumatoid arthritis and osteoarthritis.

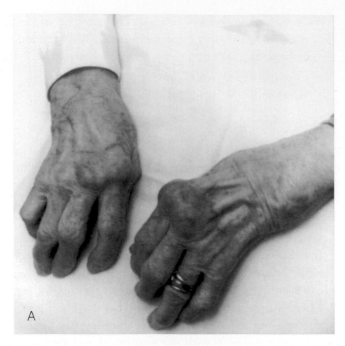

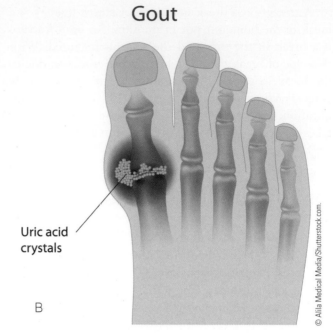

Uric acid
crystals

© Alila Medical Media/Shutterstock.com.

FIGURE 15-4 A. Arthritis of the hands. B. Gout in the big toe.

damage to cartilage, which can result in bone grinding directly on bone, which causes pain and restricts movement. If the finger joint is affected, the swelling occurs closest to the fingernail. The larger joints are the ones that cause the most pain and discomfort.

Gout is a form of arthritis that affects mainly men over the age of 40. This type of arthritis is due to the presence of too much uric acid in the client's system. The first sign of this disease is a painful big toe. It can also affect other joints such as the foot, ankle, and wrist. These areas of the body have little outpouches or protruding lesions called tophi that contain abnormal amounts of uric acid (see Figure 15-4B). The affected joint becomes extremely painful. This condition is treated with a low-purine diet, limiting the use of alcohol, and prescription drugs such as colchicine or allopurinol.

Management of Arthritis

Diet Therapy

The diet is individualized to meet the person's needs. If the client is overweight, the diet will need to be low in calories; if the client is underweight, the diet will need to be high in calories and protein. If the client has the gout form of arthritis, the client is placed on a low-purine diet. Individuals crippled with arthritis may have one or

more of the following problems that interfere with their nutritional status:

• Chronic pain
• Decreased activity can cause weight gain, immobility, and pressure sore development.
• Impaired movement may cause lack of energy for preparing foods and grocery shopping.

As a home health aide, you will most likely be employed to work in the home to assist the client with cooking, cleaning, exercising the client, and laundry duties. The client will be able to assist you to do a few of these tasks but will tire easily. You need to encourage the client to do as much as possible. Be sure you do not overtire or rush the client. The client will need a longer time to accomplish a task.

Exercise

One form of treatment for arthritis is exercise. Exercise can be passive (you do it for the client) or active (the client performs the exercise without assistance). The goals of the exercise program are to maintain complete joint movement and in some cases strengthen the muscles around the specific joint. The physical therapist will develop a care plan for your client. If the joints are very painful and swollen, the exercises should be done gently but consistently. The exercises are usually ordered three (tid) to four times (qid) a day. It is helpful to have the client take pain medication a half hour before the exercises are started. With his or her pain reduced, the client might be more willing to do the exercises. If the client does not exercise these joints, they will quickly become frozen or immobile.

Medication

The third method of treatment is through drug therapy. The specific drug used by clients will depend on many factors, such as:

- Severity of the arthritis
- Tolerance to the drug
- Cost
- Type of arthritis
- Client's response (some clients respond positively to a drug and others do not respond at all)
- Presence of other chronic diseases (e.g., if a client has a stomach ulcer, certain drugs cannot be prescribed)

The largest groups of drugs used to treat arthritis are called nonsteroidal anti-inflammatory drugs (NSAIDs), which work by decreasing pain and swelling in the joints and muscles. Some generic over-the-counter NSAIDs are ibuprofen and naproxen. Some types of NSAIDs are available only by prescription. Oral NSAIDs can cause stomach problems. NSAIDs are also available in creams or gels that can be rubbed on the joints. Another group of drugs called corticosteroids can reduce inflammation and suppress the immune system. Examples are prednisone and cortisone, which can be taken orally or given by injection. Newer drugs used to treat rheumatoid arthritis are Remicade® (infliximab), Enbrel® (etanercept), Trexall® (methotrexate), and Plaquenil® (hydroxychloroquine). These drugs are given by injection. The drugs work on the immune system in an attempt to slow down the inflammation process. All of the drugs have significant side effects, such as black stools, bloody urine, ringing in the ears, and skin bruises.

Other drugs used to treat arthritis are a group called analgesics. These drugs can help reduce pain, but have no effects on inflammation. Examples include Tylenol® (acetaminophen), Ultram® (tramadol), and narcotics such as Percocet and Vicodin.

Your case manager will inform you of the side effects to watch for in your client. More than 100 drugs are used to treat arthritis; all have different side effects.

Surgery

In the last 20 years, surgery has become successful in helping the arthritic client maintain independence. Surgeons can now replace arthritic knees, hips, and shoulders.

Surgery can also be done on the client's spine, jaw, wrist, and fingers. An aide may be employed to care for these clients on a temporary basis after they return home from the hospital. Clients will have their own individualized plan of care designed by a team consisting of the health care provider, nurse, home health aide, physical therapist, occupational therapist, and case manager.

Nursing Care After Joint Replacement Surgery

Replacement of a joint is called an arthroplasty. The surgeon removes the damaged joint such as the knee or hip and replaces the joint with artificial parts, called prostheses (Figure 15-5). The client is hospitalized for about 3 to 4 days and then sent home. At home, this client will need assistance in activities of daily living. General guidelines for caring for a client who had a total hip replacement or total knee replacement are:

- Have the client take sponge baths. Do not shower or take a tub bath until staples or stitches are removed.
- Avoid movements that twist or cause pain, such as kneeling or crossing the legs. With a hip replacement, do not bend the affected leg over 45 degrees and do not move the affected leg over the center of the body.

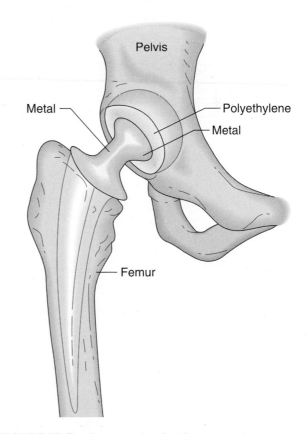

FIGURE 15-5   An example of a hip prosthesis.

- Allow only the amount of weight-bearing on the affected hip or knee as instructed by the care plan.
- Walk at least three times a day to keep the new hip or knee as mobile as possible. At first, the client will have a walker and gradually progress to the use of a cane as the mobility of the hip or knee increases.

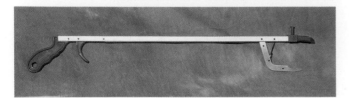

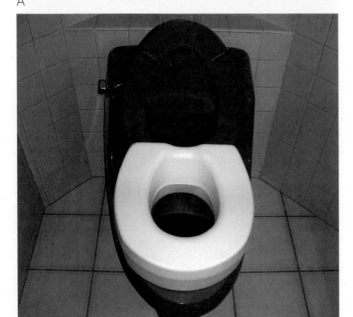

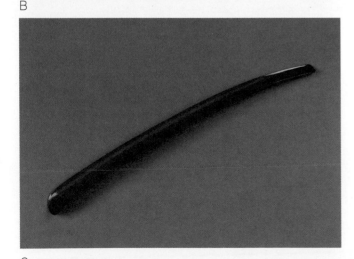

FIGURE 15-6   A. Long-handled picker-upper. B. Elevated toilet seat. C. Long-handled shoehorn.

- It is normal for the new hip or knee to be swollen and for the client to have discomfort, especially on movement. The client can take painkillers as needed and ice packs can be applied.
- Elevate the affected leg or knee when sitting in a chair to reduce swelling of the leg.
- It is helpful for the client to have a long-handled gripper (Figure 15-6A), picker-upper (Figure 15-6B), elevated toilet seat (Figure 15-6C), and a long handled shoehorn (Figure 15-7).
- The client may be sent home with an incentive spirometer, a device to help the client breathe more deeply to prevent pneumonia.
- Ice packs may be ordered to reduce swelling of the affected joint.
- Elastic stockings or TED hose may be used to help reduce swelling and the risk of blood clots in the affected joint.
- The site of the surgery will have a dressing applied and a health care provider will change this as needed. The home health aide should observe the site for an unusual amount of drainage or odorous drainage. Keep the area clean and dry.
- The aide may need to take the client to physical therapy sessions or, in some cases, the physical therapist may come to the client's home.
- Client may be on blood thinners to prevent blood clots, so watch for signs of unusual bleeding.

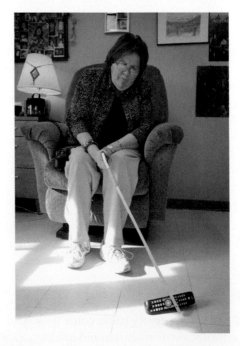

FIGURE 15-7   Client picking up TV remote with picker-upper.

Assistive Devices

An aide employed in a home with a client with arthritis will need to take special care when moving or transferring the client. It is normal for the client to be able to do everything one day but the next day very little. Encourage the client to function at the highest level of wellness possible and to be as independent as possible. Try to assist the client in making tasks as simple as possible. A suggestion might be to have Velcro closures rather than buttons on clothes. Have elastic-waist slacks rather than zipper and button closures. Bars may need to be placed by the bathroom, in the tub area, and on the bed to assist the client to get up and down. Portable whirlpool attachments can be placed in the client's tub to help soothe the client's pain. Another effective therapy is exercising or swimming in warm-water pools.

Principles of Good Body Mechanics

Each year, because of incorrect body and muscle use, millions of dollars are lost in wages and millions of dollars are spent on treatment for unnecessary injuries and disability payments. The most common injuries for the home health aide involve the muscles, ligaments, and joints of the lower back. These injuries are caused by lifting, bending, pulling, twisting, and pushing incorrectly.

New guidelines for lifting and moving are called **safe patient handling and mobility (SPHM) standards**. These guidelines are formal, systematized programs for reducing the risk of injuries and muscle disorders for health care workers, fostering a culture of safety while improving quality of care and reducing health care workers' risk of physical injury. These guidelines were written with the understanding that manual handling is hazardous and is directly responsible for musculoskeletal disorders suffered by the caregiver.

These guidelines require that a health recipient home be environmentally safe for the worker to give care. If the health recipient needs to be lifted out of bed, the home should have a ceiling or mechanical lifts, wide doorways, adequate space to maneuver portable lifts in the bathroom, and flooring that facilitates smooth movement to wheel heavy loads.

Obesity has increased among older adults. Approximately 33% of adults are obese and 7% are considered morbidly obese. These health care recipients are stressors on the health care delivery system. Due to increase of bariatric health recipients who are at particular risk for complications of immobility, new technology is being developed to deliver safe care. Ceiling lifts, lateral transfer devices, portable lifts, large electric beds, and bathing chairs are assistive devices that can assist in caring for the bariatric health recipient.

If a health care recipient is being transferred home from a long-term care or acute care facility, a home visit is made by a social worker or other health care team member to assess the home environment. The health care member will suggest changes to make to the home to make it safer to give care to the health care recipient. The home may have steps, narrow hallways, small bathrooms, or low beds and couches, which all can hinder safe care.

Standard terms and guidelines for SPHM are:

Level of Assistance—Independent: Client performs tasks safely without assistance. Stand-by-Assist: Client requires supervised cueing or coaxing.

Minimum Assist—One-person assist: Client requires transfer assistance of one caregiver with maximum force of 35 lb for lift, push/pull. Client can pivot, can bear weight on legs, and has upper body strength to hold self up and/or can help mover in bed.

Minimum Assist—Two-person assist: Client requires two caregivers—maximum 70-lb force—to assist with lifting/transferring and bed mobility.

Moderate Assist: Client requires sit-stand aid, mechanical lift and lateral transfer, and bed mobility aids.

Maximum Assistant (Total Assistance): Client requires mandatory mechanical lift and bed mobility aids.

Much of your work as a home health aide requires physical effort. To avoid injury to yourself, use good techniques when you lift a client, transfer a client between bed and wheelchair, cook meals, do laundry, or even stand, sit, or walk. All require correct, careful, and efficient use of your muscles to prevent injury and reduce fatigue.

The way in which the body moves and keeps its balance through the use of all its parts is referred to as **body mechanics**. Some muscles are better at pushing than pulling. The body organs are held in their cavities by the muscles surrounding them. When one part of the body is under strain, it may affect other parts of the body.

Your spine is like a flexible, bendable rod with a crossbar near the top where the shoulders and arms are attached. The muscles of the spine are small straps that run up and down the spine. They are designed to hold the spine steady and to bend in different directions. They are not designed to lift heavy loads. The strong muscles of

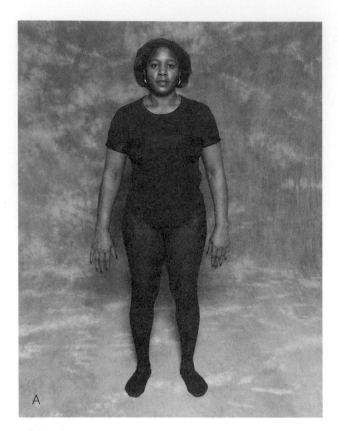

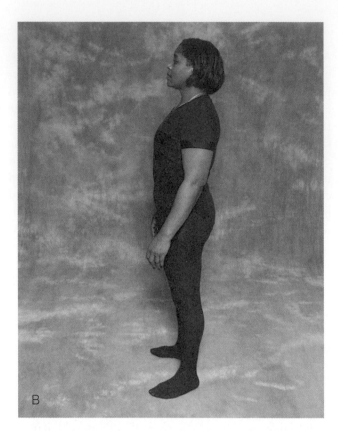

A

B

FIGURE 15-8 Correct standing position. A. Front view. B. Side view.

the hips and of the shoulders and arms are there to do the heavy work. When you lift, push, or pull, be aware of the positions of the different parts of your body. Keep your back straight and steady. Bend your knees and use the muscles of the thighs and shoulders to do the work. When you carry an object, hold it close to your body.

Good body mechanics starts with proper posture—the way you hold and position each part of your body. Correct posture means that there is a balance between your muscle groups and that the different parts of your body are in good alignment—in the correct position relative to each other (Figures 15-8A and B).

Correct posture makes lifting, pulling, and pushing easier. Correct posture is important at all times—when standing, sitting, walking, and lying. A good standing posture begins with having the feet flat on the floor, separated by about 12 inches, with the knees slightly bent, arms at the sides, and abdominal muscles tight.

Ten basic rules will help your body and muscles work well for you, prevent injury, and reduce fatigue:

1. Keep your back straight—do not twist or bend.

2. Keep your feet apart, to provide a good **base of support** (Figure 15-9).

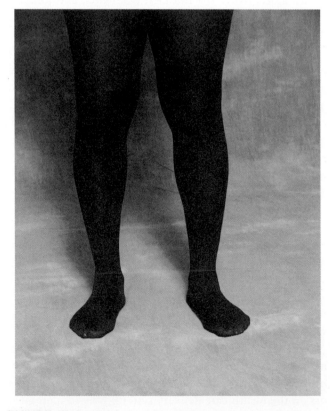

FIGURE 15-9 Keep your feet apart.

3. Bend from the knees, particularly when lifting—do not bend from the waist or spine (Figure 15-10).

4. Use the weight of your body to help pull or push an object (Figure 15-11).

5. Use the strong muscles of your thighs and shoulders to do the work (Figure 15-12).

6. Hold objects close to your body. This allows your strong shoulder and thigh muscles to work most efficiently (Figure 15-13).

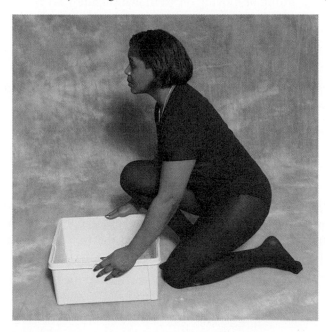

FIGURE 15-10 Bend your knees, not your back.

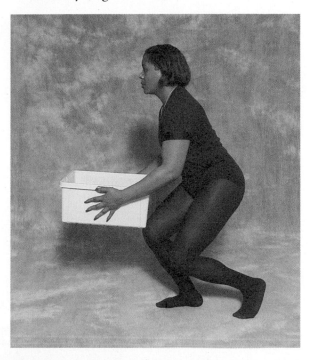

FIGURE 15-12 Use the strong muscles of your thighs and shoulders when lifting.

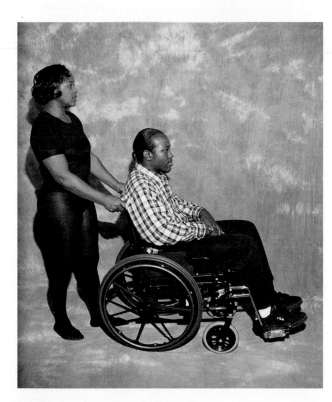

FIGURE 15-11 Push an object.

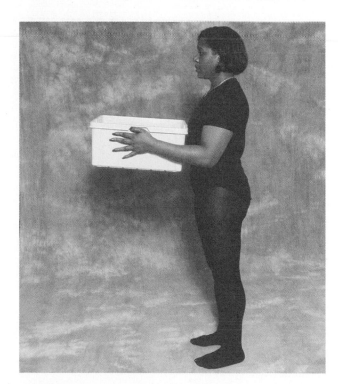

FIGURE 15-13 Hold objects close.

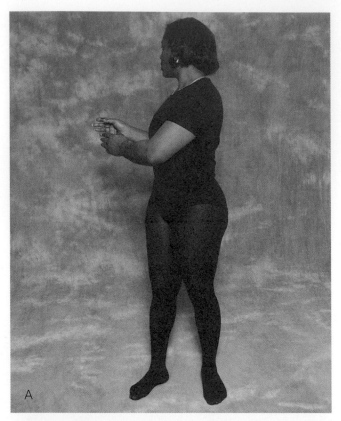

A

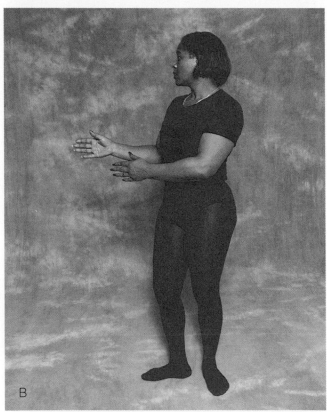

B

FIGURE 15-14 A. Avoid twisting your body. B. Pivot instead of twisting.

7. Avoid twisting your body as you work and bend. Pivot the whole body (Figure 15-14A and B).

8. Push or pull, rather than lift.

9. Always get help if you feel you cannot do the lifting or moving on your own (Figure 15-15).

10. Synchronize movements with client or others; count 1 . . . 2 . . . 3 . . . and do the job together.

Remember, it is your body, they are your muscles, and you are responsible for the way you use them.

Applications of Good Body Mechanics to Client Care

Many client care procedures require moving and turning the client. To ensure the safety of the client and to avoid self-injury, the home health aide should apply the techniques of good body mechanics to the work situation. This means that the aide should do the following:

• Stand straight, rather than slouch. Keep the back and shoulder muscles in a straight line.

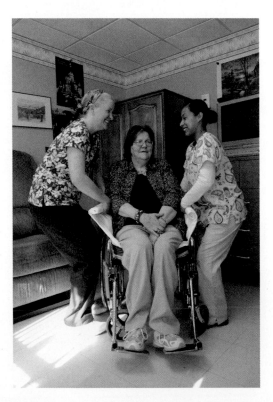

FIGURE 15-15 Determine if you can transfer alone. If not, ask for help.

- Push, pull, slide, or roll the client whenever possible. Try to avoid lifting the client.

- When turning the client, try to make the movement smooth and fluid so that the entire body shifts at the same time.

- When repositioning the client in bed, turn the client toward you rather than away from you. This lessens the danger of the client falling out of bed and keeps your weight more evenly distributed.

- When walking with the client, remain on the client's weak side. Try to stay near chairs or a couch so you can quickly seat the client if the client tires.

- If the client becomes faint while walking, help the client to sit in a chair. If there is no chair nearby, help the client slide slowly to the floor (Figure 15-16).

- When walking or transferring a client, remember to use a gait or transfer belt (Figure 15-17).

Transfer Belts

A **transfer belt** or **gait belt** is a wide canvas belt that is placed around the client's waist for the home health aide to hold onto when transferring or walking a client. The belts come in various styles and sizes. It is an assistive device used to transfer or walk clients who need help. Using the belt avoids the need to grasp the client around the ribcage or under the shoulders. It allows the aide to have more control of the transfer and keeps the client safe.

When not using the belt on the client, the aide often wears the belt around the waist. If the aide needs it, it is right there and there will be no need to look for it. Most agencies now require gait belts for all transfers. See Procedure 46, Applying a Transfer or Gait Belt, and Procedure 47, Dangling a Client.

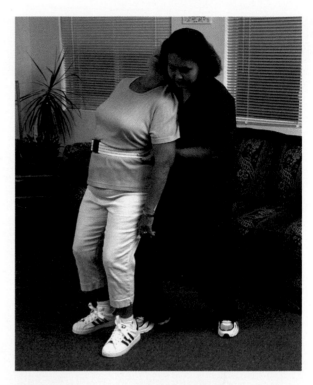

FIGURE 15-16   If an unsteady client starts to fall, slowly lower the client to the floor with a transfer belt.

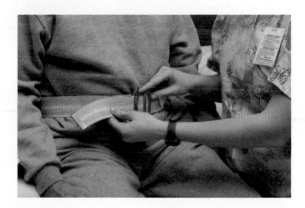

FIGURE 15-17   A transfer belt or gait belt is often used to ambulate a client who is unsteady.

PROCEDURE 46   APPLYING A TRANSFER OR GAIT BELT

Purpose

- To safely transfer a client or ambulate a client
- To prevent injury to the client's shoulder while transferring

Procedure

1. Assemble equipment:
   transfer belt
2. Tell the client what you plan to do.

(continued)

PROCEDURE 46 APPLYING A TRANSFER OR GAIT BELT (*continued*)

3. Position the client to make application of the belt possible. If the client is lying in bed, move the client up to a sitting position. If the client is sitting in a chair, ask the client to lean forward, so you can slide the belt around the client's waist.

4. Apply the belt around the client's waist over clothing, never over bare skin. It should be snug, but not too snug. Keep the belt at waist level. Buckle the belt in front by threading the belt end through the teeth side of the buckle first and then through both openings. The aide should be able to place two fingers in between the belt and the client's skin. Place the buckle side of the belt in the front.

5. When walking a client, place your hands under the belt in the back (Figure 15-18). Always walk the client holding onto the belt on the client's weak side.

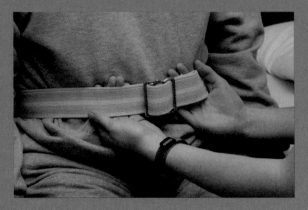

FIGURE 15-18 Proper placement of the hands on the belt when walking a client.

6. If you are using the belt to transfer the client out of bed, place both hands under the belt and support the client to stand.

7. Remove the belt after you are done transferring or ambulating (walking) a client.

PROCEDURE 47 DANGLING A CLIENT

Purpose

- To move the client's legs around to prevent blood clots
- To relieve pressure on the client's back

NOTE: This procedure is usually done after surgery before a patient is allowed out of bed.

Procedure

1. Tell the client what you plan to do.
2. Place one arm around the client's shoulder and the other arm under the knees.
3. Turn the client toward you. Once the client is in a sitting position with the legs hanging loose over the outside of the bed (dangling), ask the client to move the legs and wiggle his or her toes around for a few minutes (Figure 15-19).

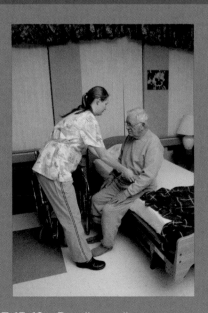

FIGURE 15-19 Dangling a client.

(*continued*)

PROCEDURE 47   DANGLING A CLIENT *(continued)*

4. Check the pulse of the client to see if it is regular and strong. If the client becomes faint, tip the client's head down for a few seconds.
5. After a few minutes, place one arm around the client's shoulder and the other arm

under the knees. Gently and slowly swing the client's legs onto the bed. Lay the client down in bed.
6. Record and document the procedure and any abnormal signs.

Positioning

Often a home health aide will need to position a client with mobility impairments. Clients who are unable to get up out of bed need to be repositioned every 2 hours. Positioning can make the client more comfortable and assist the body to function more efficiently. The correct positioning can relieve pressure on body parts, aid in breathing, and prevent injury to the client. Some clients may need your assistance in positioning so that they can engage in activities such as eating, reading, watching television, or visiting. If the client is in the sitting position, you should check to make sure that the head is erect and the spine is in straight alignment (Figure 15-20). Body weight should be evenly distributed on the buttocks and thighs. Feet should be supported by the floor with the ankles comfortably flexed. Forearms should be supported on an armrest, on the lap, or on a table positioned in front of the chair. For a side-lying position, pillows and

other positioning supports should be correctly placed (Figure 15–21). The spinal column should be in correct alignment. See Procedures 48 through 54.

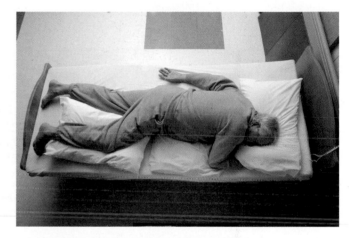

FIGURE 15-21   Check to see if the hips and knees are in correct alignment.

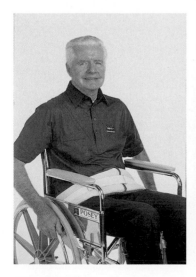
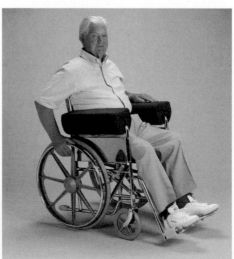
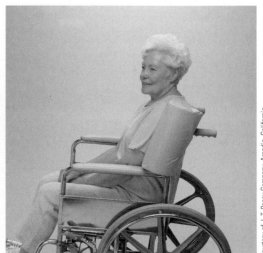

FIGURE 15-20   Postural supports help position clients and maintain body alignment without restricting movements. Clients are supported and protected without being restrained.

Courtesy of J. T. Posey Company, Arcadia, California

PROCEDURE 48 TURNING THE CLIENT TOWARD YOU

Purpose

- To make the client more comfortable
- To change the client's position
- To improve circulation and reduce skin pressure

Procedure

1. Wash your hands.
2. Tell client what you are going to do. Provide for privacy.
3. Lift the client's far leg and cross it over the leg that is nearest you.
4. Lift the far arm over the chest, bend the elbow, and bring the hand toward the client's shoulder. Position the nearest arm so that you will not roll the client on it when you turn the client.
5. Place the hand nearest the head of the bed on the far shoulder and place your other hand on the client's hip on the far side.
6. Brace your one thigh against the side of the bed and smoothly roll the client toward you. Make sure that the client's upper leg comes over and bend it at the knee to ensure that the new position is stable.
7. Go to the opposite side of the bed and place your hands over the client's shoulder and pull the client's upper body to the center of the bed. Place your hands over the client's hips and pull the rest of the client's body to the center of the bed and into good body alignment.
8. Place pillows against the client's back and secure it by pushing part of the pillow under the client's back. The client's upper arm also should be supported with a pillow.
9. Support the knee, ankle, and foot of the upper leg with a pillow, which also prevents the knees and ankles from rubbing against each other and causing skin irritation. Cover the client. You can place a chair on the side of the bed so that the client will not fall out.
10. Wash your hands.
11. Document procedure completion, time, and the client's reaction.

PROCEDURE 49 MOVING THE CLIENT UP IN BED USING A LIFT SHEET

Purpose

- To move the client up in bed with minimum discomfort
- To relieve pressure on body parts

NOTE: Very often a client will slide down in the bed away from the headboard. This is uncomfortable for the client. This procedure can be done easily in an assistive living facility, as an extra aide is readily available.

Procedure

1. Wash your hands. Provide for privacy.

2. Tell the client what you plan to do. Have your partner, a friend, a family member, or a coworker stand on the opposite side of the bed to assist you.
3. Place a pillow at the head of the bed to protect the client's head. Roll both sides of the lift sheet folded in fours toward the client. Place the client's feet 12 inches apart, so that they will not bump together as you move the client. Bend the client's knees, if possible.
4. With the hand nearest the client's feet, firmly grasp the rolled lift sheet. With the other hand, both of you cradle the client's

(continued)

PROCEDURE 49   MOVING THE CLIENT UP IN BED USING A LIFT SHEET (*continued*)

head and shoulders and firmly grasp the top of the rolled lift sheet.

5. Turn your body and feet toward the head of the bed. Keep your feet about 12 inches apart and bend your knees slightly to achieve good body mechanics as you lift the client.

6. Coordinate your lift—on the count of three, together lift the lift sheet and the client up toward the head of the bed without dragging the client (Figure 15-22). Align the client's body and limbs so that the client is straight and comfortable.

7. Place the pillow back under the client's head, and tighten the lift sheet. Replace the covers and make the client comfortable.

8. Wash your hands.

9. Document completion of the procedure, time, and the client's reaction.

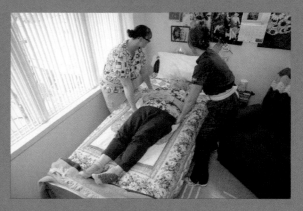

FIGURE 15-22   Be sure to position the client's head comfortably. Lifting a client up in bed using a lift sheet.

PROCEDURE 50   LOG ROLLING THE CLIENT

Purpose

- To ensure the spinal column is kept straight because of special medical conditions such as spinal injury and hip fractures

NOTE: It takes a minimum of two people to do this procedure. You will need to instruct family member or others on what you want them to do.

Procedure

1. Wash your hands.

2. Tell the client what you plan to do and provide for privacy.

3. With both you and your helper on the same side of the bed, remove the top covers.

4. Place your hand and arm under the client's head and shoulders to stabilize the neck. Your helper places her arms under

the client's body and legs. On the count of three, roll the client toward you as a single unit.

5. Do not allow the client to bend and use good body mechanics yourselves by bending your knees and keeping your backs straight (Figure 15-23A).

6. Place a pillow lengthwise between the client's thighs and legs and fold the client's arms over the chest (Figure 15-23B).

7. Go over to the other side of the bed. You are in a position to keep the shoulders and upper body straight and your helper is positioned to keep the client's lower body, hips, and legs straight. Reach over the client and roll the lift sheet firmly against the client. On the count of three, the client is rolled toward you in a single movement, keeping the

(*continued*)

PROCEDURE 50   LOG ROLLING THE CLIENT (*continued*)

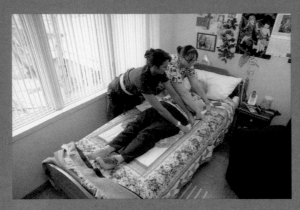

FIGURE 15-23A   With two aides using a lift sheet, roll the client as a unit toward both of you.

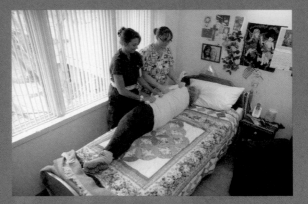

FIGURE 15-23B   A lift sheet can be used to turn a client on her side.

client's head, spine, and legs in a straight position.

8. To maintain the client's new position and alignment, place pillows against the spine and leave the pillow between the client's legs. Other small pillows or folded towels can be placed under the client's head and neck and under the arms for support.

9. Make sure the client's alignment is straight and that the client is comfortable. Arrange covers for the client. A chair may be placed on the side of the bed to prevent the client from falling out of bed.

10. Wash your hands.

11. Document the repositioning, time, and any observations you made.

PROCEDURE 51   POSITIONING THE CLIENT IN SUPINE POSITION

Purpose

• To make the client more comfortable
• To assist the body to function more efficiently
• To relieve pressure on body parts

Procedure

1. Wash your hands.
2. Tell the client what you plan to do. Provide for privacy.
3. Place a pillow under the client's head, so that the client's head is about 2 inches above the level of the bed. The pillow

should extend slightly under the shoulders (Figure 15-24).

4. Have the client's arms extended straight out with the palms of the hands flat on the bed. The arms can be supported by pillows or covered foam pads placed under the forearms and extending from just above the elbows to the ends of the fingers.

5. Place a small pillow or rolled towel along the side of the client's thighs and tuck part of the support under the thigh, ensuring that the part under the thighs is smooth. This maintains alignment of the hips and

(*continued*)

PROCEDURE 51   POSITIONING THE CLIENT IN SUPINE POSITION (*continued*)

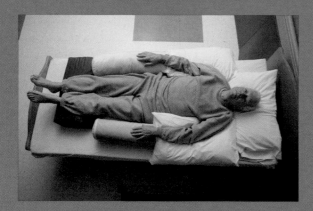

FIGURE 15-24   A client in supine position. The head of the bed may be elevated slightly with a pillow and the arms and hands may be elevated with a pillow.

thighs and helps prevent the hips from rotating outward or externally.

6. Place a small pillow or towel under the back of the ankle to relieve pressure on the heels.
7. Wash your hands.
8. Document the time, position change, and the client's reaction.

PROCEDURE 52   POSITIONING THE CLIENT IN LATERAL/SIDE-LYING POSITION

Purpose

- To provide for client comfort and change of position
- To relieve pressure on body parts

Procedure

1. Wash your hands.
2. Tell the client what you plan to do. Provide for privacy.
3. Go to the opposite side of the bed from the direction you are planning to turn the client toward.
4. Cross the client's arms over the chest. Place your arm under the client's neck and shoulders. Place your other arm under the client's midback. Move the upper part of the client's body toward you.
5. Place one arm under the client's waist and the other under the thighs. Move the lower part of the client's body toward you.
6. Turn the client to the opposite side. Pull the shoulder that is touching the bed slightly toward you. Pull the buttock that is touching the bed slightly toward you. Place a pillow under the back and buttocks. Place the bottom leg in extension and flex the upper leg. Place a small folded blanket or pillow between the upper and lower leg (Figure 15-25A).

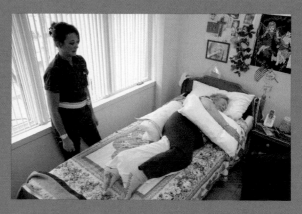

FIGURE 15-25A   Lateral/side-lying position.

(*continued*)

PROCEDURE 52   POSITIONING THE CLIENT IN LATERAL/SIDE-LYING POSITION (*continued*)

7. Place a pillow under the client's head. Rotate the arm up to bring it up to the pillow with the palm facing up. Place the other arm on a pillow that extends from above the elbow to the fingers. Extend the fingers.
8. Check the client's position to see if the body is in good vertical alignment (Figure 15-25B).
9. Wash your hands.
10. Document time, change of position, and the client's reaction.

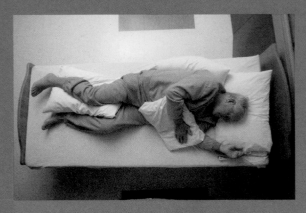

FIGURE 15-25B   Side-lying position—note the placement of pillows.

PROCEDURE 53   POSITIONING THE CLIENT IN PRONE POSITION

Purpose

- To relieve pressure on body parts
- To provide for client comfort and position

NOTE: Older adult clients are not able or do not like to be in the prone position for long because it is uncomfortable and, in some cases, makes it very difficult for the client to breathe. Never leave an older client in this position for more than 15 to 20 minutes.

Procedure

1. Wash your hands.
2. Tell the client what you plan to do. Provide for privacy.
3. Check to see that the client's arms are straight down at the sides of the bed. Turn the client on his or her abdomen. Check to see if the spine is straight and that the face is turned to either side.
4. The client's legs are extended. The arms are flexed and brought up to either side of the head.
5. A small pillow can be placed under the abdomen. (For women, this will reduce

pressure against the breasts.) An alternate method is to roll a small towel and place it under the shoulders to reduce pressure.
6. Place another pillow under the lower legs to prevent pressure on the toes (Figure 15-26).
7. Wash your hands.
8. Document time, change of position, and the client's reaction.

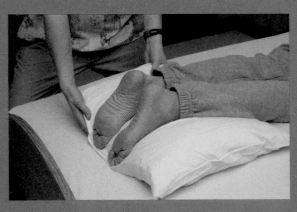

FIGURE 15-26   Place a pillow under the lower legs to relieve pressure on the toes.

PROCEDURE 54   POSITIONING THE CLIENT IN FOWLER'S POSITION

Purpose

- To provide client comfort
- To aid in breathing
- To position the client in Fowler's position so the client can engage in activities such as eating, reading, working on a laptop computer, watching television, and visiting

Procedure

1. Wash your hands.
2. Tell the client what you plan to do. Provide for privacy.
3. Check to see if the client's spine and legs are straight and in the middle of the bed.
4. Support the client's head and neck with one, two, or three pillows. If client has a hospital bed, raise the bed to a 45° angle.
5. The knees may be flexed and supported with small pillows (Figure 15-27).
6. Pillows may be placed under each arm from the elbows to the fingertips to support the shoulders.

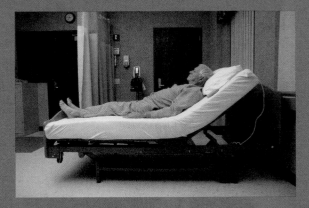

FIGURE 15-27   A client position in Fowler's position.

7. Place a pillow or padded footboard against the feet.
8. Wash your hands.
9. Document time, position change, and the client's reaction.

Transfers

Often an aide will be asked to transfer a client who has difficulty standing or bearing weight on the lower extremities. Using the proper transfer techniques will ensure that the client is moved safely from one location to another. Before assisting a client to stand, make sure the client is wearing shoes. If the bed is adjustable, make sure it is at a safe level. See Procedures 55 through 61.

PROCEDURE 55   ASSISTING THE CLIENT FROM BED TO WHEELCHAIR

Purpose

- To move client from one location to another safely and with little discomfort

Procedure

1. Wash your hands.
2. Tell the client what you plan to do.
3. Assemble needed equipment.

4. Place the chair so that the client moves toward the client's strongest side. Set the chair at a 45° angle to the bed. Lock the wheels. Move the footrests out of the way.
5. Assist the client to sit at the edge of the bed, as close to the edge of the bed as possible. Never pull on the client's arms or under the client's shoulders. Use verbal cues if necessary during transfer.

(continued)

PROCEDURE 55   ASSISTING THE CLIENT FROM BED TO WHEELCHAIR (*continued*)

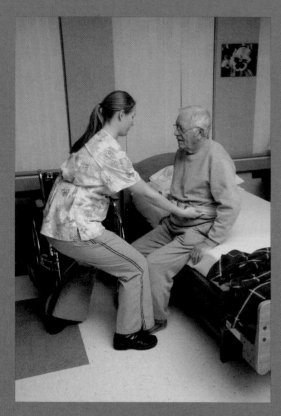

FIGURE 15-28A   A transfer belt is applied to the client.

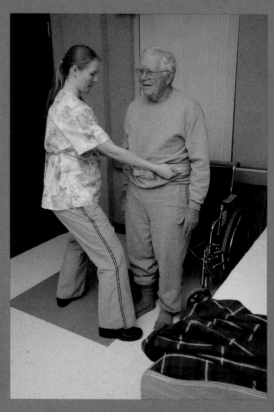

FIGURE 15-28B   An aide places fingers under the belt and assists the client to stand.

6. Wait a few seconds to allow the client to adjust to a sitting position. Assist the client to put on socks and shoes.

7. Apply the transfer belt (Figure 15-28A). Make sure the belt is not too tight or too loose.

8. Spread your feet apart and flex your hips and knees, aligning your knees with the client's.

9. Grasp the transfer belt from underneath with both hands. Rock the client up to standing on the count of three, while straightening your hips and legs, keeping your knees slightly flexed (Figure 15-28B).

10. If the client has a weak leg, press your knee against it or block the client's foot with

yours to prevent the weaker leg from sliding out from under the client.

11. Instruct the client to use the armrest on the chair for support, and be sure to flex your hips and knees while lowering the client into the chair. Remove the transfer belt (Figures 15-28C).

12. Check the alignment of the client in the chair and make adjustments accordingly. The feet of the client are placed on the footrest (Figure 15-28D).

13. Wash your hands.

14. Document time, position change, and the client's reaction.

(*continued*)

PROCEDURE 55 ASSISTING THE CLIENT FROM BED TO WHEELCHAIR (*continued*)

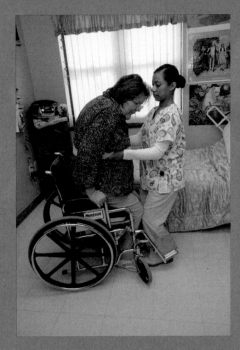

FIGURE 15-28C The client is lowered into a wheelchair, which is locked.

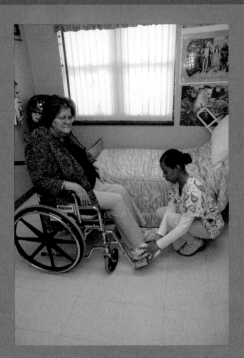

FIGURE 15-28D The feet are positioned on the foot rest.

PROCEDURE 56 TRANSFER WITH PIVOT DISC

Purpose

- To transfer client from bed to chair

Equipment

- Transfer belt and pivot disc

The pivot disc is designed for use by clients who are able to stand but cannot readily move their legs. This disc is used in conjunction with a transfer belt. The disc is placed on the floor with the top facing downward. The disc is "locked" in place when the aide places his or her heel on the floor and the rest of the aide's foot firmly on the place between the feet of the client. The client's feet are placed on the disc. The handle of the pivot disc should be placed facing the client, to prevent interfering with the feet of the aide. The aide should place a foot on the disc to safely monitor and control the transfer. The client with his or her feet on the disc can easily be transferred from a sitting position on the edge of the bed to a chair. After use of the pivot disc it should be removed from the floor.

PROCEDURE **57**   ASSISTING THE CLIENT FROM WHEELCHAIR TO BED

Purpose

- To change the client's position
- To transfer the client safely from one location to another

Procedure

1. Wash your hands.
2. Tell the client what you plan to do.
3. Position the client with his or her strong side toward the bed with the wheelchair at a 45° angle. Lock the wheels (Figure 15-29).
4. Apply the transfer belt and place both hands on the back of the belt. Have the client slide forward in the chair as far as possible; this will make it easier for the client to stand up. Instruct the client, if able, to put his or her feet flat on the floor and hands on the chair. On the count of three, have the client push up to a standing position. While standing, have the client pivot (turn) on his or her strong leg toward the bed. Have the client lower him- or herself to the bed to a sitting position.

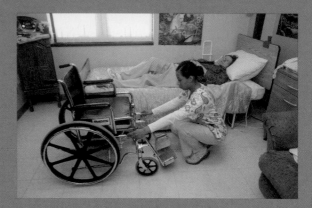

FIGURE 15-29 Lock the wheels of the wheelchair before transferring the client.

5. Assist the client to a lying position. Position the client comfortably and in good alignment. Remove the client's shoes and socks, and remove the transfer belt.
6. Wash your hands.
7. Document time, change of position, and the client's reaction.

PROCEDURE **58**   TRANSFERRING THE CLIENT FROM WHEELCHAIR TO TOILET/COMMODE

Purpose

- To enable the client to sit on the toilet for normal excretion of body wastes

NOTE: It is essential to have grab bars, preferably secured to the wall, but they can be attached to the toilet seat. A walker can also be placed in the bathroom backwards over the toilet to be used as support when sitting or standing on the toilet.

Procedure

1. Wash your hands.
2. Tell the client what you plan to do and provide for privacy.

3. Have the client in a wheelchair with his or her strong side nearer to the toilet or commode.
4. Lock the wheelchair. Apply the transfer belt. Lift the foot pieces out of way.
5. Loosen clothing on the client, but not so loose that the slacks fall while transferring.
6. Have the client slide forward in the chair and place the feet apart. Place your hands on the back of the transfer belt. Have the client place his or her hands on the arm pieces and on the count of three push up.

(continued)

PROCEDURE 58   TRANSFERRING THE CLIENT FROM WHEELCHAIR TO TOILET/COMMODE (*continued*)

7. Stand the client up and have the client place his or her strong arm on the grab bars. As you continue to hold onto the transfer belt, pull the client's pants down and slowly lower the client onto the toilet or commode. Have the client hold onto grab bars while you lower the client's pants.

8. Remove the belt and move the wheelchair out of the way.
9. Provide privacy for the client. Give the client toilet paper.
10. Check often to see if the client is all right.
11. Assist the client as needed to return to the wheelchair and assist back to prior activity.
12. Wash the client's hands and your hands.

PROCEDURE 59   TRANSFERING THE CLIENT USING A MECHANICAL LIFT

Purpose

- To transfer the client from one place to another, usually from bed to chair
- To safely transfer a client who is heavy or has no weight-bearing ability

NOTE: Check slings, chains, and straps for frayed areas or defective hooks. Two types of slings are supplied with the Hoyer lift: hammock style and two-piece canvas strips. The hammock type of sling is better for clients who are weak and need support (Figure 15-30). If you need to lift more than 35 pounds, always use a lift. The canvas strips can be used for clients with normal muscle tone.

Procedure

1. Wash your hands and assemble equipment.
2. Tell the client what you plan to do. Provide for privacy.
3. Position the chair near the bed and allow adequate room to maneuver the lift. Be sure the chair has adequate padding before transfer.
4. Roll the client away from you.
5. Place the hammock sling or canvas strips under the client to form a seat (Figure 15-31A); with two canvas pieces, the lower edge fits under the client's knees (wide piece) and the upper edge goes under the client's shoulders (narrow piece).

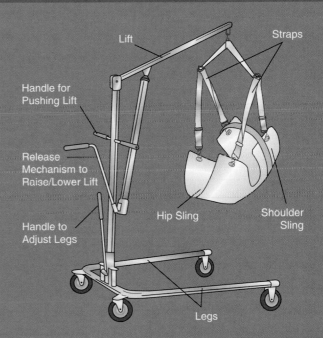

FIGURE 15-30   Mechanical lift.

6. Go to opposite side of bed, roll client away from you and straighten hammock or strips through (Figure 15-31B).
7. Roll the client supine into the canvas seat.
8. Place the lift's horseshoe bar under the side of the bed (on the side with the chair). Have the base of the lift in maximum open position and lock (Figure 15-31C).

(*continued*)

PROCEDURE 59   TRANSFERING THE CLIENT USING A MECHANICAL LIFT (*continued*)

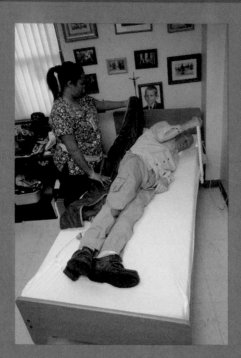

FIGURE 15-31A   Place the canvas lift under the client.

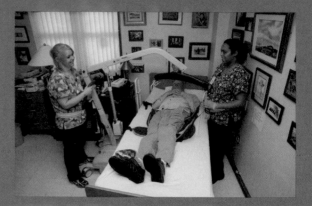

FIGURE 15-31C   Place the mechanical lift over the client in bed.

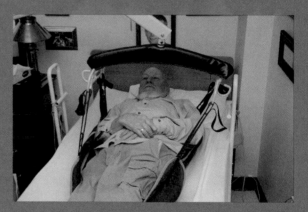

FIGURE 15-31D   Attach the canvas to the mechanical lift.

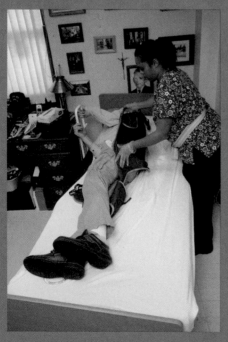

FIGURE 15-31B   Turn the client to the other side and pull the canvas lift through.

9.   Lower the horizontal bar to sling level by releasing the hydraulic valve. Lock the valve.
10. Attach the hooks or strap (chain) to the holes in the sling. Short chains/straps hook to top holes of the sling; lower chains hook to the bottom of the sling. Point the hooks to the outside when attaching (Figure 15-31D).
11. Fold the client's arm over the chest.
12. Pump the handle until the client is raised free of the bed, but no higher than necessary (Figure 15-31E).

(*continued*)

PROCEDURE 59   TRANSFERING THE CLIENT USING A MECHANICAL LIFT (*continued*)

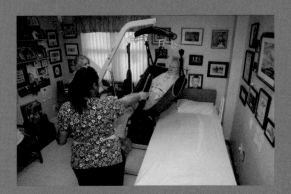

FIGURE 15-31E   Lift the client off of the bed using the mechanical lift.

13. Use the steering handle to pull the lift from the bed and maneuver to the chair.
14. Roll the base around the chair. Slowly release the check valve and lower the client into the chair (Figure 15-31F).
15. Check to see if the client is positioned correctly. Unhook the chains or straps and remove the lift.
16. If a canvas sheet was used, it can be removed (Figure 15-31G). If the hammock sling was used, the sling will remain underneath the client so it is in position for transfer back to bed.
17. Wash your hands.
18. Document transfer, time completed, and the client's reaction.

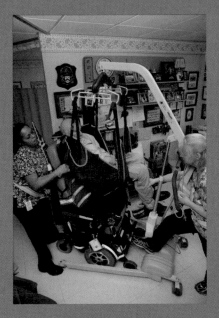

FIGURE 15-31F   Place the client over the wheelchair and slowly lower the client into the chair.

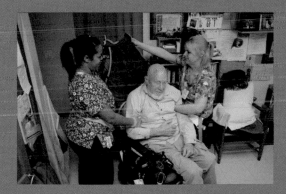

FIGURE 15-31G   Remove the canvas lift sheet.

PROCEDURE 60   TRANSFERRING A CLIENT USING A STAND LIFT

Purpose
- To safely transfer a client from bed to chair
- To safely ambulate a client

Procedure
1. Assemble equipment.
2. Bring the stand lift to the side of the wheelchair (Figure 15-32A).

(*continued*)

PROCEDURE 60 TRANSFERRING A CLIENT USING A STAND LIFT (*continued*)

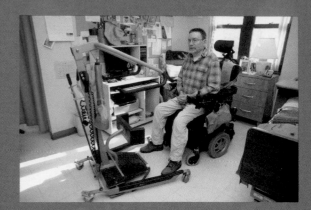

FIGURE 15-32A Stand lift.

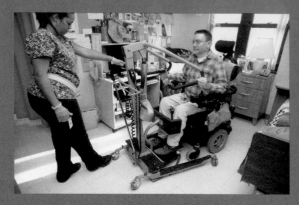

FIGURE 15-32B Remind the client to hold onto the handles.

3. Tell the client what you plan to do.
4. Dress the client and be sure the client is wearing a good pair of shoes with nonskid soles that will give support while walking or transferring.
5. Position the harness around the upper body of the client, so the sides of the harness are between the client's upper body and arms, resting 2 to 3 inches below the underarm.
6. For the safety of the client, securely fasten the safety strap around the client's torso.
7. Secure the buckle and pull the strap to tighten.
8. Spread the legs of the stand lift and place the stand lift directly in front of the client.
9. Have the client place his or her feet on the foot plate and secure the shin strap around the client's legs (Figure 15-23B).
10. Position the client's arms on the outside of the harness and the client's hands on the handles (Figure 15-32C).
11. With the lift arm in the lowest position, attach the harness to the hooks at the end of the stand lift arms, using the loops at the end of the harness. To ensure comfort and safety, use the same size loop on each side. Lock the wheels on the lift (Figure 15-32D).
12. Use the hand controls to raise the lift. Stop lifting when the client is in a standing position.
13. With the client in a standing position, transfer the client to the desired location (Figure 15-32E).

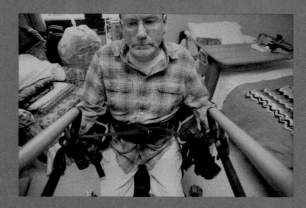

FIGURE 15-32C Position client's arms on the outside of the harness.

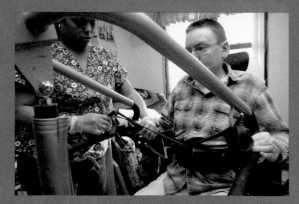

FIGURE 15-32D Attach the loops to the stand lift.

14. When lowering the client to the chair, use the leg spreader bar to open the legs to go around the chair. Lower the client onto the seating position by pushing the **DOWN** button of the control. The aide should stand beside the client.

(*continued*)

PROCEDURE 60   TRANSFERRING A CLIENT USING A STAND LIFT (*continued*)

15. When the client is seated, lower the stand arm until there is enough slack to unhook the harness loops from the arms. Unfasten the buckle that is across the client's torso. Release the shin strap on the client's leg.
16. Move the lift away from the client. Remove the harness from behind the client by grasping the center harness handle.
17. Return equipment to storage area.
18. Document completion of the procedure and any abnormal reactions.

NOTE: There are many different types of stand lifts, each one somewhat different from the next one. For safety reasons, do the procedure first with your case manager or a home health aide before doing it alone. All stand lifts run on batteries and needs to be charged at a designated time, usually at night.

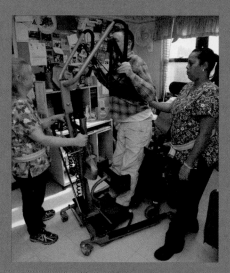

FIGURE 15-32E   Stand the client up and walk the client to his destination.

PROCEDURE 61   SLIDING BOARD TRANSFER

Purpose

• To transfer client from bed to chair

Equipment

• Sliding board and transfer belt

Procedure

1. Inform the client of what you plan to do. Provide for privacy.
2. Gather supplies: wheelchair, transfer belt, and board.
3. Position the wheelchair parallel to the bed. The bed needs to be the same height as the wheelchair seat.
4. Remove the arm of the wheelchair closest to the bed.
5. Apply a transfer belt to the client.
6. Assist the client to move close to the edge of the bed.
7. Tell the client to lean away from the wheelchair. Place the sliding board under the client's buttocks, with the beveled side of the board face up and the opposite end of the board well onto the seat of the wheelchair.
8. Have the client push up with his or her hands, lock his or her elbows, and slide across the board. Repeat until the client is seated in the chair with one buttock on the board. Assist the client by grasping the transfer belt with an underhand grasp and sliding laterally when the client pushes down on the bed.
9. Support and move the client's legs with the your hands.
10. Instruct the client to lean away from the bed. Remove the board and replace the armrest.
11. Remove the transfer belt and replace or fold down the foot rest.
12. Document the transfer and the client's response.

Cast Care

Casts are used to immobilize extremities or joints following trauma or fractures, or to correct a bone/joint defect. Casts may be applied to an extremity or to the entire body. Casts may be made of two main types of material: fiberglass or plaster of Paris. The fiberglass casts are lighter and more durable. Air can circulate more freely inside a fiberglass cast. The plaster casts are easier to mold for some uses than fiberglass, and are also cheaper. Casts promote healing and protect the injury as it heals. See Procedure 62, Caring for Casts.

PROCEDURE 62   CARING FOR CASTS

Purpose

- To prevent complications after application of a cast to a body part.
- Keep the client has comfortable as possible after application of a cast.

Procedure

1. Elevate the entire new cast on pillows and expose to air. For the first 48 to 72 hours after the cast is applied, an icepack loosely covered in a thin towel may be applied around the cast. Apply ice to the cast—not the skin—for 20 minutes every 2 hours. Generally, it is not allowed to have the client lie on the injured side. Instruct the client to frequently wiggle the toes or fingers on the casted extremity. Do not cover the casted extremity and keep it dry (Figure 15-33).

2. Observe the new cast every 2 to 3 hours for the first 2 days and then four times daily. The following signs and symptoms should be reported to the case manager.
   - Cyanosis (blue coloring) below the cast, unusual coldness, and any unusual odor
   - Numbness below the cast
   - Edema (swelling) at either end of the cast
   - Increased pain and tightness in the injured area

3. Observe the cast daily for roughness around the edges, as this may cause skin irritation. Rough edges may be filed, covered with soft padding, or covered with plain white tape. This is called petaling.

4. Observe the cast itself, noting any redness that may indicate bleeding or drainage from under the cast. Circle the area with a marker, noting the date and time that you first noticed the redness.

5. To relieve itching of underlying skin, set a hair dryer on a cool setting and aim it under the cast. An ice pack covered with a thin towel can be applied to the area of itching. Never stick anything down the inside of the cast.

6. When the cast is near the perineal area, protect it from moisture. Ask your case manager for special instructions on which waterproof or protective device to use. Protect the cast and skin by preventing any dirt, sand, or small particles from getting inside the cast, which could cause an infection under the cast.

7. Ask the client if he or she has pain in any particular area under the cast. This may indicate a pressure point and skin breakdown under the cast. Note this area. Be sure to position your client correctly. Figure 15-34 shows several types of commonly applied casts.

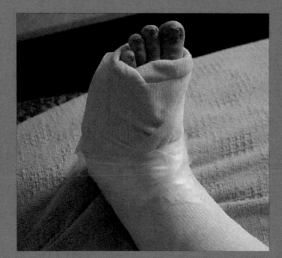

FIGURE 15-33   Frequently check the client's toes for warmth, color, and response to touch.

(continued)

PROCEDURE 62   CARING FOR CASTS (*continued*)

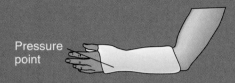

Pressure point

A. THUMB CAST

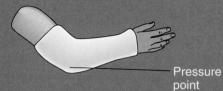

Pressure point

B. LONG ARM CAST

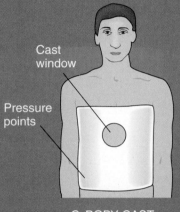

Cast window

Pressure points

C. BODY CAST

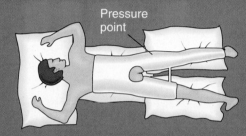

Pressure point

D. HIP SPICA CAST

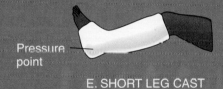

Pressure point

E. SHORT LEG CAST

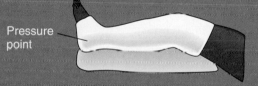

Pressure point

F. LONG LEG CAST

FIGURE 15-34   Casts that are frequently applied.

8. Check the care plan for specific orders for passive range-of-motion exercises. A physical therapist or occupational therapist may come to assist the client with specific exercises.

Safety for the Client with a Cast

1. Check the house for throw rugs or objects on the floor. Remove any hazard that could cause the client to fall. Remind the client to leave a night-light on to prevent a fall in the middle of the night.

2. Remember that at first the client may not have a good sense of balance and may be unsteady in walking. Arrange the furniture so that the client may hold on to furniture or handrails while walking.

3. Assist the client in making changes in eating, dressing, writing, toileting, and walking.

Application of Cold

Cold applications are ordered to promote comfort and healing. Cold applications can ease pain and decrease the swelling of localized areas. The care plan will tell the aide when to apply ice and how to do it. All ice applications must be covered with a cloth. Never apply ice directly to the skin. A towel, face cloth, or fitted cover should be used against the skin. If using commercial ice packs have a minimum of two, so you can rotate their use. Ice packs can be bought in many different sizes. Some are very firm on the outside, whereas others are soft and flexible. They should be placed in the freezer until needed. See Procedure 63, Applying a Cold Application to the Client's Skin.

Personal Care

Some clients with functional or cognitive impairments may need assistance with personal care, such as dressing and undressing. See Procedure 64, Dressing and Undressing the Client.

PROCEDURE 63 APPLYING A COLD APPLICATION TO THE CLIENT'S SKIN

Purpose

- To ease pain
- To decrease swelling of localized area

Procedure

1. Assemble equipment: ice pack and cover.
2. Wash your hands.
3. Tell the client what you plan to do.
4. Cover the ice pack with a thin covering of cloth.
5. Give the ice pack to the client to apply to the affected area.
6. Leave the ice pack on for 20 minutes and remove. Check for signs of redness, whiteness, or cyanosis (blue color).

7. Remove the ice pack, wipe with alcohol wipes, and place in freezer.
8. Document completion of procedure and if the application of ice benefited the client. Occasionally, instead of lessening the client's discomfort, cold may increase the pain.
9. Wash your hands.

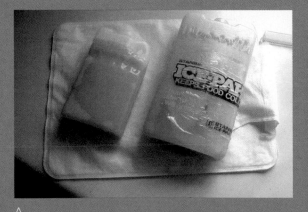

A

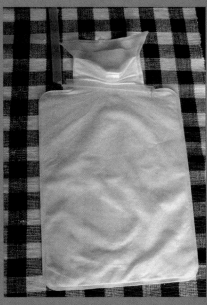

B

FIGURE 15-35 A. Commercial ice packs. B. Refillable ice pack.

PROCEDURE 64 DRESSING AND UNDRESSING THE CLIENT

Purpose

- To keep the client clean and comfortable
- To increase the client's self-image and well-being
- To reduce the client's discomfort and reduce the client's risk of strain or injury

NOTE: Do not allow the client to remain in night-clothes during the day (unless the care plan states it is all right). The client needs to know that it is daytime and needs to dress accordingly.

Procedure

1. Wash your hands and tell the client what you plan to do.
2. Assemble clean items and provide for privacy.
3. If the client is able, help the client to sit at the edge of the bed and dangle his or her legs. If the client is too weak to sit up, have the client lie flat on the bed. Place a sheet or robe over the client to avoid embarrassing or chilling the client.
4. Assist the client to put on undergarments. (A front-closing bra is very convenient for women with limited movement in their arms.) If the client has a weak leg, place the weak leg in first, then the other leg. Then put on clothing in the same manner. If the client can stand, pull the pants or slacks up to the waist. If the client must remain on the bed, ask the client to press the heels into the bed and raise the buttocks. While the client is in this position, quickly slide the pants or slacks up to the waist. If the client is unable to lift buttocks up, roll the client from side to side as you raise the slacks over the hips. Slacks with an elastic waist are preferred, as they are put on more easily than pants with zippers and buttons. Cotton jogging suits are becoming a popular option for elderly clients or those with disabilities. They are warm, easy to get off and on, and attractive. They also launder easily.
5. Assist the client to put on a shirt by placing the weaker arm in the sleeve first. Pull the shirt around for the client to place the other arm in the sleeve.
6. When removing a shirt, remove the sleeve of the strongest arm first, followed by the weaker arm. Encourage the client to do as much as he or she is able.

Mobility and Exercises

Individuals who become immobile due to illness are very vulnerable to complications. Common effects of immobility are blood clots, pneumonia, kidney stones, atrophy (wasting away) of the muscles, contractures (shortening of the muscles), and loss of motion in the joints of the body. Range-of-motion exercises are performed on clients to prevent these complications. If the client can do the exercises without the assistance of the aide or another person, they are called active range-of-motion exercises. If they are done with the support of another person, they are called passive range-of-motion exercises. There are special terms used to describe the movements that you will be doing when exercising the client. The following is a list of some of the common terms used in regard to movement of the body:

Abduction—to move a part away from the midline of the body

Adduction—to move a part toward the midline of the body

Dorsiflexion—bending the foot toward the ankle

Extension—straightening out a joint

Flexion—bending a joint

Opposition—touching each fingertip with the thumb

Internal rotation—turning a joint inward

External rotation—turning a joint outward

Plantar flexion—bending the foot downward

Pronation—turning the palms downward

Rotation—turning a joint in a circle

Supination—turning the palms upward

Guidelines for doing range-of-motion exercises include:

1. Do only the joints that are ordered to be exercised. Be sure to check the care plan. It is common for the physical therapist to record (on video or DVD) how the exercises should be done for the client and leave the recording at the client's home. This is a great tool for aides to see how the exercises should be performed.

2. Do the exercises only to the point of pain. It is a good idea to have the client take pain medication 30 minutes before doing the exercises, if indicated.

3. Do not exercise the head, unless the care plan states you should.

4. Start with the larger joints and work down to the smaller joints (e.g., start with the shoulder joint and end with the fingers).

5. Do one side of the body first and then repeat on the opposite side.

6. Provide privacy for the client and expose only the part of the body being exercised.

7. Do each movement at least three to five times.

8. The exercises can be incorporated when doing other client care procedures such as bathing or walking.

9. Exercise the client's body part in a smooth, gentle, but firm style.

10. Support the extremity above and below the joints being exercised.

11. Exercises can be done either in the bed or a chair. See Procedures 65 and 66.

PROCEDURE 65   PERFORMING ACTIVE RANGE-OF-MOTION EXERCISES

Purpose

- To increase muscle tone and strength in the client's body
- To restore function to injured parts of the body
- To prevent joint stiffness, contractures, and other complications of immobility

The following are stretch exercises the client can do without the assistance of an aide. The client may need to be reminded to do them. They should be done a minimum of three to five times on each extremity.

1. Chest stretch: Place both hands on the forehead with the arms bent at the elbow, bring the elbows forward, touching each other, then repeat (Figure 15-36A).

2. Shoulder stretch: Take one arm and stretch it over the opposite shoulder and hold for 10 seconds, then bring the arm to the side in extension. Do the same with the other arm (Figure 15-36B).

3. Rotation: Start with the arm in extension on the side of body, then bring the arm up and make circle with the arm. Do the same with the other arm (Figure 15-36C).

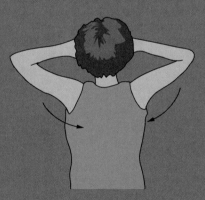

FIGURE 15-36A   Chest stretch.

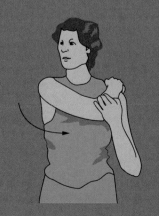

FIGURE 15-36B   Shoulder stretch.

(continued)

PROCEDURE 65   PERFORMING ACTIVE RANGE-OF-MOTION EXERCISES (*continued*)

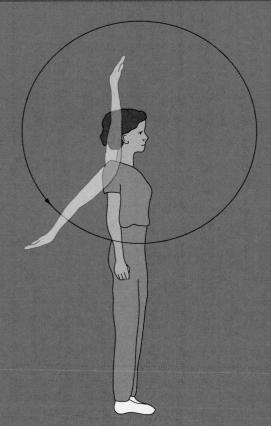

FIGURE 15-36C   Rotation of the arm.

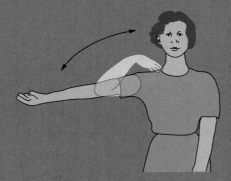

FIGURE 15-36E   Extension/flexion.

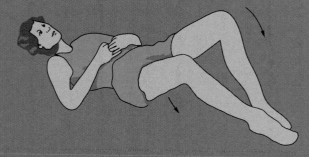

FIGURE 15-36F   Hip adduction.

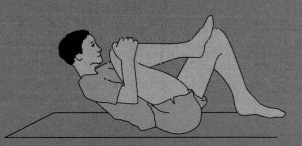

FIGURE 15-36G   Upper thigh stretch.

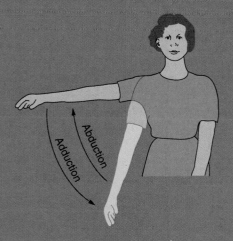

FIGURE 15-36D   Abduction/adduction.

4. Adduction/abduction: With the arm in extension, bring the arm toward the midline of the body, then bring the arm straight out to the side of the body, keeping the arm straight (Figure 15-36D). Be sure to do both arms.

5. Extension/flexion: Extend the arm straight out on the side of body, bend the elbow. and touch your shoulder with your hand. Then switch arms and do the opposite arm (Figure 15-36E).

6. Hip adduction: While lying on your back with the feet together, try to raise your buttocks by bending the knees, then try to hold buttocks up for 10 seconds (Figure 15-36F).

7. Upper thigh stretch: While lying down, hold on to one knee using both hands, bend your knee and try to bring your nose to your knee, and hold for 10 seconds (Figure 15-36G). Then do the opposite leg.

(*continued*)

PROCEDURE 65   PERFORMING ACTIVE RANGE-OF-MOTION EXERCISES (*continued*)

8. Hamstring stretch: Sit down on a bench and with the leg stretched out, bend the knee toward the upper body as far as you can; hold for 10 seconds (Figure 15-36H). Then do the other leg.

9. Quadriceps stretch: While facing the wall, place one hand on the wall, bring back the opposite leg as far as you can, and hold for 10 seconds (Figure 15-36I). Then do the other leg.

10. Calf stretch: While facing the wall, place both arms on the wall, bring one leg back about 3 feet from the wall with the arms stretched out, and hold this position for 10 seconds (Figure 15–36J). Repeat with the opposite leg.

11. Lower back stretch: While lying on the back, bring up one knee as far as you can, and hold for 10 seconds (Figure 15–36K). Repeat with the opposite leg.

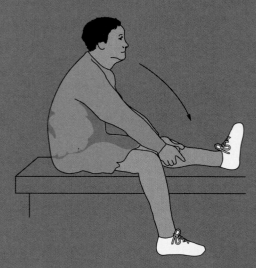

FIGURE 15-36H   Hamstring stretch.

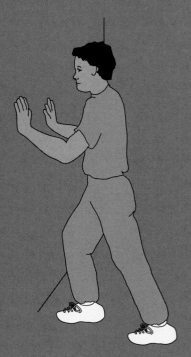

FIGURE 15-36J   Calf stretch.

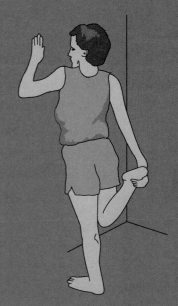

FIGURE 15-36I   Quadriceps stretch.

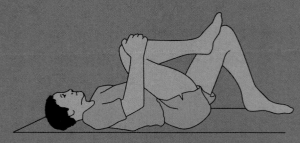

FIGURE 15-36K   Lower back stretch.

PROCEDURE 66 — PERFORMING PASSIVE RANGE-OF-MOTION EXERCISES

Purpose

- To increase muscle tone and strength in the client's body
- To restore function to injured parts of the body
- To prevent joint stiffness and contractures

Procedure

1. Wash your hands.
2. Read any special instructions for these exercises for the client on the care plan.
3. Tell client what you plan to do. Ask the client to assist as much as possible. Provide for privacy.
4. Exercise the shoulder. Turn the shoulder; arm bent, move hand toward head—outward rotation (Figure 15-37A). Turn shoulder; arm bent, move hand toward waist—inward rotation (Figure 15-37B).
5. Move arm in circle—rotation (Figure 15-38).
6. Bend elbow—flexion (Figure 15-39A).
7. Straighten elbow—extension (Figure 15-39B).
8. Turn lower arm, palm up—supination (Figure 15-40A).
9. Turn lower arm, palm down—pronation (Figure 15-40B).
10. Straighten wrist—extension (Figure 15-41A).
11. Bend wrist—flexion (Figure 15-41B).
12. Bend fingers—flexion (Figure 15-42A).
13. Straighten fingers—extension (Figure 15-42B).
14. Move fingers apart—abduction (Figure 15-43A).
15. Move fingers together—adduction (Figure 15-43B).

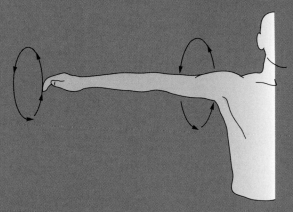

FIGURE 15-38   Move arm in circle—rotation.

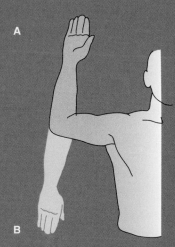

FIGURE 15-37   Exercise the shoulder. A. Turn shoulder; arm bent, move hand toward head—outward rotation. B. Turn shoulder; arm bent, move hand toward waist—inward rotation.

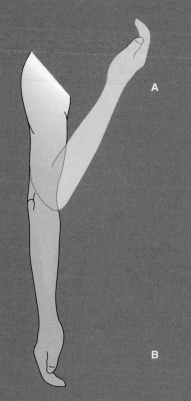

FIGURE 15-39   A. Bend elbow—flexion. B. Straighten elbow—extension.

(continued)

PROCEDURE 66 PERFORMING PASSIVE RANGE-OF-MOTION EXERCISES (*continued*)

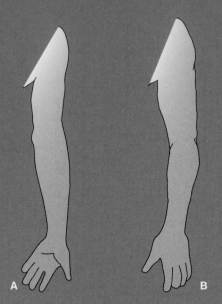

FIGURE 15-40 A. Turn lower arm, palm up—supination. B. Turn lower arm, palm down—pronation.

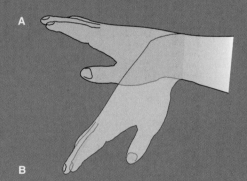

FIGURE 15-41 A. Straighten wrist—extension. B. Bend wrist—flexion.

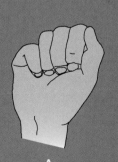

FIGURE 15-42 A. Bend fingers—flexion. B. Straighten fingers—extension.

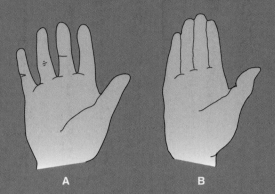

FIGURE 15-43 A. Move fingers apart—abduction. B. Move fingers together—adduction.

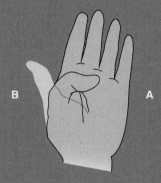

FIGURE 15-44 A. Bend thumb—flexion. B. Straighten thumb—extension.

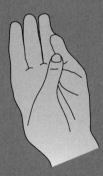

FIGURE 15-45 Touch thumb to fingers—opposition.

16. Bend thumb—flexion (Figure 15-44A).
17. Straighten thumb—extension (Figure 15-44B).
18. Touch thumb to fingers—opposition (Figure 15-45).
19. Bend hip—flexion (Figure 15-46A).
20. Straighten hip—extension (Figure 15-46B).

(*continued*)

PROCEDURE 66   PERFORMING PASSIVE RANGE-OF-MOTION EXERCISES (*continued*)

21. Roll leg inward—inward rotation (Figure 15-47A).
22. Roll leg outward—outward rotation (Figure 15-47B).
23. Bend ankle, foot upward—dorsiflexion (Figure 15-48A).
24. Bend ankle, foot downward—plantar flexion (Figure 15-48B).
25. Bend toes—flexion (Figure 15-49A).
26. Straighten toes (Figure 15-49B).
27. Go to the other side and repeat the movements for each joint.
28. Wash your hands.
29. Document completion of exercises and the client's reactions.

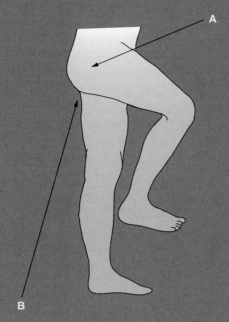

FIGURE 15-46   A. Bend hip—flexion. B. Straighten hip—extension.

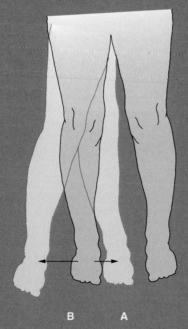

FIGURE 15-47   A. Roll leg inward—inward rotation. B. Roll leg outward—outward rotation.

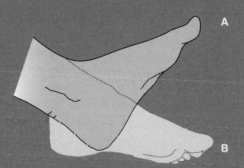

FIGURE 15-48   A. Bend ankle, foot upward—dorsiflexion. B. Bend ankle, foot downward—plantar flexion.

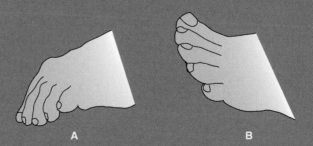

FIGURE 15-49   A. Bend toes—flexion. B. Straighten toes.

Rehabilitation

Part of the care plan for a client may include **rehabilitation**, which is the restoring of physical abilities to the highest level possible. Most rehabilitation is planned by the physical or occupational therapist. When a physical ability or skill has been lost, the client must relearn it or adjust to coping without it. A client who is blind must be taught self-feeding and learn how to become more independent. A stroke victim must again learn to use parts of the body that may be paralyzed. Range-of-motion exercises, speech therapy, and other kinds of rehabilitation may be needed. In most cases the home health aide will be involved in the rehabilitation program. A physical therapist will determine when the client is ready to begin walking again and what types of assistive devices may be necessary to maintain the client's safety. There are three basic walking patterns: nonweight-bearing, partial weight-bearing, and weight-bearing. With a nonweight-bearing pattern, all the weight is placed on the arms and uninvolved leg. A partial weight-bearing pattern means that minimal weight is placed on the toes. However, most weight is still on the arms and the uninvolved leg. To walk in a nonweight-bearing pattern the client uses crutches (Figure 15-50). The physical therapist measures the client to select the correct length of crutches and also teaches the client how to walk with the crutches.

To walk in a partial weight-bearing pattern the client can use crutches or a walker. A walker is a curved metal aid that gives maximum stability as the client moves. The client steps forward while holding onto the walker with both hands. Some walkers have wheels so that the client does not have to lift up the walker between steps (Figure 15-51). The wrists of the client should be even with the handgrips when the client's arms hang at the side. The client's arms should be slightly bent at the elbows when the client's hands are on the grips.

To walk with full weight bearing is the ability to use both legs when walking. A cane is used when the client is strong enough to bear full weight on both legs. It helps with balance as the client regains strength and mobility. The client holds the cane on the unaffected side. Many different types of canes are available. A standard cane is used for minor support. A special cane with four short legs, called a quad cane, is designed to bear a small amount of weight only (Figure 15-52). A cane is primarily used for balance.

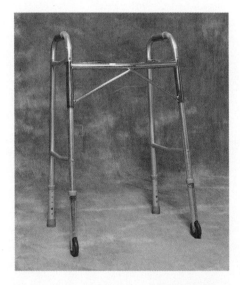

FIGURE 15-51   Roller walker.

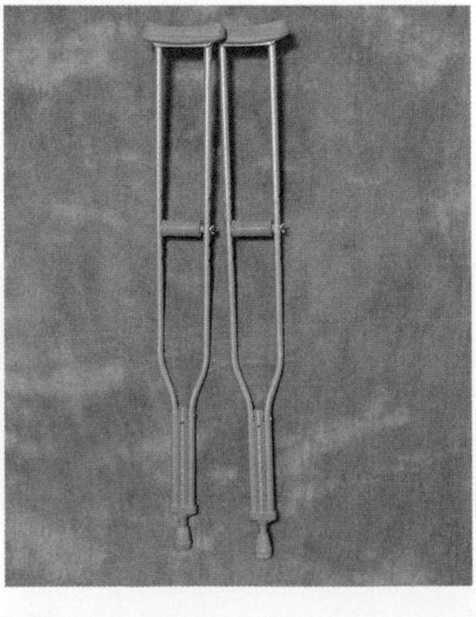

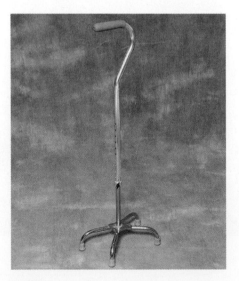

FIGURE 15-50   Crutches.

FIGURE 15-52   Four-point adjustable cane.

Check the rubber tips on the canes, walkers, and crutches because they wear out quickly if used on sidewalks.

Always have the client wear good supportive shoes with nonskid soles. Instruct clients to pick up their feet and not to look at their feet but to look straight ahead when ambulating.

See Procedure 67, Assisting the Client to Walk with Crutches, Walker, or Cane.

PROCEDURE **67** ASSISTING THE CLIENT TO WALK WITH CRUTCHES, WALKER, OR CANE

Purpose

• To provide support and maintain balance as client walks

Procedure

1. Apply the transfer belt unless care plan states not to.
2. Always walk on the client's weak side.
3. Walk slightly behind the client, holding onto the transfer belt from behind.
4. For the client using crutches, hold onto the transfer belt if the client feels uncomfortable using the crutches (Figure 15-53).
5. For the client using a walker, instruct the client to place the walker firmly before walking (Figure 15-54). If the client is strong enough, the walker and the weaker leg can be moved forward at the same time.
6. Stand lifts van be used to walk clients that are unable to use a walker or cane (Figure 15.55A). For the client using a cane (Figure 15-55B), instruct the client to hold the cane in the hand opposite the weaker leg. If the right ankle has been injured, the client should hold the cane in the left hand. The weak leg should move forward at the same time as the cane.
7. Balance is a judgmental situation. If the client has poor balance, the aide should support the weak side and use a transfer belt for safety reasons.
8. Document how far the client walked and the client's reaction.

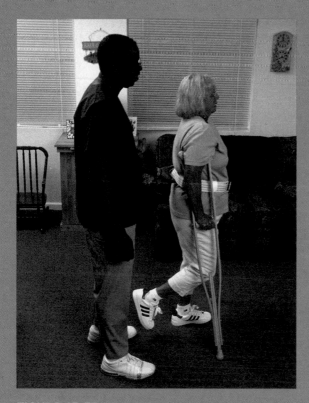

FIGURE 15-53 Walking with crutches.

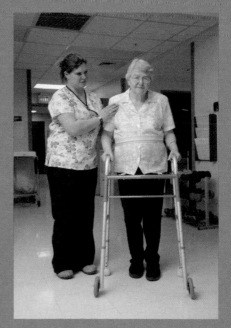

FIGURE 15-54 Walking with a walker.

(continued)

PROCEDURE 67 ASSISTING THE CLIENT TO WALK WITH CRUTCHES, WALKER, OR CANE (*continued*)

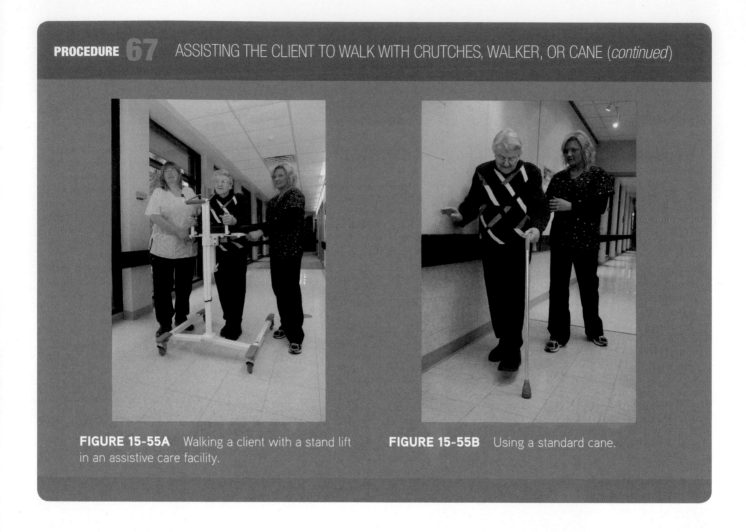

FIGURE 15-55A Walking a client with a stand lift in an assistive care facility.

FIGURE 15-55B Using a standard cane.

Emotional Aspects of Rehabilitation

While recovering from an illness, clients sometimes become discouraged and depressed and fear they will never feel better. A home health aide must give positive reinforcement to the client, but not raise the client's expectations beyond a reasonable level. It is better to emphasize the client's "abilities" rather than "disabilities." It is important to set realistic daily goals while at the same time working toward a long-term level of physical rehabilitation that can be reasonably expected. If, for instance, a client is relearning to walk after an accident or stroke, the client should be praised and consistently given positive feedback for being able to take one more step than the client took the day before. The aide and client could set a goal of walking from the chair to the door by the end of the week, for example. If that goal is reached, the client will be very happy. If, on the other hand, the goal is not quite reached, the aide can point out how much closer the client is than the client had been the week before. This is an example of positive reinforcement.

If an aide were working with a young person recovering from a fractured leg and the client claimed the exercises planned by the physical therapist were too painful and refused to do them, what would the aide do? A home health aide's job is to encourage the client and explain that although there is pain, it is best to follow a daily plan. Let the client know that he or she is responsible for his or her own recovery. Suggest that a little pain now is better than permanent stiffness, which can lead to permanent disability.

A person with a disability may have lost an ability many of us take for granted. However, he or she can be quite capable in other areas. The loss of sight, which makes assistance with bill paying necessary, for example, does not mean that a person cannot make correct decisions about his or her money. A person unable to walk is still quite capable of making choices or to direct his or her own care. The home health aide should treat every client, no matter his or her ability, with dignity and respect, enabling the client's right to make decisions, to maximize and support the physical, cognitive, and emotional abilities that do exist.

The aide should document the client's lack of motivation or interest. This may be a sign of depression that can be treated. The case manager may have some tips on ways to motivate this individual or may want to involve family members in supporting and motivating the client.

The important fact to know about rehabilitation is that the client's condition will determine the extent of rehabilitation possible. A blind person will probably never be able to see again. A client with crippling arthritis will probably never regain full use of the hands or feet. The aide's job is to assist clients to regain as much use of the body as is possible under a given set of circumstances. The aide should remember to give honest praise when a client is making progress and encourage a client who is reluctant to even try to help him- or herself.

Activities for the Client While Rehabilitating

The care plan is developed to make the client comfortable and to work toward recovery or to regain as much ability as possible. Several factors influence the care that is planned. The case manager and the home health aide must consider the person's age, condition, abilities, areas where assistance is needed, and personal interests before the accident or illness occurred. The personal habits and the client's personality also enter into the total care plan. The possibilities for activities are unlimited. A recreational or activity therapist can recommend activities geared to the abilities and interests of the client.

The value of activity must not be overlooked. Activities are useful in helping a person relearn skills that may have been lost because of the illness or accident. They also provide meaningful activity to a person who may be depressed due to the illness. An appropriate activity reminds a person of what he or she is still able to do. Activities are not just structured arts and crafts or music, but also include sorting socks, washing dishes, planning a meal, answering e-mails, playing card games on the computer, reading a newspaper, watching a movie, and sorting photos for a photo album, for example. A younger client is very computer literate and can be entertained all day using the computer. An older client may not be computer literate, and will need other activities to keep the mind active (Figure 15-56A, B, and C).

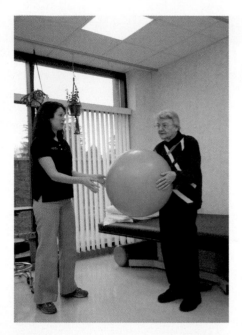

FIGURE 15-56A   Exercising with a large ball.

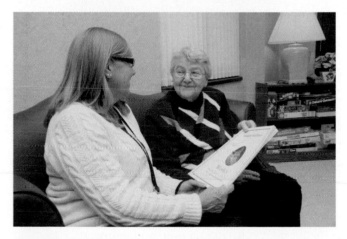

FIGURE 15-56B   Sharing photos.

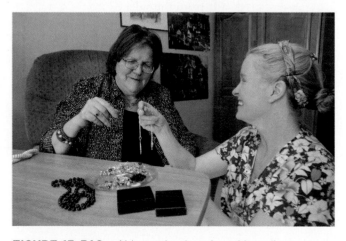

FIGURE 15-56C   Aide sorting jewelry with a client.

WORKBOOK REVIEW

Go to the workbook and complete the review exercises and activities for Unit 15.

REVIEW

1. You are going to pick up the laundry basket; you should do which of the following?
   a. Use only one hand for lifting.
   b. Flex your knees.
   c. Bend over at the waist.
   d. Keep your feet close together.

2. When lifting a client, you should keep your _____ straight.
   a. back
   b. hips
   c. knees
   d. thighs

3. When walking a client with a transfer belt,
   a. use an underhand grasp.
   b. use an overhand grasp.
   c. stand behind the client.
   d. lift from the side.

4. T   F   There are three basic walking patterns: nonweight-bearing, partial-weight-bearing, and weight-bearing.

5. T   F   With a nonweight-bearing person, all of the weight is placed on the arms and the involved leg.

Fill in the blanks for the following two questions:

6. Ligaments connect _____ to _____.

7. Tendons connect _____ to _____.

8. Match the term in Column I with the description in Column II.

    Column I

    _____ 1. plantar flexion

    _____ 2. dorsiflexion

    _____ 3. extension

    _____ 4. opposition

    _____ 5. adduction

    _____ 6. abduction

    _____ 7. flexion

    Column II

    a. bend

    b. straighten

    c. bend foot downward

    d. bend foot upward

    e. touch thumb with fingers

    f. bring arm toward the midline

    g. bring arm away from the body

9. Fill in the blank: If a person does the exercises without any assistance, they are called _____ range-of-motion exercises.

10. When dressing a client with right-sided weakness, do you place the *strong* or *weak* arm in a shirt first?

11. Fill in the blank: Arthroplasty is _____.

12. Arthritis can be treated by which of the following methods?

    a. Drug therapy

    b. Exercise program

    c. Surgery

    d. All of the above

Case Studies

13. Your client has a severe form of arthritis. The physical therapist has developed a care plan for your client; however, when you ask the client about it she tells you "it hurts too much to exercise." What three steps could you take to ensure that your client completes her exercises?

14. Your client, Mr. Clark, is a 78-year-old man with left-side weakness due to a stroke. He uses a walker when up. You need to transfer him from the bed to his recliner. How would you transfer him?

UNIT 16
Nervous System

KEY TERMS

amyotrophic lateral
  sclerosis (ALS)

aneurysm

aphasia

arteriogram

carotid arteries

carotid ultrasound

cerebrovascular
  accident (CVA)

computerized
  tomography (CT)

embolus

epilepsy

expressive aphasia

hemiplegia

hemorrhage

hypertension

magnetic resonance
  imaging (MRI)

multiple sclerosis (MS)

muscular dystrophy

neurologist

occupational therapist

paraplegia

Parkinson's disease

quadriplegia

receptive aphasia

seizures

thrombus

transient ischemic attack
  (TIA)

LEARNING OBJECTIVES

After studying this unit, you should be able to:

- List three functions of the nervous system

- Define paraplegia, hemiplegia, and quadriplegia

- Discuss the later signs and symptoms of Parkinson's disease

- Discuss the disease multiple sclerosis and its signs and symptoms

- Discuss the disease amyotrophic lateral sclerosis and its signs and symptoms

- Discuss epilepsy and two different types of seizures

- Explain how to care for a client having a generalized seizure

- Discuss the disease muscular dystrophy, its major signs and symptoms.

- List risk factors for stroke

- List two causes of a stroke

- List three signs or symptoms of TIA.

- Discuss long-term effects of a stroke

- List two types of aphasia

- Discuss the role of the aide in assisting a client recovering from a stroke

- Demonstrate the following:

  PROCEDURE 68   Caring for a Client Having a Seizure

Nervous System

The brain, spinal cord, and nerves make up the nervous system. This system is the communication center that sends messages to all parts of the body. It is the system that enables the body to see, hear, smell, taste, and touch. Sight, sound, taste, smell, and touch are known as the five body senses. The brain (Figure 16-1) is the master control or main switch of the nervous system. Messages are relayed to the brain from all parts of the body. The brain decides how to respond to each message (or stimulus) sent by the nerves. Each area of the brain performs a specialized duty. The brain alerts other control centers in the body so that the body correctly responds to a message.

The spinal cord can be compared to the electrical wiring system in a house. All the major nerves of the body are bound together in the spinal cord and lead into the brain. The spinal cord is protected by the spinal column. If the spinal column is damaged or diseased, the spinal nerves may be affected. For example, if a person suffers a broken back and the spinal cord is cut or damaged, the nerves below the cut can no longer send messages up to the brain. The parts of the body below the cut can no longer feel pain and the muscles would no longer move.

Paraplegia refers to paralysis of the lower part of the body and both legs. **Quadriplegia** refers to paralysis of both arms and both legs. Both paraplegia and quadriplegia can result from disease or injury to the brain or spinal cord. **Hemiplegia** is a paralysis of one side of the body. Figure 16-2 illustrates the portion of the body affected by hemiplegia, quadriplegia, and paraplegia. It is frequently the result of a **cerebrovascular accident (CVA)**, or stroke.

The nerves radiate from the spinal cord to all parts of the body, forming a network. The nerve endings might be compared to the electrical outlets in the house. In the body, the nerves are usually ready to receive stimuli. For instance, the hand touches a hot surface, the nerve sends the message to the spinal cord, and it goes to the brain. The brain sends back the message to move the hand off the hot surface. This entire process takes place in an instant so that one is only aware of the result. The time it takes to respond to a stimulus is known as reaction time. As the human body ages, reaction time often slows down a great deal. It also is affected when part of the brain has been damaged, as with a stroke.

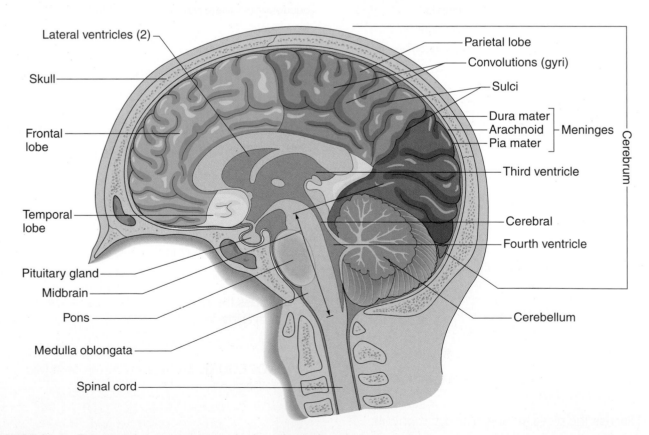

FIGURE 16-1 The central nervous system—brain and spinal cord.

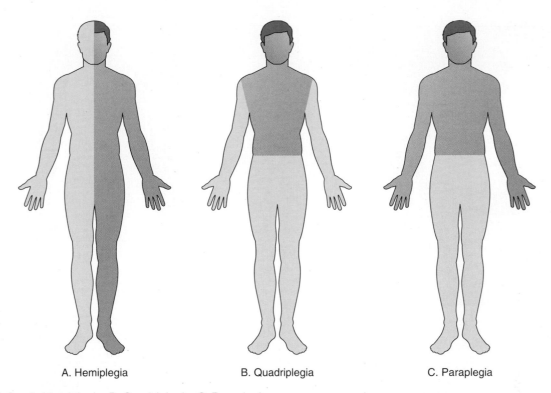

A. Hemiplegia   B. Quadriplegia   C. Paraplegia

FIGURE 16-2   A. Hemiplegia. B. Quadriplegia. C. Paraplegia.

Disorders of the Nervous System

Disorders of the nervous system can be the result of disease or injury to the brain or spinal cord. Many of these disorders cause mobility and cognitive problems. For example, shakiness in the extremities (tremors), difficulty walking, and mental changes are common symptoms of nervous system disorders. The home health aide can assist the client who has a nervous system disorder by being aware of the client's limitations, encouraging the client to complete the assigned exercises, and observing and reporting changes in the client's health status and functioning levels to the health care team.

Parkinson's Disease

Parkinson's disease, first documented by James Parkinson in 1817, is a progressive degeneration of nerve cells in the area of the brain that controls muscle movements. The disease results from the inability of these nerve cells to produce dopamine, which is necessary for the transmission of signals within the brain.

Parkinson's disease often starts in middle or late life and is progressive in nature, with symptoms worsening over time. At first the signs and symptoms are manageable with medication and exercise. As the disease progresses the signs and symptoms are more evident and less controlled by medication. Characteristics signs and symptoms of Parkinson's disease in the later stages are shakiness of the hands at rest (resting tremors), pill-rolling movement of thumb and fingers, reduced facial expressions (mask-like expression), very slow movements, slurred and poorly spoken speech, stiffness and rigidity of limbs, stooped posture, drooling of salvia, difficulty in swallowing food, and incontinence of bowel and bladder (Figure 16-3).

In its most severe form, the individual becomes incapacitated by rigidity and tremors (Figure 16-4). Personality and behavioral changes are common among individuals diagnosed with this disease, as is depression.

Treatment for Parkinson's disease involves drug therapy to restore the brain's supply of dopamine to reverse problems of the disease involving walking, movement, and tremors. The drugs do help in relieving the tremors. Common drugs used to treat this disease are Artane®, Cogentin®, and Sinemet®. Clients should be monitored for serious side effects such as involuntary movements, nausea, dizziness, and mental changes so that medications can be adjusted to suit the client. Timing of the medication is important, as a client may be having severe tremors, but an hour after taking the medication, the tremors may subside. This is the ideal time to bathe and feed the client. Eating a well-balanced, nutritious diet is very beneficial. In the later stages of the disease, food thickeners are

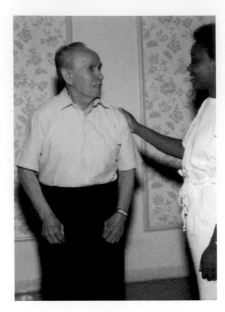

FIGURE 16-3 A characteristic symptom of Parkinson's disease is a flat, mask-like facial expression.

use to help the client swallow liquids. Regular exercise is another critical part of treatment. However, clients with Parkinson's disease will require many rest periods because their energy levels may go up and down throughout the day. Surgery can relieve some of the shaking and tremors in some cases. Participation in support groups and physical therapy programs can play an important role in helping the client maintain a positive mental attitude and avoid depression.

Multiple Sclerosis

Multiple sclerosis (MS) is a disease affecting the central nervous system, and is generally seen in young adults. In most cases, the disease begins with episodes that last only weeks or months that are separated by periods of remission (absence of symptoms). The cause of MS is not clearly understood. Multiple sclerosis produces a wide variety of symptoms, including poor coordination of muscle movement, numbness or tingling sensations, vision problems, such as blurred or double vision, paralysis of lower extremities, problems with bowel and bladder control, and problems with mental functions. Individuals with MS also suffer from a lack of energy and fatigue easily.

Currently there is no cure for MS; however, most people with MS live very productive lives and are able to work. Three prescription drugs that can be used to treat this disease are Tysobril®, Betaseron®, and Copaxone®. Corticosteroid drugs are also used to treat this disorder. Plasma exchange is a new method of treating the disease. Physical and occupational therapy are also an important

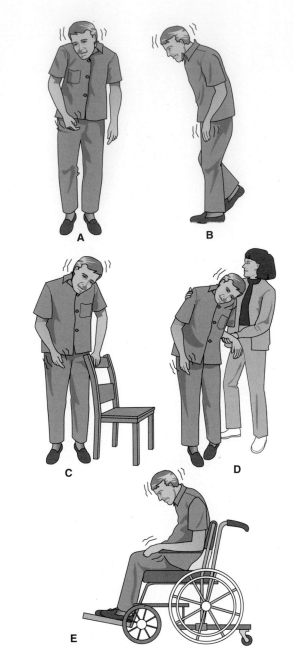

FIGURE 16-4 Progression of Parkinson's disease. A. The person leans slightly forward and develops flexion of an affected arm. B. The person stoops forward and walks with a shuffling gait. C. The person tends to shuffle faster and faster, leaning forward until he falls on his face. D. The disease progresses to the point of needing assistance for ambulation. E. The person has profound weakness and severe tremors. Ambulation becomes impossible.

part of an MS treatment plan. At first, people with MS are capable of doing all of their activities of daily living (ADLs), but as the disease progresses they may need total assistance in most ADLs. The average life expectancy is 35 years after the onset of the disease.

Amyotrophic Lateral Sclerosis

Amyotrophic lateral sclerosis (ALS) is more commonly known as Lou Gehrig's disease, after the famous baseball player who died from ALS. ALS is a progressive degeneration of the nerve cells in the brain and spinal cord that control the voluntary muscles. Its cause is unknown.

The signs and symptoms of ALS include slow loss of strength and coordination in one or more limbs, muscle twitches, and cramps; increasingly stiff, clumsy gait; and difficulty with swallowing, speaking, or breathing. The onset of ALS begins gradually, first affecting one upper limb and then the next one. Additional muscle areas then become affected and complete paralysis may result. The person's mind stays alert while his or her body wastes away, which is very hard for the family to witness. Following diagnosis, a person generally lives only 2 to 6 years.

Epilepsy

Epilepsy is a chronic brain disorder characterized by a sudden episode of intense electrical activity in the brain, which results in seizure activities. Epilepsy takes different forms, with various types of seizures. **Seizures** are classified as partial or generalized. Partial seizures do not involve the entire brain, only part of the brain. A client having this type of seizure may just stare into space or smack the lips, or pick on clothing. There is no loss of consciousness when having an attack, but the client does not remember doing the particular behavior. An example of the second type of seizure (generalized) is a grand mal seizure. In this type of seizure, the attack begins with a loud cry (aura), followed by the client falling to the ground and becoming unconscious. The entire body becomes stiff, followed by shaking of the entire body with foaming from the mouth due to overproduction of saliva. Fecal and urinary incontinence may also occur. The attacks last only 1 to 2 minutes. After an attack the client may be confused, drowsy, and weak, and may complain of having a headache. There are many drugs available to treat seizures and most are very effective, if the right medication is ordered for the right type of seizure. It is also important that the client take the seizure medication as prescribed. Some common seizure drugs are Dilantin®, Tegretol®, and Carbatrol®. If a client refuses to take the seizure medication, be sure to notify the case manager. A client with this diagnosis should also wear a Medic Alert bracelet or necklace. See Procedure 68, Caring for a Client Having a Seizure.

PROCEDURE 68   CARING FOR A CLIENT HAVING A SEIZURE

During the Seizure

1. Gently roll the client onto one side.
2. Keep the client safe. Removing any objects that the client may strike when thrashing about is the number one objective.
3. Support the head with something small that is nearby—such as a jacket or small pillow.
4. Keep calm and stay with the client.
5. Time the seizure with a watch and note the details of the seizure.
6. Don't try to restrain the client.
7. Loosen clothing around the client's neck.
8. Do not put your fingers or anything else in the client's mouth.
9. Clear the area of any danger—such as a chair or table.

After the Seizure

1. If the client has never had a seizure before, if the client has hurt him- or herself, if the seizure lasts more than a few minutes, or if the seizure recurs, call your agency immediately.
2. Always respect the dignity of the client. The client is often embarrassed when he or she regains consciousness.
3. Once the seizure is over, position the client on his or her side. This will allow for normal breathing and for any vomitus, saliva, or blood to drain from the mouth.
4. Confusion may be present for a period of time. Watch the client until there is complete return of mental function. A client may feel very tired after a seizure.
5. Treat any bumps, bruises, or cuts that may have resulted from the seizure. The client may have become incontinent during the seizure and will need to be cleaned up.
6. Document the details of the seizure for the health care provider. It is important to note the duration of the seizure, extremities involved, precipitating factors, and any other characteristics noted.

Muscular Dystrophy

Muscular dystrophy is a progressive disease caused by insufficient nourishment of the muscles. The lack of a key protein essential to muscle function causes the muscles to decrease in size and grow weaker. Muscular dystrophy is a rare disease that is inherited. The disease usually strikes at an early age, usually before 3, and affects only boys. Muscular dystrophy ultimately cripples the person entirely.

Signs and symptoms of the disease are muscle weakness, lack of coordination, clumsy gait, inability to lift the arms over the head, and progressive crippling resulting in a loss of mobility. By the teenage years, most clients require a wheelchair. Many persons with muscular dystrophy die before adulthood. There is no cure. The best treatment regimen involves physical therapy to help minimize deformities.

Spinal Cord Injuries

A spinal injury can cause loss of sensation and function in body parts below the spinal injury. Most spinal cord injuries are the result of traffic or industrial accidents, falls, gunshot wounds, and sports and war injuries. The extent of impairment will depend on where the spinal cord was severed. Many of these clients will spend the remainder of their lives in a wheelchair, with little hope of ever walking again.

Cerebrovascular Accident (CVA) or Stroke

Stroke is the common term for cerebrovascular accident (CVA). The blood flow to a specific area of the brain is interrupted, resulting in sudden acute symptoms such as paralysis, vision disturbances, language problems, mental confusion, or a combination of these.

Stroke is caused by a lack of oxygen and nutrients to the brain cells. This interruption of blood to the brain may be due to one of the following three reasons: an **aneurysm** (a ballooning out of the wall of an artery) that breaks open and causes a **hemorrhage**, an **embolus** (a moving blood clot) that causes complete blockage of an artery, or a **thrombus** (a blood clot that forms inside an artery) that can cause a blockage of blood flow to the brain cells (Figure 16-5). Brain cells deprived of circulation for even a few seconds stop functioning. If the circulation stops for a few minutes, brain cells die. Once brain cells are dead, they cannot be brought back to life. Unlike other cells in the body, new brain cells do not form to replace damaged ones.

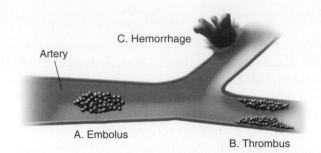

FIGURE 16-5 A. Embolus. B. Thrombus. C. Aneurysm that has broken open, causing a hemorrhage.

Risk Factors for Stroke. Often, long before a stroke occurs, there are conditions that are now recognized as associated with an increased risk of stroke. These are:

- **Hypertension**—sustained, elevated blood pressure
- Over the age of 55
- Personal or family history of stroke, heart attack, or **transient ischemic attack (TIA)**
- High cholesterol
- Cigarette smoking or exposure to secondhand smoke
- Diabetes
- Obesity
- Overuse of alcohol or illicit drugs
- Physical inactivity

An individual who has one or more of these conditions or habits has a greater risk of developing a stroke than those without them.

Diagnostic Tests for a Stroke. Clinical evaluation of the stroke client usually includes an examination by a **neurologist** (a doctor specializing in diseases of the brain). A **carotid ultrasound** may show narrowing or clotting of the carotid arteries (Figure 16-6). An **arteriogram**, in which the doctor inserts a catheter in the groin, followed by injection of dye into the carotid artery, provides x-ray images of the arteries. In **magnetic resonance imaging (MRI)**, a strong magnetic field and radio waves are used to generate a 3-D view of the brain. This test can detect brain tissue damaged by an ischemic stroke. A **computerized tomography (CT)** scan provide 3-D images of blood vessels of the neck and brain and show hemorrhages.

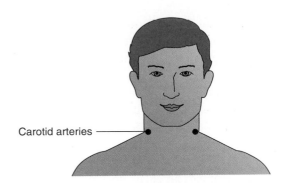

FIGURE 16-6 The carotid arteries are located on both sides of the neck.

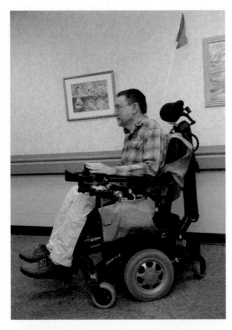

FIGURE 16-7 A client with a right-sided stroke operating a motorized wheelchair.

Possible Effects After a Stroke. Stroke can affect an individual in many different ways, depending on which part of the brain has been damaged. Among the possible deficits and problems are:

- Physical deficits
  - Paralysis or complete loss of strength or mobility in a part of the body, usually the arm, leg, and face on one side.
  - Pain and numbness or other strange sensations in parts of the body affected by the stroke
  - Loss of sensation (feeling) in parts of the body, usually on one side
  - Loss of bladder and bowel control
  - Difficulty in eating and swallowing
  - Loss of coordination, such as unsteady gait
- Perceptual/cognitive (thinking) deficits
  - More withdrawn and less social
  - Speech and language disability—difficulty thinking of and saying words or difficulty using or understanding words
  - Denial or neglect of the right or left part of the body and environment
  - Very sensitive to temperature changes
  - Difficulty performing tasks in proper sequence
  - Disrupted sleep–wake cycles
  - Uncontrolled laughter or crying (labile)
  - Confusion, forgetfulness, memory loss, impaired judgment
- Personal/family problems
  - Loss of job
  - Inadequate financial resources
  - Loss of independence
  - Loss of sexual capacity
  - Loss of self-esteem
- Psychological problems (mood)
  - Depression, apathy
  - Anger, hostility
  - Euphoria
- Environmental problems
  - Architectural barriers in the home
  - Lack of accessible transportation

Not all of these problems happen to each individual. When any of them do happen, there are degrees of difficulty. Most of these problems can be improved over time. However, after a stroke, the person will always have limitations (Figure 16-7).

Treatment Immediately After a Stroke. An aspirin is usually given to a client who apparently just had a stroke to restore blood flow to the brain. A new drug called tissue plasminogen activator (TPA) can be injected through a vein to help the client recover more fully. This drug needs to be injected within a 4- to 5-hour window of the stroke occurring, which is done in an emergency room

When a stroke is occurring, remember **BE FAST**:

B = Sudden loss of coordination and **B**alance
E = Sudden loss of vision or double vision (**E**yes)
F = Weakness on one side of the **F**ace
A = **A**rm or leg weakness on one side
S = Difficulty speaking or understanding **S**peech
T = **T**ime symptoms started

If a client experience any of these, call 911 and have the ambulance come.

Rehabilitation After a Stroke.   A care plan will be developed by the home health team for each individual client. The plan will be implemented once the client has returned home. The goal of the plan is to have the client return to the highest level of function as possible. The client will need to be encouraged continuously to do as much as possible with as little assistance as possible from others. At times it may be easier for an aide to dress or feed the client, but it must be remembered that the goal of care is to have the client do it, not the aide.

After a stroke the client will most likely have one-sided weakness. The client will need to do exercises to regain strength and function to the side of the body that is weak. If the client is unable to do the special exercises, called range-of-motion exercises, the aide will need to assist the client in doing the exercises. The case manager or physical therapist will train the aide to do the exercises. Exercises will be helpful in the prevention of further immobility and will improve the client's self-image.

Ambulation is important in the rehabilitation of a person after a stroke. The client may need to have a brace applied to the weak leg for support before ambulating. Check to see that the brace fits properly and does not cause skin irritation. Occasionally a client's sight may be affected after a stroke. Be sure when you walk a client there is a clear pathway without obstacles in the way. You, the home health aide, may see these obstacles, but your client may not. Another example would be that the client only sees half of his plate of food and not the whole plate; the aide may need to turn his plate around once he finishes one side.

Dressing is another area in which the client may need assistance. If you need to assist the client to put on a shirt, remember to put the shirt on the weak arm first and then the strong arm. If the client is unable to button the shirt, Velcro closures can be substituted in place of buttons. Elastic-waist slacks will be easier to slip on and off than pants with belts and zippers.

Oral care is of special importance for the client with a stroke. Before mealtime, it is important to do routine oral care, and if the client has dentures, encourage the client to wear them. The client may need assistance in eating or the client may need to use one of the many assistive feeding devices now available. An occupational therapist may work with the client in restoring the ability to eat without the assistance of others. It will be the home health aide's job to follow through with the plan designed by the occupational therapist. Be sure to check the inside of the weak side of the mouth for food particles after the client has finished eating. The client does not have feeling on the paralyzed side and often food becomes lodged in the cheek and the client may not know it.

Bowel and bladder retraining may also be part of the rehabilitation of a stroke client. The aide should follow the schedule on the care plan.

Communication Problems.   The client with a stroke often has a great deal of trouble communicating. Aphasia is a condition in which the ability to speak is impaired. Aphasia is common after a client has had a stroke. Aphasia can affect the ability to talk, listen, read, or write. The client's speech may be slurred, distorted, and slowed. A client who has receptive aphasia does not understand the words someone else says. In this case, it may be better to have a communication board to point to (Figure 16-8). In a few cases the client might understand all words coming into the brain, but he is unable to respond appropriately. An example of this might be when an aide asks him if he is hungry and he responds with "no" and in reality he wanted to say "yes" but the answer came out just the opposite of what he wanted. This is extremely frustrating to both you and the client. This type of aphasia is called expressive aphasia because the client is unable to express himself correctly. The care plan will state how to communicate more effectively. Sometimes the only words a stroke client uses are curse words or nonsense syllables. This is called automatic speech (involuntary speech). The client's use of curse words can be somewhat embarrassing, as the client may have never used these words before he or she had a stroke. If your client does use curse words, do not take it seriously because the client has no knowledge of what he or she is saying. In speaking to a stroke client, the aide should use simple sentences that require only short and simple answers from the client. Speaking clearly and simply aids the client's understanding.

Clients who normally wear glasses should continue to wear them even if their sight has been affected by the stroke. This makes the client feel less changed in outward appearance. The same is true if the client wears dentures or a hearing aid.

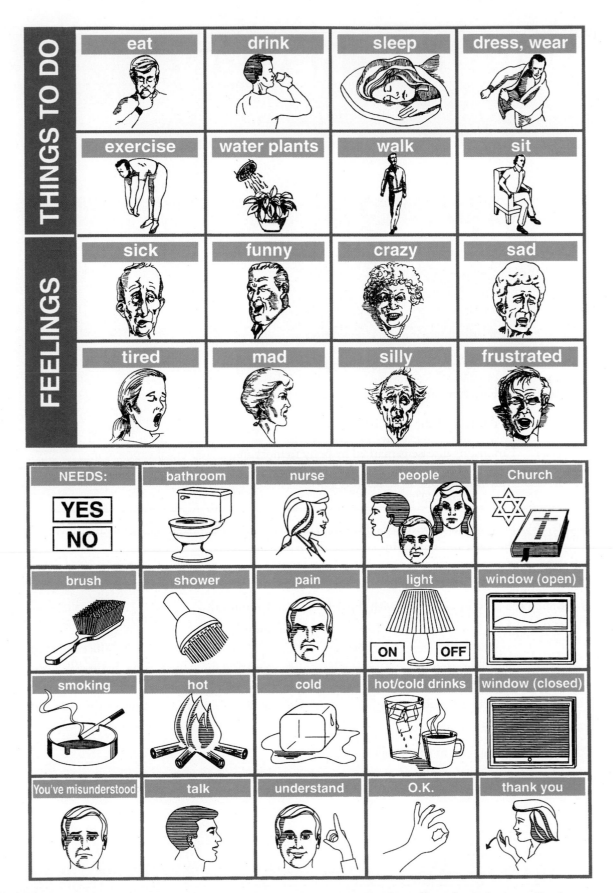

FIGURE 16-8   A communication board is often used to increase communication with a client who has aphasia.

WORKBOOK REVIEW

Go to the workbook and complete the review exercises and activities for Unit 16.

REVIEW

Fill in the blanks for the following three questions:

1. Paralysis of the lower part of the body and both legs is called _____.

2. Paralysis of both arms and both legs is referred to as _____.

3. Paralysis of one side of the body is known as _____.

4. T   F   Parkinson's disease is marked by body tremors and a fixed facial expression.

5. T   F   Amyotrophic lateral sclerosis is a disease where there is slow loss of strength and coordination in one or more limbs.

6. T   F   In multiple sclerosis, the disease is characterized by periods of remission and then periods when the signs and symptoms are very much evident.

7. T   F   Muscular dystrophy strikes only males.

8. Match the term in Column I with the definition in Column II.

   Column I
   ____ 1. amyotrophic lateral sclerosis
   ____ 2. multiple sclerosis
   ____ 3. Parkinson's disease
   ____ 4. muscular dystrophy
   ____ 5. seizures

   Column II
   a. inability of nerve cells to produce dopamine
   b. electrical discharges of the brain cells disorganized
   c. Lou Gehrig's disease
   d. double vision and tingling of the extremities
   e. a rare disease that is inherited in many cases

9. List four warning signs of a stroke.

   _____
   _____
   _____
   _____

10. A client who has had a stroke or CVA has difficulty speaking, a disorder that is called
    a. aphasia.
    b. lethargy.
    c. paraplegia.
    d. mutism.

11. Mr. Kane has had a stroke. Which of the following signs would you expect Mr. Kane to display?
    a. Aphasia
    b. Hemiplegia
    c. Lip drooping on one side of the face
    d. All of the above

Case Studies

12. While you are visiting Ms. Jones at her home, she has a seizure. What steps should be taken to ensure that she does not hurt herself during the seizure? What should you observe about the seizure? What steps should you take after the seizure has subsided?

13. Ms. Hoff, age 79, just returned home from the hospital after having a right-sided stroke. Her speech is slurred, distorted, and slow, and she answers questions incorrectly. She walks with a four-point cane, using her left arm. What type of aphasia does she have—receptive or expressive? On what side of her body would you stand if you were going to assist her to walk?

UNIT 17
Circulatory System

KEY TERMS

activities of daily living
  (ADLs)
anemia
angina pectoris
angiogram
arrhythmias
arterial insufficiency
arteriosclerosis
arteries

blood tests
catheterization
collateral circulation
congestive heart failure
  (CHF)
echocardiogram
electrocardiogram (EKG)
gangrene
hemophilia

hypotension
iron deficiency anemia
ischemia
leukemia
magnetic resonance
  imaging (MRI)
myocardial infarction
myocardium
nitroglycerin

pernicious anemia
phlebitis
pulmonary embolus
sickle cell anemia
sublingually
thrombophlebitis
venous insufficiency

LEARNING OBJECTIVES

After studying this unit, you should be able to:

- Name the main function of the heart

- Name three types of blood vessels

- List at least six risk factors for heart problems

- Describe an angina attack and when it usually occurs

- List four tests used in diagnosing heart conditions

- Describe the signs and symptoms of a myocardial infarction

- Describe signs and symptoms of congestive heart failure

- Describe phlebitis and venous insufficiency

- Describe arterial insufficiency

- Describe three ways the aide can assist in the care of a client with venous insufficiency.

- List six blood disorders

- Demonstrate the following:

  PROCEDURE 69   Applying Elastic Stockings

The organ that provides power to the body system is the heart. The heart is a hollow muscular organ about the size of a closed fist (Figure 17-1). Although it is one of the most important organs in the body, it has only one job—to pump blood throughout the body. From the time the fetus is 3 1/2 months old, the heart continues to pump until death.

Circulatory System

The heart has four chambers, the right and left atria and the right and left ventricles. The right atrium receives oxygen-poor blood from the tissues. This blood is pumped to the lungs by the right ventricle, where carbon dioxide is exchanged for oxygen from the lungs. The oxygenated blood is received by the left atrium, which then pumps it to the left ventricle; it is then pumped out to all parts of the body (Figure 17-2).

Connected to these chambers are the largest blood vessels in the circulatory system. There are three kinds of blood vessels. The arteries carry blood away from the heart to the body cells. The arteries join the tiny blood vessels, called capillaries. The capillaries meet the veins. The veins carry the blood back to the heart. It takes 1 minute for blood to leave the heart; travel through the arteries, capillaries, and veins; and return to the heart. This is a cycle that continues each minute of the day.

As the heart contracts (squeezes together) and expands (relaxes), it pushes the blood into the arteries. The arteries contract and expand in the same rhythm as the heart. The pulse measured at the wrist is the expansion of the radial artery. The blood carried in the arteries is a rich, bright red color. Venous blood is a darker red because it is low in oxygen. There are many age-related changes that affect the cardiovascular system. Heart muscle fibers become calcified and thick. The valves of the heart stiffen and become more rigid. The blood vessels become less flexible. These changes can increase the risk for older adults to develop heart disease.

Risk Factors

Because of the number of deaths due to heart problems, many research studies have been conducted on individuals

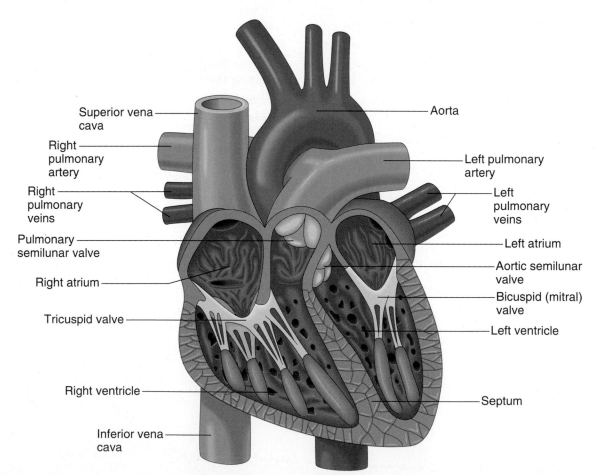

FIGURE 17-1   The heart is a hollow muscular organ about the size of a closed fist.

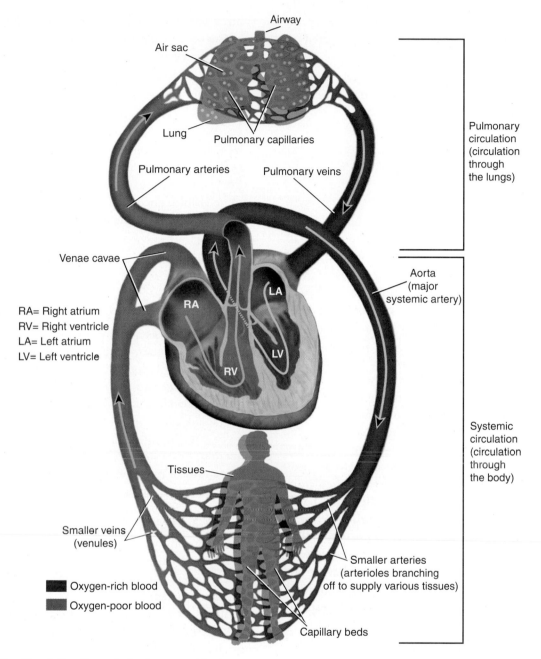

FIGURE 17-2 Circulation through the lungs and body.

with heart problems. Research has documented the following as major risk factors in heart disease:

- Heredity—Children of parents with heart problems have a greater risk of developing heart conditions.

- Male sex—Men have greater risk than women and have heart attacks earlier in life.

- Age—The majority of heart attacks occur in individuals who are 64 or older.

- Smoking—Long-time smokers have twice as many heart attacks as nonsmokers.

- High blood pressure—High blood pressure increases the heart's workload and weakens the heart and also the blood vessels in the brain, which eventually can cause either a heart attack or stroke.

- High cholesterol levels—As cholesterol levels increase, the risk of having heart disease increases.

- Diabetes—People with diabetes have a greater incidence of heart attacks.

- Obesity—Individuals who are 30% overweight have a greater incidence of heart disease.

- Physical inactivity—Inactive individuals are nearly twice as likely to develop heart problems compared to those who are active.
- Stress—Stress and anxiety can trigger the arteries to tighten. This can raise the blood pressure and increase the risk of heart attack.

Heart and Circulatory System Disorders

The number one killer of individuals in the United States is heart disease. Circulatory problems affect people of all ages. Cardiovascular disease refers to heart and blood vessel disorders including coronary artery disease (CAD) and heart valve disease, abnormal rhythms (arrhythmias), heart conditions present at birth (congenital defects), congestive heart failure (CHF), and other heart conditions. The majority of individuals who survive after a heart attack will need continuous medical care and a few will need assistance with activities of daily living (ADLs). A home health aide has an important role to play in the recovery of these clients. Some of these clients will need assistance with ADLs for the rest of their lives.

In many cases, disorders of the heart and circulatory system force people to change their lifestyles. Many people become very frightened when a heart or circulatory condition is diagnosed. The emotional effects can be almost as crippling as the illness itself. People may think they will be permanently disabled or wonder how they can support themselves and their families. People who have had one heart attack may be afraid of having another heart attack. As a result, they often avoid moving about or doing any exercise. Inactivity usually leads to boredom, irritability, and depression.

Tests Used to Diagnose Heart Conditions

- Blood tests—A blood test to diagnose congestive heart failure is called a BNP. If the heart is overworked, this hormone in the blood will be elevated. Blood tests can also measure the cholesterol level and cardiac enzymes of the client.
- Chest x-ray—An x-ray of the chest will show the size and shape of the client's heart.
- Echocardiogram—This test uses sound waves to produce a detailed video image of the heart's size, structure, and function. This test can determine how the heart is pumping and what areas are not pumping,

- Stress test—In a stress or exercise test, the client exercises on a treadmill and the heart rate is monitored while the client is exercising.
- Electrocardiogram (EKG)—This test measures the electrical impulses given off by the heart.
- Angiogram—This test is also called a coronary catheterization (a tube is placed in a blood vessel to visualize the heart). A catheter is placed into a blood vessel in the groin. The catheter is guided into the heart. A dye is injected into the arteries to make the arteries more visible. The test will show where the arteries are narrowed and how the heart is pumping.
- Magnetic resonance imaging (MRI)—This test uses magnetic fields and radio waves to show detailed images of the heart.

Angina Pectoris

Angina pectoris is a symptom of a condition called myocardial ischemia, which occurs when the heart muscle (myocardium) does not get an adequate supply of blood and oxygen to do its work. Lack of blood supply is called ischemia. Angina pectoris is a mild pain in the chest radiating to the left arm and up through the neck area; or a feeling of fullness, pressure, aching, burning, squeezing, or painful feeling in the chest, back, or jaw. This condition results from lack of oxygen in the heart muscle due to constricted blood vessels. An attack can last from a few seconds to several minutes. It may occur after physical exertion or it may occur after eating, excitement, and exposure to cold. The client becomes pale and ashen and the body stiffens. Blood pressure increases dramatically (hypertension). The client becomes flushed and perspires heavily.

Immediate treatment for angina is physical rest. If this is not the first angina attack, the client is likely to have nitroglycerin on hand to take immediately. A common emergency medication used for angina is nitroglycerin. Nitroglycerin may be taken sublingually, in which case the tablet is placed under the tongue. A spray is also available that can be sprayed under the tongue. Nitroglycerin can also be applied topically in the form of a nitro-patch placed on the skin (Figure 17-3). The nitroglycerin is absorbed through the skin; a patch provides 24 hours of medication. Old nitroglycerin patches should be removed and the area of skin under the patch cleansed before a new patch is applied. This is to prevent a buildup effect from residual nitroglycerin. Application sites should be alternated daily to prevent skin irritation.

Nitroglycerin opens the blood vessels to increase the blood flow. The effects of the drug occur within 2 to

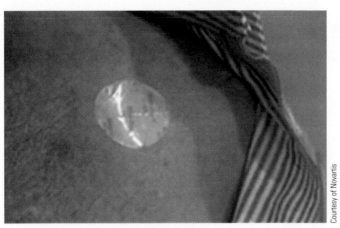

FIGURE 17-3 The client may receive nitroglycerin through the skin by means of a transdermal patch.

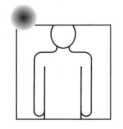

The symptoms are:

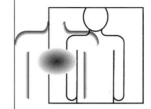

An uncomfortable feeling in your chest —
- Heaviness
- Pressure
- Tightness
- A squeezing sensation

It can spread to your left arm, sometimes to both arms and to your neck and jaw.

You may also get sweaty, feel like vomiting and have trouble breathing.

Take action:

Go to the nearest hospital emergency room, or call 911 if you're too sick to go on your own. Do it right away! New treatments can save your life and help you recover. But you must act quickly. The quicker you act the better your chances. Every minute counts.

FIGURE 17-4 Symptoms of a heart attack.

3 minutes. The pain from angina is usually relieved in 5 to 10 minutes. If three tablets taken over a time span of 15 minutes do not provide relief, emergency care is required.

Myocardial Infarction

Myocardial infarction is more commonly known as a coronary, or a major, heart attack. A myocardial infarction is a condition in which a blood vessel of the heart muscle closes or is blocked by a blood clot. The size and location of the incident determines the seriousness of the attack. There can be permanent damage to the heart. In the case of permanent damage, parts of the heart muscle die and **collateral circulation** may develop. This means that other small blood vessels take over the job of bringing blood to the heart muscle. These smaller vessels actually become enlarged so they can carry the required amount of fresh, oxygenated blood to the heart muscle. The symptoms of a heart attack are shown in Figure 17-4.

The client may go into shock and collapse. Prompt emergency treatment is needed and is begun in the ambulance and continued in the hospital.

Congestive Heart Failure (CHF)

Congestive heart failure is a condition in which the heart does not pump effectively. This condition can affect the right or left side of the heart, or even both sides at the same time. This is most often caused by heart muscle damage. Thus, the heart's pumping action is weakened. The signs and symptoms of congestive heart failure include a cough, shortness of breath (dyspnea), bluish-tinged skin and nails (cyanosis), dizziness, weakness, rapid and irregular heartbeat, and retention of fluid (edema). Fluid (frothy pink sputum) may accumulate in the lungs, causing pneumonia.

Clients with congestive heart failure are encouraged to stay in an upright or semi-upright position (head higher than feet). The client will need to have activities spaced throughout the day to prevent becoming overly fatigued. When sitting in a chair, the client will need to have the legs slightly elevated and never crossed.

Refer to Figure 17-5 for a summary of the effects of congestive heart failure.

Arteriosclerosis

Arteriosclerosis is a condition in which the **arteries** become hard and lose their soft, rubber-like stretchiness. It is caused by a buildup of fatty deposits on the inside walls of the blood vessels. This disease takes many years to develop and once symptoms appear, the disease is fairly well advanced. Individuals who smoke and have high cholesterol and high blood pressure are at the greatest risk. A client who has high cholesterol can be

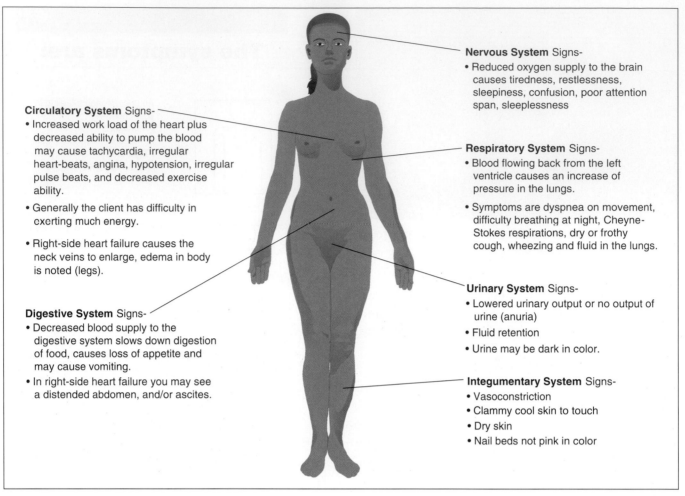

Nervous System Signs-
- Reduced oxygen supply to the brain causes tiredness, restlessness, sleepiness, confusion, poor attention span, sleeplessness

Circulatory System Signs-
- Increased work load of the heart plus decreased ability to pump the blood may cause tachycardia, irregular heart-beats, angina, hypotension, irregular pulse beats, and decreased exercise ability.
- Generally the client has difficulty in exerting much energy.
- Right-side heart failure causes the neck veins to enlarge, edema in body is noted (legs).

Respiratory System Signs-
- Blood flowing back from the left ventricle causes an increase of pressure in the lungs.
- Symptoms are dyspnea on movement, difficulty breathing at night, Cheyne-Stokes respirations, dry or frothy cough, wheezing and fluid in the lungs.

Urinary System Signs-
- Lowered urinary output or no output of urine (anuria)
- Fluid retention
- Urine may be dark in color.

Digestive System Signs-
- Decreased blood supply to the digestive system slows down digestion of food, causes loss of appetite and may cause vomiting.
- In right-side heart failure you may see a distended abdomen, and/or ascites.

Integumentary System Signs-
- Vasoconstriction
- Clammy cool skin to touch
- Dry skin
- Nail beds not pink in color

FIGURE 17-5   Congestive heart failure—systems involved.

placed on one of the newer anticholesterol drugs such as Lipitor® (atorvastatin), Zocor® (simvastatin), and Pravachol® (pravastatin).

Phlebitis

Phlebitis occurs when the lining of a vein becomes inflamed, causing a clot to form in the vein. This usually occurs in one leg, which may become swollen and painful to touch. The area may feel warm. The health care provider may order elastic bandages to be applied to the affected leg or to both legs.

Venous Insufficiency

Venous insufficiency is due to damage of the veins that return blood to the heart. The symptoms are chronic aching, edema, and discoloration of the lower extremities. The client may develop leg ulcers due to lack of oxygen available to these tissues. Clients with venous insufficiency are at risk of developing **thrombophlebitis**, which occurs when the vein becomes inflamed and a clot forms. The signs and symptoms of this condition are tenderness, redness, warmth over the vein, and pain in the calf of the leg when the client flexes his or her foot. As part of the treatment for this condition the aide may have to assist clients with the application of elastic stockings, which promote venous blood return. The client should be discouraged from standing or sitting for any prolonged period of time. It is important to have the legs elevated when the client is sitting to help lessen pain and edema, and to increase venous flow. A serious complication of thrombophlebitis is a **pulmonary embolus**, which is a clot that has broken away and traveled to the lungs. The symptoms of pulmonary embolus are shortness of breath, chest pain, and increased heart rate. This is a life-threatening condition that requires immediate medical attention.

Elastic Hose

Support hose are ordered for post-surgical client and clients who have swelling of their legs and ankles. Apply the stockings with the client lying down. The stockings are usually applied before the client gets up in the morning and removed before going to bed. Elastic hose come in a variety of sizes and lengths. They need to be supportive but not too tight. If they are too loose, they lose their effectiveness. The nurse usually measures the client's legs and orders the stockings. The stockings are usually washed by hand and placed in the bathroom to dry overnight. Do not wash in hot water, as that will damage the elasticity of the stockings. Other names for this type of stocking are TEDS® hose and Ace stockings. See Procedure 69, Applying Elastic Stockings.

PROCEDURE 69   APPLYING ELASTIC STOCKINGS

Purpose

- To prevent swelling of the feet and ankles
- To prevent formation of blood clots in the legs
- To increase blood circulation in the legs

Procedure

1. Wash your hands.
2. Tell the client what you plan to do. Provide for privacy.
3. With the client lying down, expose one leg at a time.
4. Turn the stocking inside out to the heel by placing your hand inside the stocking and grasping the heel (Figure 17-6A).
5. Position the stocking over the foot and heel of the client, making sure the heel of the stocking is in the proper place. If the client just had a bath, apply a thin coat of powder on the legs to make application easier (Figure 17-6B).
6. Slide the remaining stocking over the foot and heel (Figure 17-6C).
7. Continue to pull the stocking over the calf or thigh. The stocking can be either full length to the thigh or knee length, which ends just above the knee (Figure 17-6D).
8. Check to be sure the stocking is applied evenly and smoothly and there are no wrinkles.
9. Repeat the procedure on the opposite leg.
10. Wash your hands.
11. Document completion of the procedure and any unusual observations such as swelling of the ankle.

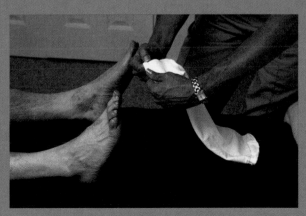

FIGURE 17-6A   Turn stocking inside out to the heel.

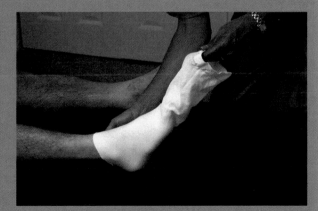

FIGURE 17-6B   Position the stocking over the foot and heel of the client, making sure the heel of the stocking is properly placed.

(continued)

PROCEDURE 69 APPLYING ELASTIC STOCKINGS (*continued*)

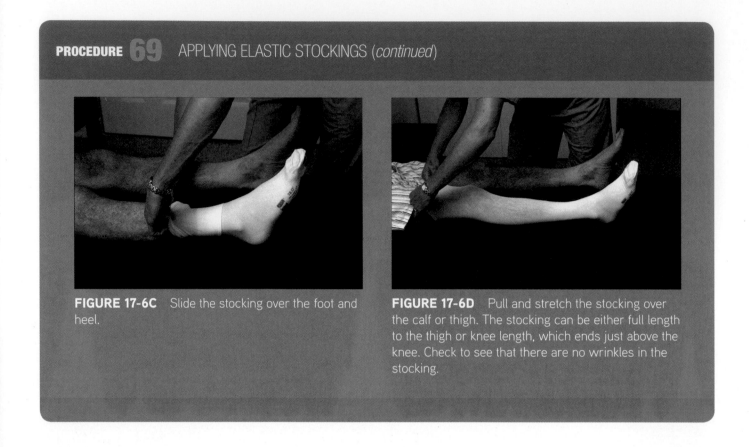

FIGURE 17-6C Slide the stocking over the foot and heel.

FIGURE 17-6D Pull and stretch the stocking over the calf or thigh. The stocking can be either full length to the thigh or knee length, which ends just above the knee. Check to see that there are no wrinkles in the stocking.

Arterial Insufficiency

Arterial insufficiency results from a narrowing of the arteries that deliver blood to the lower extremities. When a client walks any distance, exercise increases the demand for oxygen to the tissues and muscles of the legs. Because of the narrow arteries, the blood flow is not sufficient to meet the demand. The client experiences cramping pain in the calf of the leg or thigh. This pain should subside after the client rests for a few minutes. Treatment for mild symptoms is to encourage the client to lose weight if obese, to avoid smoking, and to walk daily up to the point where pain is experienced, and then to rest.

Gangrene

Gangrene is death of body tissue brought on by lack of adequate blood supply to the area. Signs of gangrene are fever, pain, darkening of the skin, and unpleasant odor. Those at risk for developing this infection include diabetics and other people with poor circulation. The lower extremities are most often affected. The home health aide must look carefully for any signs of skin breakdown, especially in diabetics, and report any sign of skin breakdown to the case manager.

Blood Disorders

Blood is the life stream of the human body. Blood performs many tasks, and no part of the body can live without it. Blood supplies the cells of the body with the food and oxygen they need for work and growth. It carries waste products to specific organs that remove them from the body, or breaks them down into harmless substances. Blood also fights germs that enter the body. Blood has four main parts:

1. Plasma (the liquid part of the blood)

2. Red blood cells (carry oxygen and carbon dioxide to and from the lungs and body tissues)

3. White blood cells (fight infections)

4. Platelets (help to clot the blood)

Disorders of the blood can occur as a result of a malformation or malfunction of a part of the blood.

Diagnostic Tests

A blood test called a complete blood count (CBC) shows the percentages of red and white blood cells. A bone marrow biopsy is done to see if the body's blood factory is working correctly.

Anemia

Anemia occurs when there are not enough red blood cells. It may result from an excessive loss of blood, from malformation of blood cells, or from a lack of essential nutrients. If blood loss is excessive, **hypotension** (low blood pressure) may occur.

Iron Deficiency Anemia. **Iron deficiency anemia** causes shrinkage of the red blood cells, leading to weakness, headaches, loss of color, and loss of concentration. Iron deficiency is the most common nutrient deficiency in the world. Treatment includes taking an iron supplement or eating iron-rich foods such as red meats, beans, dark leafy vegetables, and fortified breads and cereals.

Pernicious Anemia. **Pernicious anemia** is a vitamin B_{12} deficiency caused by the body's inability to produce the intrinsic factor, which helps with vitamin B_{12} absorption. Red blood cells and the nervous system can be damaged with this anemia. Extreme weakness, numbness, and tingling in the extremities, anorexia, and weight loss may occur. Treatment involves a monthly injection of vitamin B_{12}.

Sickle Cell Anemia. With **sickle cell anemia** the client's red blood cells are crescent shaped, like a sickle. The cells do not carry enough oxygen in them, causing anemia. This is an inherited disease for which there is no cure. It is characterized by joint pain, thrombosis, fever, and chronic anemia. This disease is more prevalent in African Americans.

Leukemia

Leukemia, or cancer of the blood, is a condition in which there are too many immature white blood cells. These excess white blood cells block the normal transport of oxygen to the body's tissues. They may also affect production of new red blood cells. Signs and symptoms are fever or chills, tiredness, swollen lymph glands, and bone pain or tenderness. Leukemia clients are very prone to infections and must be protected from outside sources of infection such as crowds of people and especially those with colds.

Hemophilia

Hemophilia is a hereditary disease characterized by spontaneous hemorrhages due to a deficiency of a clotting factor in the blood. The classic form of the disease affects males only. If an individual starts to bleed, a special preparation can be given to stop the bleeding. These individuals must be protected from injury by use of helmets, elbow pads, and kneepads.

WORKBOOK REVIEW

Go to the workbook and complete the review exercises and activities for Unit 17.

REVIEW

1. List six risk factors that would make a client more susceptible to having a heart attack.

_____

_____

_____

_____

_____

_____

2. List three signs that a client may have if suffering a heart attack.

_____

_____

_____

3. As a home health aide caring for a client with congestive heart failure (CHF), which of the following would *not* be in the care plan?
    a. Low-salt, low-fat diet
    b. Scheduling all activities for the morning
    c. Observing for shortness of breath and retention of fluid
    d. Application of elastic hose.

4. T   F   The drug nitroglycerin may be used by clients with heart problems.

5. T   F   A client with a diagnosis of angina pectoris will often have mild chest pain after exercising or eating a large meal.

6. You are working with a client who has thrombophlebitis. Which one of the following symptoms would necessitate that you seek immediate medical attention for your client?
    a. Lower extremity edema
    b. Redness and warmth over vein
    c. Shortness of breath
    d. Pain in the calf of the leg when the foot is flexed

7. Name two blood disorders caused by a malformation of the red blood cells.

_____

_____

8. Describe the appearance of gangrene in the big toe.

9. A condition in which there are too many immature white blood cells is called
    a. anemia.
    b. hemophilia.
    c. leukemia.
    d. all of the above.

Case Studies

10. Your client, Mr. Jones, is a 60-year-old man who recently had a heart attack and bypass surgery. His hospitalization went well and he seems to be recovering very well. On release from the hospital he was given a special diet to follow, new medications to take, and an exercise plan. When you arrive at his home, you discover that he has not been exercising and appears irritable and depressed. What steps can you take to properly care for Mr. Jones? What are some of the emotional factors that might have an impact on Mr. Jones's recovery?

11. Mr. Swing is a 78-year-old man with a history of angina. He insists on shoveling snow after a snowstorm. He goes without a jacket because he says he gets too warm with a jacket on. After 20 minutes he comes into the house complaining of chest pain. He takes his nitroglycerin medication. What should you observe him for? Would you suggest that he rest for a while?

UNIT 18
Respiratory System

KEY TERMS

asthma

chronic bronchitis

chronic obstructive
  pulmonary disease
  (COPD)

emphysema

expectorate

hypostatic

Jet nebulizer

pneumonia

pneumonia vaccine

respiratory system

LEARNING OBJECTIVES

After studying this unit, you should be able to:

- Discuss the basic function of the respiratory system.

- Name the major organs of the respiratory system.

- List four tests used to diagnose respiratory conditions.

- Define and list common signs and symptoms of pneumonia, chronic bronchitis, asthma, and emphysema.

- Describe two devices used to administer oxygen.

- Demonstrate the following:

PROCEDURE 70   Collecting a Sputum Specimen

PROCEDURE 71   Assisting with Cough and Deep-Breathing Exercises

PROCEDURE 72   Assisting the Client with Oxygen Therapy

The **respiratory system** consists of the nose, pharynx, larynx, trachea, bronchi, and lungs (Figure 18-1). Through effective air distribution and gas exchange, the respiratory system helps maintain a constant balance in the body, enabling the cells to function properly.

Respiratory System

The respiratory system is closely linked to the circulatory system. Blood is supplied with fresh oxygen by means of this system. Fresh air is inhaled into the body and carried to the lungs. The oxygen from the air is carried to all parts of the body by the circulatory system. As oxygen is delivered to the cells of the body, waste gases are picked up and carried back to the lungs, where they are exhaled from the body. The most plentiful waste gas is carbon dioxide. In short, oxygen is inhaled and carbon dioxide is exhaled. In addition to the functions just described, the respiratory system filters, warms, and humidifies the air we breathe.

Diagnostic Tests

- Arterial blood gas analysis measures how well the lungs bring oxygen into the body and remove carbon dioxide from the blood.

- The pulmonary (lung) function test helps determine the condition of the extent of lung disease.
- Sputum examination aids in identifying infection and detecting cancer (see Procedure 70, Collecting a Sputum Specimen).
- A chest x-ray assesses heart size and position and the presence of fluid or changes in the lung.

Treatment of Respiratory Conditions

- If the client has a respiratory infection like pneumonia, an antibiotic may be ordered. If the infection is a viral infection, an antibiotic will not be given.
- Bronchodilators are drugs that make the alveoli and bronchi of the lung larger and are given by a nebulizer. A nebulizer is a device used to administer medication in the form of a mist into the lungs. The most common type is a **Jet nebulizer**, which is connected by tubing to a compressor that causes compressed air or oxygen to flow through a liquid medication into an aerosol, which is inhaled by the client. Other types of nebulizers are handheld and portable nebulizers (Figures 18-2 and 18-3). A respiratory therapist or nurse will train the client on the proper use of equipment and medication.

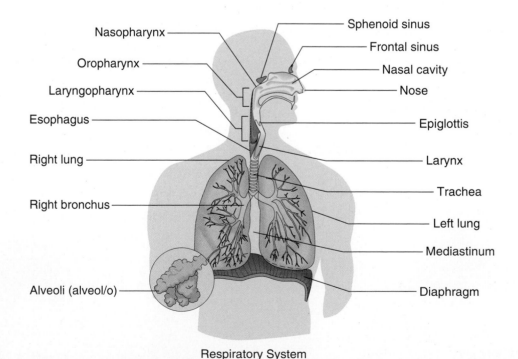

Respiratory System

FIGURE 18-1 The respiratory system. The primary organs of the respiratory tract are the nose, pharynx, trachea, bronchi, and lungs. The upper respiratory tract refers to anything outside the chest cavity. The lower respiratory tract refers to within the chest cavity.

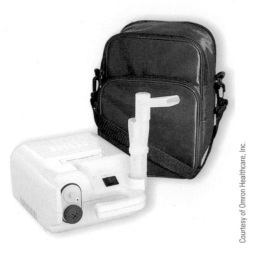

FIGURE 18-2 Portable nebulizer.

Courtesy of Omron Healthcare, Inc.

The home health aide may coach the client through a breathing treatment or simply be supportive of the client who is self-administering a breathing treatment (Figure 18-4). It is important to observe and report to the team if a client has breathing difficulties. Although the home health aide is not allowed to give the treatment, the aide can assist the client to gather the equipment needed for the treatment.

- Corticosteroid medication is given through an inhaler for lung conditions. Be sure to give the client something to rinse the mouth out after treatment, as this drug leaves a bad aftertaste in the mouth.

- Oxygen therapy is given to clients with breathing difficulties, but usually in low amounts (e.g., 2- to 3-liter flow).

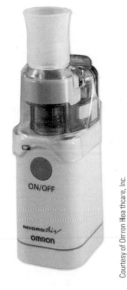

FIGURE 18-3 Handheld nebulizer.

Courtesy of Omron Healthcare, Inc.

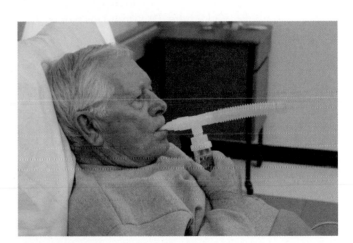

FIGURE 18-4 A client using a nebulizer.

PROCEDURE 70 COLLECTING A SPUTUM SPECIMEN

Purpose

- To provide a sputum specimen for a diagnostic test
- To monitor the client's ongoing condition

NOTE: Do not have the client use mouthwash before collecting a sputum specimen. The specimen should be from the lungs and not saliva from the client's mouth. The best time to collect sputum is early in the morning.

Procedure

1. Assemble supplies:
   disposable gloves
   specimen container, cover with label completed, and laboratory slip
   tissues
   disposable biohazard plastic bag
   mask (optional)
2. Wash hands and apply gloves. Wear a mask if the client has an infectious disease.

(continued)

PROCEDURE **70** COLLECTING A SPUTUM SPECIMEN (*continued*)

3. Ask the client to cough deeply and bring up sputum from the lungs. Have the client expectorate (spit) into the container. Collect 1 to 2 tablespoons of sputum unless otherwise directed. Be sure to have the client cover his or her mouth with tissue to prevent the spread of droplets in the air. If excess sputum contaminates the outside of the container, wipe it off right away.

Cover the specimen container and place it in a biohazard plastic bag and attach the laboratory slip.

4. Remove gloves and wash hands. Take the specimen to the designated area to be transferred to the laboratory.

5. Document the collection of sputum and when transported to the laboratory.

Pneumonia

Pneumonia is an inflammation of the lungs due to an infection by bacteria or viruses. The incidence of pneumonia increases in infants and adults. Pneumonia is named after the part of the lung that is affected, such as right lower bronchial pneumonia or right lower lobar pneumonia. If caused by bacteria, pneumonia can generally be treated using antibiotics. The type of pneumonia seen in the frail elderly and postsurgical clients is called **hypostatic** pneumonia. This type of pneumonia is due to inactivity of the lungs. If a patient has surgery, doing deep-breathing exercises can prevent this type of pneumonia.

Pneumonia is a leading cause of death in the United States. Because many elderly persons already have preexisting conditions and chronic illnesses, they are more vulnerable. It is critical to understand that many older adults do not always have severe early symptoms, but then can become acutely ill very quickly. This puts them in danger because of the chance for delayed or missed diagnosis. Signs to look for (but not always present in older adults) are fever, productive cough with thick phlegm, sharp chest pains, rapid respirations, nausea, vomiting, and fatigue. The care plan may include rest, fluids (intravenous or oral), respiratory therapy with oxygen, antibiotics, and good nutrition. It is recommended that older adults get a flu vaccine every year, because the flu can lead to pneumonia. Another preventive measure is to get the **pneumonia vaccine**, which will protect the elderly from a common type of pneumonia called pneumococcal pneumonia.

Chronic Bronchitis

Chronic bronchitis often occurs in middle-aged or elderly persons. It can result from a number of acute conditions, such as asthma, bronchitis, cigarette smoking, and air pollution.

Bronchitis is an inflammation of the bronchi. This condition is seen most often in the elderly, people who are obese, and smokers. This includes, in particular, elderly individuals with a history of chronic lung disease.

Signs and symptoms include fever (usually low grade) with coughing spells that produce thick, white, greenish, or yellowish phlegm, and lethargy, malaise, and breathlessness. Treatment includes rest, fluids, and cough medication to loosen secretions. Medications to dilate the bronchi and facilitate more effective breathing are also ordered. Encourage clients to elevate both the head and chest to facilitate better breathing. See Procedure 71, Assisting with Cough and Deep-Breathing Exercises.

Asthma

Asthma is a condition that affects the bronchial tubes or airways of the lungs. It is usually caused by an allergic reaction, although there are other causes. Often the specific substance causing the asthma cannot be determined. Signs and symptoms may include coughing, difficulty breathing, wheezing, and a feeling of tightness in the chest.

Primarily asthma is associated with constriction of the large and small airways, causing spasms. Swelling in the airway and increased mucous productivity result in these symptoms: severe difficulty breathing, wheezing, sweating, feelings of suffocation, and anxiety. The care plan includes resolving immediate respiratory distress, taking medications as ordered, and encouraging the client to inhale through the nose and exhale through pursed lips. Have client avoid the potential allergens (the substances causing allergic reactions) if they are known.

PROCEDURE 71   ASSISTING WITH COUGH AND DEEP-BREATHING EXERCISES

Purpose

- To prevent congestion or infections in the client's lungs
- To expand the lung capacity

Procedure

1. Wash your hands.
2. Explain the procedure to the client.
3. Assemble equipment:
   disposable gloves—optional
   pillow case—covered pillow
   tissues
   optional: incentive spirometer
4. Have the client in a sitting position.
5. If the client has recently had surgery, a pillow placed over the incision site may reduce muscle movement in the area and reduce discomfort.
6. Ask the client to take as deep a breath through the nose as possible and hold it for 5 to 7 seconds and then exhale slowly through pursed lips—like a whistle.
7. If using an incentive spirometer, have the client inhale air through the mouthpiece of the incentive spirometer and try to get the yellow ball up as far as he or she can, hold it for 6 to 7 seconds, and then exhale slowly after removing the mouthpiece (Figure 18-5).
8. Repeat the exercise about five times.
9. Give the client tissues and instruct the client to take a deep breath and cough forcefully twice with the mouth open. Collect any secretions that are brought up in tissues. Protect yourself from secretions and droplets.
10. Slip on gloves if you will be touching or handling the tissues.
11. Dispose of the tissues in a plastic bag and assist the client to a comfortable position.
12. Remove gloves and wash hands.
13. Document the procedure completed, your observations, and the client's reaction.

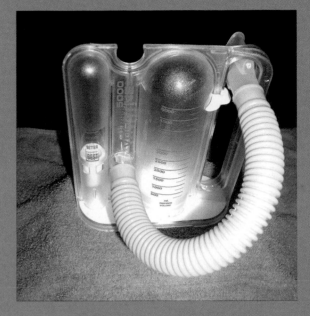

FIGURE 18-5   Incentive spirometer.

Emphysema

Emphysema is a lung condition in which the air sacs within the lung lose their elasticity. Breathing is difficult for the client affected by this disease. Medications can relieve the symptoms of emphysema, but there is no cure. The typical emphysema client is a smoker 50 to 80 years of age, and may continue to smoke. As the lung loses elasticity, it results in altered oxygen and carbon dioxide exchange and increased airway resistance from severe narrowing or collapse of the airways. Signs and symptoms include shortness of breath that gradually worsens, pursed-lip breathing, and increased effort to breathe, with use of accessory muscles such as the diaphragm. Later symptoms include barrel chest (Figure 18-6), headache, irritability, possible confusion due to poor air exchange, and leaning forward in posture. Treatment includes giving oxygen as ordered to facilitate breathing and use of a nebulizer. A position used often by emphysema clients is to sit up in a lounge chair with a small table placed across the chair with pillows on top of the table. Emphysema clients often sleep in this position because they have problems breathing in a supine position in bed.

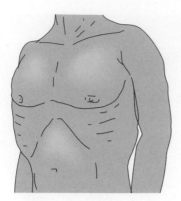

FIGURE 18-6 Barrel chest.

Chronic Obstructive Pulmonary Disease (COPD)

Chronic obstructive pulmonary disease (COPD) is the occurrence of chronic bronchitis or emphysema and a pair of co-existing diseases of the lungs such as pneumonia where the client's airway becomes narrowed. This leads to a limitation of flow of air to and from the lungs, causing shortness of breath (dyspnea). Other signs and symptoms of COPD are wheezing, production of large amount of mucus or sputum, chest tightness, and bluish color to the lips. Clients with breathing difficulties will need more frequent rest periods because they tire easily. In addition, they will need more time to accomplish their activities. Often, clients who experience difficulty breathing will be anxious, which makes breathing even more difficult. As the disease progresses, the client will need assistance in all activities of daily living (ADLs).

Use of Oxygen in the Home

Oxygen is available in a tank or reservoir. If it is a tank, the smaller the tank, the less oxygen it contains. An oxygen reservoir contains larger amount of oxygen. An oxygen concentrator (Figure 18-7) removes the oxygen from the air. Always check the meter of the oxygen tank or reservoir. If low, check to see if there is a spare tank. If there is not a spare tank, call for a replacement. Oxygen is delivered to the client by either a mask or nasal cannula (Figure 18-8). Both of these devices are connected to the oxygen by use of tubing. Often a long tube is connected to the device, giving the client greater freedom of movement, but watch that the client doesn't trip over it. Oxygen is delivered in liter flow. The care plan will state the liter flow to be administered to the client. A typical order would look like this: O_2 @ 4L prn—O_2 is the abbreviation for oxygen, L is the abbreviation for liter, and prn means as needed. The home health aide should read the care plan to verify the correct flow of oxygen is

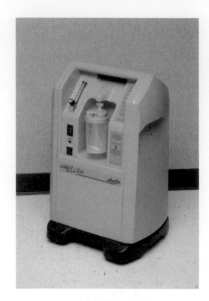

FIGURE 18-7 Oxygen concentrator.

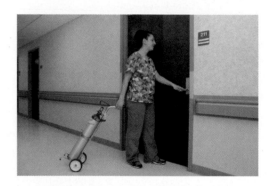

FIGURE 18-8 Portable oxygen tank being delivered to a room in an assistive living facility.

being delivered to the client. If incorrect, notify the case manager.

See Procedure 72, Assisting the Client with Oxygen Therapy.

Safety Precautions While Oxygen Is Being Administered

- Do not smoke in a room where a client is receiving oxygen. Post "No Smoking" sign, if necessary, to warn visitors not to smoke.

- Do not use matches, candles, or open flames where oxygen is used or stored.

- Do not use electrical appliances during oxygen therapy. Avoid sparks. If you need to shave the client, turn off the oxygen while using the electric razor, or use a disposable razor.

PROCEDURE 72   ASSISTING THE CLIENT WITH OXYGEN THERAPY

Purpose

- To assist the client to receive the correct amount of oxygen
- To avoid misuse of oxygen equipment and careless practices that risk causing fires, explosions, or injury
- To increase oxygen intake for the client

Procedure

1. Wash your hands.
2. Check to see if the client's oxygen mask or cannula is placed properly (Figures 18-9A and B). The straps on the cannula should be secure but not too tight. Check the top of the ears for signs of irritation. Check for signs of irritation where the prongs touch the client's nose. Be sure both prongs are in the client's nose. If a mask is being used, check to see whether the mask is over both the nose and mouth. If the inside of the mask is wet, remove it and dry the inside.
3. Check the gauge to see if the oxygen is being given at the correct amount of liter flow (Figures 18-10).
4. Check the client's position. If in bed, elevate the head with two or three pillows to assist the client in breathing.
5. Do frequent mouth care for clients receiving oxygen therapy. The client's mouth can become dry and have an unpleasant taste. Apply water-soluble lubricant to the lips and nose, if they become dry.
6. Wash your hands.
7. Document the liter flow and the device being used, your observations, and the client's breathing pattern.

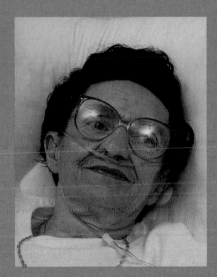

FIGURE 18-9A   If the client is receiving oxygen through a nasal cannula, be sure both nosepieces are in the nose.

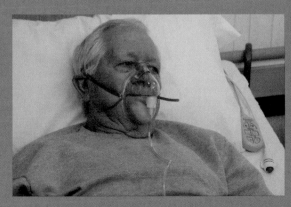

FIGURE 18-9B   A client receiving oxygen through a mask.

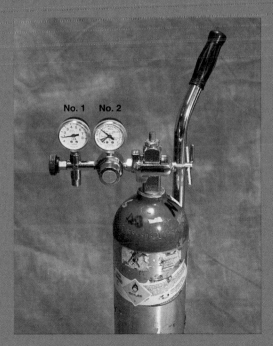

FIGURE 18-10   The No. 1 gauge notes the liter flow. The No. 2 gauge notes the amount of oxygen left in the tank.

WORKBOOK REVIEW

Go the workbook and complete the review exercises and activities for Unit 18.

REVIEW

1. Name the major organs of the respiratory system.

2. List the purposes of the respiratory system.

_____

_____

3. T F A person with emphysema can never receive "too much" oxygen.

4. T F The only reason to collect a sputum specimen is to see what the sputum looks like.

5. T F Asthma is a lung condition in which the air sacs lose their elasticity.

6. T F Oxygen is given by liter flow.

7. T F Avoid doing oral care on clients receiving oxygen.

8. T F Deep-breathing exercises can prevent pneumonia from occurring.

9. T F Expectorate means to exhale.

Case Studies

10. Mr. Paulson has emphysema, and even with oxygen running, he is unable to sleep in bed. What position would you suggest he sleep in?

11. Mrs. Coleman is an 82-year-old client of yours. You are to ambulate her with oxygen and give her a shower. She becomes very short of breath while you are walking her. What actions can you take to complete the tasks as ordered?

UNIT 19

Reproductive System

KEY TERMS

cervix

chlamydia

dysmenorrhea

ectopic pregnancy

estrogen

fallopian tubes

genital herpes

genital warts

genitalia

gonorrhea

gynecologist

menopause

menstruation

nongonococcal
  urethritis

ovaries

pelvic inflammatory
  disease (PID)

penis

progesterone

scrotum

sexually transmitted
  diseases (STDs)

syphilis

testes

testosterone

urethra

uterus

vagina

vaginitis

vulva

LEARNING OBJECTIVES

After studying this unit, you should be able to:

- Identify the male and female reproductive organs

- Describe the functions of each major organ

- List and describe male and female hormones and their functions

- Name three common disorders of the reproductive system

- List five sexually transmitted diseases and their signs and symptoms

- Discuss how sexually transmitted diseases can be prevented

Reproductive System

The reproductive system consists of the external and internal sex organs of the male and female. The male organs include the scrotum, a saclike organ that contains the testes and other tubules; the testes, which produce sperm, the hormone testosterone and fluid; and the penis, which contains the urethra for transporting urine and sperm (Figure 19-1).

The female external organs are the genitalia (vulva) and breasts. The internal organs include the vagina, which functions as the birth canal and leads to the cervix and uterus; the cervix, which is the mouth of the womb; the uterus, located behind the urinary bladder (which functions as the womb that receives the fertilized egg and developing fetus); the ovaries, located on either side of the lower abdomen, which produce estrogen and progesterone hormones as well as egg cells; and the fallopian tubes, which carry the egg cells from the ovaries to the uterus (Figures 19-2 and 19-3).

The female has a menstrual cycle approximately every 28 days, by which the uterus is prepared to nurture the fertilized egg into a viable fetus. However, if the egg cell that is produced midcycle is not fertilized by the sperm cell, the uterine lining is sloughed off, and bleeding occurs for approximately 3 to 5 days. This is called menstruation.

The reproductive system is important in maintaining sexual characteristics. The hormones that produce male characteristics (such as broad shoulders and facial, chest, and pubic hair) and female characteristics (such as rounded hips, enlarged breasts, and pubic hair) are also thought to help maintain function in other systems of the body. Illness or malfunction of the reproductive system can cause emotional and physical problems. In giving care, it is important to treat the client with understanding and consideration and to give the client opportunities to express feelings about illness.

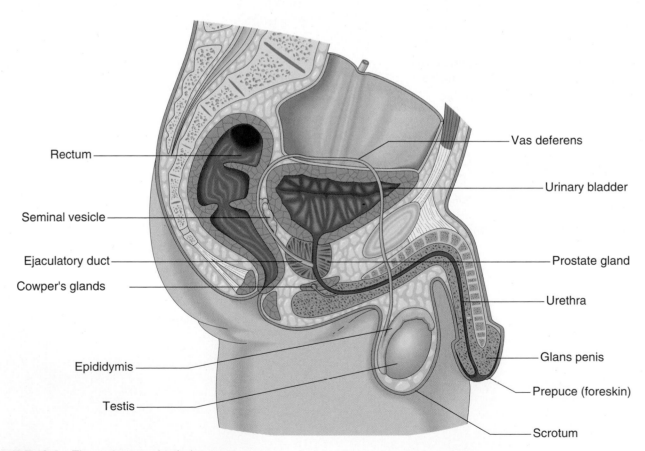

FIGURE 19-1 The male reproductive system.

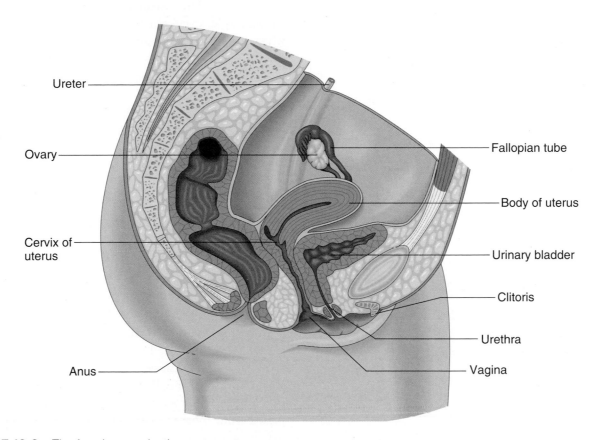

Ureter

Ovary

Cervix of
uterus

Anus

Fallopian tube

Body of uterus

Urinary bladder

Clitoris

Urethra

Vagina

FIGURE 19-2 The female reproductive system.

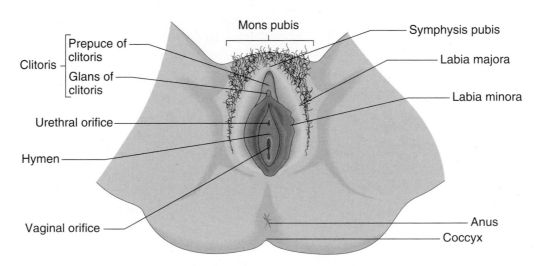

Clitoris
Prepuce of
clitoris
Glans of
clitoris

Urethral orifice

Hymen

Vaginal orifice

Mons pubis

Symphysis pubis

Labia majora

Labia minora

Anus

Coccyx

FIGURE 19-3 The female external genitalia.

Common Disorders of the Reproductive System

Some common disorders of the reproductive system include dysmenorrhea, vaginitis, and sexually transmitted diseases. Many of these disorders may be caused by infections or sexual activity with an infected person, and may require medication for treatment.

Dysmenorrhea

Dysmenorrhea refers to pain that sometimes accompanies the menstrual flow. Although a large percentage of women experience some minor discomfort during menstruation, it should be emphasized that menstruation is a normal process. Women with this problem are recommended to take nonsteroidal anti-inflammatory drugs (NSAIDs) such as ibuprofen—Advil®, Ibuprin®, or Motrin®—for relief of discomfort. However, any severe cramping or persistent pain should be reported to a gynecologist, a health care provider specializing in women's reproductive health.

Vaginitis

Vaginitis is an infection of the vagina (birth canal), which may be caused by bacteria, viruses, or yeast, or may result from changes in vaginal secretions after menopause (the permanent end of menstruation). There is usually a whitish, odorous discharge with itching and burning. Treatment consists of wearing cotton underwear, avoiding garments that hold heat and moisture, eating yogurt, and treating the infectious organisms with drugs. In older women, vaginal creams containing estrogen may be used.

Sexually Transmitted Diseases (STDs)

Infections spread by sexual intercourse are called sexually transmitted diseases (STDs). These are common worldwide, especially among young adults. Many county health departments offer free screening for STDS.

Common signs and symptoms of sexually transmitted diseases occur in or near the vagina or penis and include unusual discharge; lumps, bumps, or rashes; sores that are painful, itchy, or painless; itchy skin; and burning on urination. In most cases both partners need to be tested and treated.

Prevention of STDs

To prevent STDs, sexually active people should, ideally, have a single sexual partner, always use a latex condom when engaged in penetrative sex, and avoid practices that could damage the delicate lining of the vagina or anus. People with signs or symptoms of an STD or who are being treated for an STD should abstain from sex, and their partners should be checked for infection and also treated. If only one person is treated, that person can be reinfected again if his or her partner is not treated.

Chlamydia

Chlamydia is a disease caused by bacteria that is spread when infected fluid from the sex organ or rectum contacts the penis, vagina, mouth, or anus. Women may have an inflammation of the cervix with a foul-smelling discharge, burning on urination, and itching around the sex gland. Men have similar symptoms. Chlamydia may also have a silent beginning, whereby there will be no symptoms exhibited until the infection has spread to the pelvic area and causes pelvic inflammatory disease (PID). It is the most common cause of STDs and is a common cause of infertility. Chlamydia can be treated with antibiotics. If left untreated in a pregnant woman, the disease can be passed from mother to infant during birth. The infant may have eye, lung, or other health problems.

Pelvic Inflammatory Disease

Pelvic inflammatory disease (PID) is an infection of the upper female reproductive tract. Bacterial organisms such as *Chlamydia* or gonorrhea cause the disorder. Diagnosis is based on analysis of the cervical or vaginal secretions. It can be treated with antibiotics. If not treated, PID can cause severe damage and scarring of the reproductive tract. Complications include chronic pelvic pain, infertility, and abnormal menstruation. Scarring in the fallopian tubes can block passage of the fertilized egg, increasing the risk of an ectopic (tubal) pregnancy, a condition in which the egg implants outside the uterine cavity.

Nongonococcal Urethritis

Nongonococcal urethritis, also known as nonspecific urethritis, is urethral inflammation caused by an infection other than gonorrhea. This infection is among the most prevalent of all STDs. Signs and symptoms usually start 1 to 3 weeks after exposure. In women, the main sign is abnormal vaginal discharge. Men, as a result of inflammation of the urethra, commonly experience discharge from the penis and pain when urinating. Infection may cause scrotal pain and swelling. Treatment consists of antibiotics.

Gonorrhea

Gonorrhea, a bacterial infection, causes a discharge of pus from the penis or sometimes the vagina, and pain on urination. The main sites of infection are the urethra and, in women, the cervix; organisms can then spread to the uterus, fallopian tubes, and ovaries. The rectum can also be affected. A pregnant woman risks passing the infection to her baby during childbirth. In men, it infects the urethra, and then spreads to the testes and prostate. This can cause pain, swelling, and scarring. Gonorrhea is treated by antibiotics.

Syphilis

Syphilis is a bacterial disease. Syphilis progresses in three stages and becomes more severe in each stage. The earliest sign of syphilis is usually an ulcer (chancre) on the genitals. However, an ulcer can also develop in the mouth or on the anus. A rash, mouth ulcers, and enlargement of the lymph nodes follow. Later effects include brain, heart, and bone disorders. A pregnant woman can pass the infection to her baby. It is treated with antibiotics.

Genital Herpes

One of the most common STDs is **genital herpes**, and its reported incidence has increased over recent years. Caused by an organism known as herpes simplex virus, genital herpes tends to recur. The first episode is the most severe, with subsequent occurrences decreasing in severity and frequency.

During an episode, crops of small blisters form on the penis or around the vagina, then develop into shallow, painful ulcers. The first attack of herpes may be accompanied by headache, fever, and pain in the groin, buttocks, and legs.

There is no cure for genital herpes. Painkillers and keeping lesions clean and dry, as well as not scratching them, can relieve symptoms. Certain drugs can provide pain relief and speed healing during an attack. Prolonged use of the antiviral drug Zovirax® (acyclovir) may reduce the number and frequency of occurrences.

Genital Warts

Viruses cause **genital warts**. These warts may appear as bumps or small pink or red growths, or be flat and difficult to see. They can be painful and irritating. The warts can grow in, on, or near the penis, vagina, cervix, rectum, or throat. Treatment with chemicals, freezing, or laser therapy can remove them. More than one treatment is usually needed. These warts can continue to reappear, and just removing them does not mean the disease is cured. Even when condoms are used during sex, the virus can be spread through contact with the skin of the infected partner, which the condom does not cover.

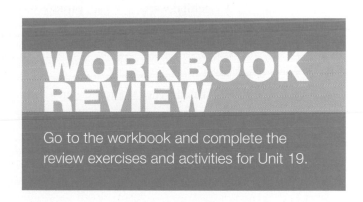

WORKBOOK REVIEW

Go to the workbook and complete the review exercises and activities for Unit 19.

REVIEW

1. The male reproductive system includes which of the following?
   a. Scrotum, testes, and penis
   b. Uterus and cervix
   c. None of the above
   d. All of the above

2. The female fallopian tubes
   a. produce estrogen and progesterone.
   b. carry egg cells from the ovaries to the uterus.
   c. slough off during menstruation.
   d. none of the above.

3. The acronym STD stands for
   a. short-term disability.
   b. sanitize to disinfect.
   c. sexually transmitted disease.
   d. all of the above.

4. Match the term in Column I with the definition in Column II.

   Column I
   _____ 1. uterus
   _____ 2. scrotum
   _____ 3. vaginitis
   _____ 4. menstruation
   _____ 5. testosterone
   _____ 6. genital herpes

   Column II
   a. sloughing off of uterine lining
   b. male hormone
   c. sexually transmitted disease
   d. receives fertilized egg and developing fetus
   e. infection of the vagina
   f. saclike organ that contains testes and other tubules

5. Match the term in Column I with the definition in Column II.

   Column I
   _____ 1. genital warts
   _____ 2. chlamydia
   _____ 3. PID
   _____ 4. gonorrhea

   Column II
   a. pink or red lesions around genital areas
   b. most common cause of STDs
   c. discharge of pus from the penis
   d. major cause of infertility in women

6. T F   Dysmenorrhea is another term for painful menstruation.

7. T F   The ovaries produce estrogen and progesterone.

8. T F   A gynecologist is a health care provider specializing in women's reproductive health.

9. T F   Pelvic inflammatory disease affects male and female reproductive systems.

Case Studies

10. John, a 23-year-old man, was recently involved in a motorcycle accident where he sustained multiple injuries and now requires the services of a home health aide. Prior to his accident, he was sexually active, with multiple partners. Now he is complaining of painful urination and unusual drainage from his penis. The home health aide suspects a sexually transmitted disease is the cause. What should the home health aide do next?

11. When giving an 80-year-old woman a bath, the home health aide notices that the woman has a fairly large amount of whitish, odorous drainage from the vagina. Should the aide report this drainage or is this a normal occurrence in a woman of this age? Should the aide wear gloves when bathing this client?

UNIT 20

Endocrine System and Diabetes

KEY TERMS

acidosis	ducts	glucose	hypothyroidism
blood lancet	endocrine glands	hormones	insulin
cyanotic	gangrene	hyperglycemia	insulin shock
diabetes	gestational	hyperthyroidism	neuropathy
diabetic coma	glucometer	hypoglycemia	subcutaneously

LEARNING OBJECTIVES

After studying this unit, you should be able to:

- List six glands of the endocrine system

- Discuss the importance of hormones

- List two disorders of the thyroid gland

- Name four signs and symptoms of diabetes

- List four types of diabetes mellitus

- Name three ways of controlling diabetes

- Name three long-term effects of diabetes

- List signs and symptoms for hypoglycemia and hyperglycemia and the immediate care for each

- Explain special foot care given to the diabetic client

- Describe what information should be on a Medic-Alert identification

- Demonstrate the following:

  PROCEDURE 73 Finger-Stick Blood Sugar

Endocrine System

The endocrine system is composed of many glands scattered throughout the body. The endocrine glands are ductless glands that secrete substances within the body called hormones (Figure 20-1). The glands do not have ducts (little tubes) and are therefore unlike tear and sweat glands. Hormones are chemicals that are secreted directly into the bloodstream. They are carried throughout the body to regulate and control specific body functions. They are powerful substances and direct the functions of other systems. Each hormone has a special job to do (Figure 20-2). It only takes a small amount of hormone to trigger a body reaction. Most scientists agree that the brain sends messages to the endocrine glands, and these messages cause the glands to secrete the hormones needed by the body. For instance, in a time of physical danger the adrenal gland secretes a hormone called adrenalin, which causes the heart rate to increase. This forces more blood through the body, which increases the nourishment to the muscles. Sugar is released into the body, giving it quick energy. The adrenalin release also speeds up the body's reflexes. All of these changes occur rapidly, making the body better able to react and save itself or others from harm.

The thyroid gland regulates the metabolic rate of the body. This determines the speed at which food is turned into energy.

Hyperthyroidism and Hypothyroidism

The thyroid weighs less than an ounce but all aspects of metabolism, from the rate at which your heart beats to the speed at which you burn calories, are regulated by the thyroid hormones. A person with hyperthyroidism has an overactive thyroid, which produces too much T3 and

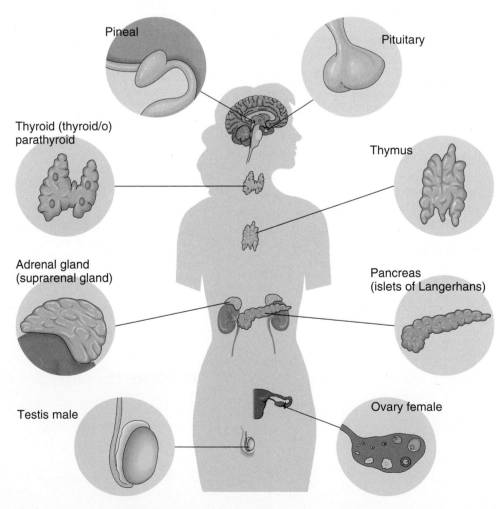

Pineal

Pituitary

Thyroid (thyroid/o) parathyroid

Thymus

Adrenal gland (suprarenal gland)

Pancreas (islets of Langerhans)

Testis male

Ovary female

FIGURE 20-1   Location of the endocrine glands.

Pituitary gland	Once called the "master gland" of the body; secretes numerous hormones that regulate many bodily processes. The pituitary is completely controlled by the hypothalamus, a part of the brain.
Thyroid gland	Helps to regulate the metabolic rate and growth processes.
Parathyroid glands	Regulate metabolism of calcium and phosphorous.
Thymus gland	Regulates immunity to infectious diseases during infancy and early childhood; becomes smaller as the body ages.
Adrenal glands	Adjust the body to crisis and stress; increase blood pressure; speed reactions; metabolize carbohydrates and proteins.
Pineal gland	Regulates the secretion of the hormone melatonin. Light inhibits melatonin secretions, whereas darkness stimulates melatonin production. This hormone regulates sleep and waking cycles.
Pancreas	Produces insulin needed to burn sugar in the body. (Too little insulin causes diabetes; too much insulin causes hyperglycemia.) Also produces glucagon to raise blood sugar.
Ovaries	Produce ovum (egg) for reproduction; secrete estrogen and progesterone that develop and maintain secondary sexual characteristics (breasts, pubic and underarm hair, etc.).
Testes	Produce sperm to fertilize ovum; secrete male hormone testosterone.

FIGURE 20-2 Functions of the glands of the endocrine system.

T4 hormones. Signs and symptoms of this condition are an increase or decrease in appetite, insomnia, heat intolerance, muscle weakness, fatigue, and thinning of hair. This condition can be readily treated. Treatment options are: (1) Radioactive iodine treatment, which shrinks the thyroid; (2) anti-thyroid medication called methimazole (Tapazole®); (3) surgery, a thyroidectomy, but this is not as common as the other two options.

Hypothyroidism is a condition that usually comes on slowly. The cause of this disorder is a decrease in the production of thyroid hormones. Early signs and symptoms of an underactive thyroid, such as sluggishness and fatigue, are often very vague. As the metabolism continues to slow, signs such as chronically cold hands or feet, constipation, pale and dry skin, a puffy face, and hoarse voice may develop. There may be some weight gain but usually not more than 10 to 20 pounds, plus an increase in cholesterol levels. This disorder can be readily treated with a daily dose of thyroid drug.

Diabetes Mellitus

Diabetes mellitus is a chronic disease that affects the way your body metabolizes glucose (sugar). The disease is primarily managed through diet, exercise, and drug therapy.

The pancreas either does not produce any or produces an inadequate amount of a hormone called insulin.

The functions of insulin are to enable the body to use glucose (sugar), to aid in the storage of nutrients, and to make possible the metabolism of carbohydrates and protein. When insulin is not manufactured or cannot be used correctly, a condition called diabetes develops. In diabetes, the person's blood sugar level is elevated (hyperglycemia) because the sugar remains in the blood instead of being absorbed into the cells and used for food. The buildup of sugar in the blood is unhealthy for a number of reasons. It disturbs the fluid balance in the body because it causes problems with the filtering system of the kidneys. Diabetes suppresses the immune system, and this allows infections to flourish. Sugar buildup in the blood vessels results in restricted circulation because of damage to the blood vessels. The lack of adequate blood supply to certain body areas causes many problems in the brain, extremities, eyes, kidneys, and heart.

Risk Factors

- Age—the risk of diabetes increases as one gets older, usually over 45 years of age.
- Weight—overweight is one of the main risks. If your body stores weight in the abdomen, the risk of

diabetes is greater than if the body stores weight in the hips and thighs.

- Family history—the chances increase if one has a close relative, parent, or sibling with diabetes.
- Race—African Americans, Hispanics, Asian Americans, and Native Americans are particularly prone to the disease.
- Inactivity—the less physically active you are, the greater the risk of developing the disease.
- Prediabetes—this occurs when a person's blood sugar is higher than normal but not high enough to be classified as type II diabetes, increases risk for developing diabetes.

Classifications

Diabetes can be classified into several types:

- Insulin-dependent diabetes mellitus (IDDM)—type I diabetes: usually occurs before age 25. The pancreas no longer produces any insulin and this person needs daily insulin injections.
- Non-insulin-dependent diabetes mellitus (NIDDM)—type II diabetes: usually develops after the age of 45 and is commonly seen in older adults. Insulin is produced, but may be insufficient or ineffective in preventing hyperglycemia. This person is unable to use the insulin effectively to change glucose (sugar) into energy. People with type II diabetes may need to use insulin, but usually take oral diabetic medication.
- **Gestational**—type III diabetes: Occurs during a woman's pregnancy when the blood sugar levels are elevated; the blood sugar levels usually return to normal after delivery. However, women with gestational diabetes often will develop diabetes later in life unless changes are made in diet and exercise. If the baby weight was more than 9 pounds at birth, the mother is at risk for type II diabetes.
- Type III diabetes also includes other types that are associated with hormonal changes, pancreatic diseases, and adverse effects of drugs.

Signs and Symptoms

Signs and symptoms of diabetes can come on slowly and can only be verified by a physical evaluation and blood tests. Some of the signs and symptoms to watch for are:

- Weakness
- Sudden weight loss
- Unusual thirst

- Frequent need to urinate
- Increase hunger with weight loss
- Blurred vision
- Sores that do not heal
- Repeated infections

Diagnostic Testing

Common tests used in the diagnoses and care of diabetes are:

- Fasting blood sugar (FBS): Blood is tested for sugar content; normal range is between 70 and 110 mg.
- Urinalysis: Urine sample is tested for presence of sugar or ketones.
- Glucose tolerance tests: Series of tests done on blood within designated time periods. Blood is tested while fasting and then after drinking a high-glucose solution at different time periods.
- Glycosylated hemoglobin (A1C): Blood test that will give the average blood sugar level over a period of 2 to 3 months.

Treatments and Drugs

Diet

Diet is the cornerstone to the management of diabetes. The diet should contain necessary elements of good nutrition, maintain blood sugar levels, and be acceptable to the client's preferences. The diet consists of plenty of fruit, vegetables, and grains, and limited amounts of carbohydrates. Animal products and sweets are limited. The food intake should be distributed throughout the day and accommodate the client's lifestyle, activity, and diabetic medication. A diabetic client also needs to remember to eat meals and snacks at the same time every day. Of all the different components of a client's diet—carbohydrates, fats, and proteins—carbohydrates have the greatest effects on blood sugar levels.

An important duty of the aide is to prepare meals using the diet prescribed by the dietitian. The diabetic MyPlate method is an easy way for the home health aide and the client to put a meal together. The aide needs to encourage and reinforce the importance of abiding by this diet. Occasionally the client will try to deny the disease and not follow the prescribed diet. There is little you can do in the client's own home to force the individual to eat the correct foods. Many times the client will eat the correct foods when you are there, but when you leave he or she does not follow the prescribed diet. If you become aware of this, it is important to document it and inform your case manager.

Obesity and poor nutrition are two common problems in diabetes. Most diabetics who stick to a diet, take medication, and exercise moderately have fewer health problems. The diabetic client who does not follow the health care provider's orders risks serious health problems.

Exercise

Regular exercises are often recommended in the daily routine of clients with diabetes. The benefits of exercise are many. Exercise can improve the client's circulation, assist in maintaining ideal weight, increase the client's well-being, and improve control of glucose in the body. A home health aide should encourage and assist the client in doing exercises.

Blood Sugar Testing

Once diagnosed with diabetes, clients are taught how to test one's blood for sugar. Testing the blood gives a reading of what the blood sugar value is at the moment. Blood sugar testing equipment (**glucometer**) has been greatly improved in the last few years, is very reasonable in cost, and is user-friendly. Testing procedures for blood sugar vary according to the type of glucometer the client has purchased. The instructions must be followed carefully to avoid an inaccurate reading. It is also important if you assist with the procedure that you follow standard precautions. Some machines have the ability to talk the client or the caregiver through the procedure with recorded instructions. It is important to know when the blood sugar reading is high or low, and often the care plan will have this information in it. Be sure to check the expiration date on the blood strips. Store the strips in the original vial in a cool, dry place. Do not store in a humid place, such as the bathroom. Always keep the vial capped tight. Dispose of the blood lancet in a "sharps" container. When pricking the finger, rotate fingers and use the side of the finger that has less use. See Procedure 73, Finger-Stick Blood Sugar.

PROCEDURE 73   FINGER-STICK BLOOD SUGAR

Purpose

- To monitor the blood sugar level

Procedure

1. Gather necessary equipment:
   - disposable gloves
   - blood glucose meter and corresponding blood strips (Figure 20-3A)
   - blood lancet (needle)
   - alcohol swab (optional)
   - sharps container
2. Wash hands and apply gloves.
3. Insert strip into meter.
4. Have the client massage the site to increase blood flow and wipe the finger with an alcohol wipe (optional); then have the client squeeze and pierce the side of the finger with the lancet (Figure 20-3B) and place a hanging drop of blood onto the strip (Figure 20-3C).

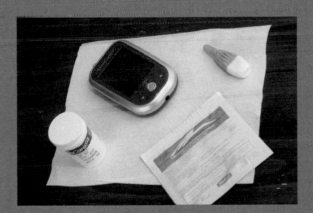

FIGURE 20-3A   Diabetic blood testing equipment: glucometer, lancet, gauze, and blood testing strips.

5. When the meter makes an audible beep the blood sugar value is displayed on the screen for about 5 seconds.
6. Discard the lancet in the sharps container.

(continued)

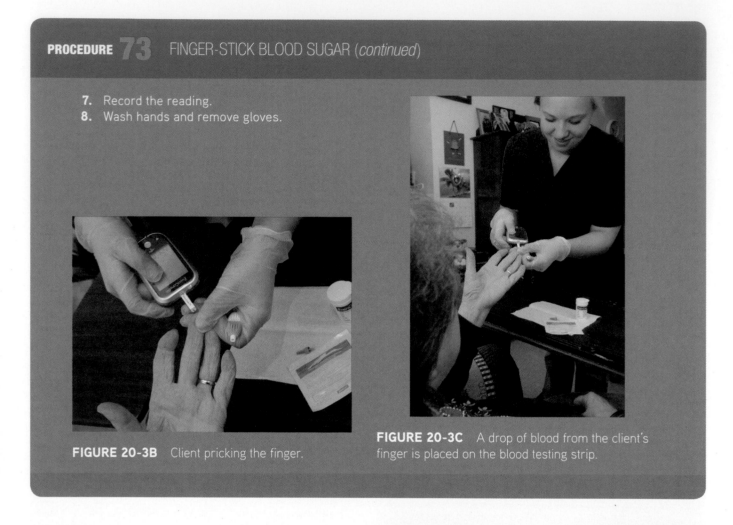

7. Record the reading.
8. Wash hands and remove gloves.

FIGURE 20-3B   Client pricking the finger.

FIGURE 20-3C   A drop of blood from the client's finger is placed on the blood testing strip.

Drug Therapy

Type I Diabetes.   Type I diabetes is treated with a drug called insulin, which needs to be injected **subcutaneously** (under the skin). It cannot be taken orally because the stomach juices will dissolve the drug before it can be effective. The client with diabetes is taught where, when, and how to inject the medication (Figure 20-4). If a diabetic client is unable to self-inject, another member of the family might be taught to give the injections. Some diabetics are too young to give themselves injections; other clients with diabetes may have poor eyesight or be uncoordinated. Most diabetic clients, if instructed properly, are able to inject their own insulin.

Insulin Injections.   A home health aide is not permitted to inject insulin. The aide's responsibility is limited to bringing the medication and necessary supplies to the client. The aide should always check the expiration date on the insulin bottle. The insulin should not be used if it is past the expiration date because it might not be effective any longer. It is not necessary to refrigerate insulin, but it should be kept in a cool place and where

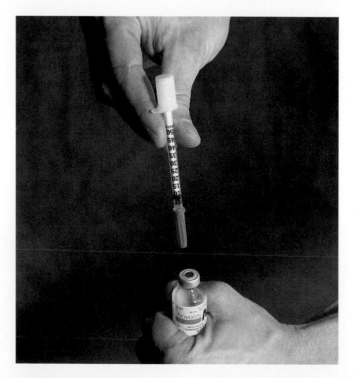

FIGURE 20-4   Bottle of insulin and insulin syringe.

the temperature stays the same. The three most important factors to remember about insulin are:

1. Measurement must be *accurate*.

2. The drug must be taken at the same time every day.

3. Sterile technique must be maintained when injecting the drug.

The health care provider may prescribe different kinds of insulin—for example, fast-acting, intermediate-acting, or slow-acting insulin. The health care provider will prescribe the type of insulin needed, as well as the frequency, time, and amount of insulin.

Sites recommended for injections include the abdomen, upper arms, buttocks, and thighs. Most clients are encouraged to rotate injection sites on a daily or weekly basis to avoid changes in the skin tissues, which can alter the rate of absorption of the drug. It is a good idea to keep a record of where the injection was given to assist the client in rotating sites (Figure 20-5).

The insulin pump is another option for delivery of insulin to the body. It is the size of a cell phone and continually delivers insulin through a tube inserted under the skin of the abdomen. This pump can lower the risk of the client's glucose level going too high or too low. Another benefit is that the client does not have to inject insulin through the skin numerous times a day. A control button or a switch allows the client to adjust the release of insulin.

Type II Diabetes. Type II diabetes can be treated in three ways. One way is by diet, and an individual with diabetes may be able to maintain his or her blood sugar level without drugs. The second way is by taking oral

hypoglycemic drugs daily. These drugs work in different ways to assist the client to regulate blood sugar. Examples of hypoglycemic drugs are:

Generic Name	Brand Name
glipizide	Glucotrol®
glimepiride	Amaryl®
glyburide	Glynase®
metformin	Glucophage®
sitagliptin	Januvia®
saxagliptin	Onglyza®
repaglinide	Prandin®

As a home health aide you need to remember to encourage your client to take the prescribed drug as ordered. Generally, the drug is taken once a day, but it is not uncommon for a health care provider to order the drug two (bid) or three (tid) times a day. You should be sure the client has an adequate supply of drugs on hand. These drugs are costly and, occasionally, a client will want to save money and stop taking the medication. If this happens, be sure to inform the case manager.

The third way of treating type II diabetes is with insulin injections, as described earlier in the chapter.

Long-Term Effects

Untreated or improperly treated diabetes can lead to many physical problems. Abnormal conditions that occur after a person develops diabetes are called diabetic complications. In some cases, even a well-cared-for diabetic may develop serious complications. The most common complications are vascular (blood vessel) disease and a high risk of infections. The most common long-term effects are described in Figure 20-6.

Neuropathy in the Diabetic

Neuropathy is defined as a destructive disorder of the nerves. Diabetic neuropathy is the loss of sensation in the nerves. Individuals with neuropathy may be unable to feel pain or differentiate between hot and cold temperatures. This can be extremely dangerous. For example, a diabetic injures a foot or leg and, because no pain is felt, continues to use the limb. An infection can occur and the diabetic does not even realize there is a problem. Cuts or wounds not felt and thus not cared for can become infected. A home health aide carefully and routinely must check the client's feet and legs for any sign of redness, any "warm" area, any swelling, or any open cuts. Many diabetics have poor eyesight, or have difficulty bending their legs, and

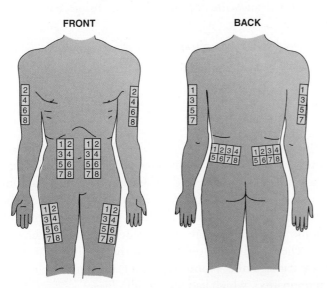

FRONT   **BACK**

FIGURE 20-5 Sites and rotation for insulin injections.

Long-Term Disorders	Cause	Signs & Symptoms	Treatment	Aide's Care
Blindness	Cataracts, glaucoma, Hemorrhage diabetic retinopathy	Partial or total loss of sight, client drops items, tumbles or falls, develops tunnel vision	Surgery for cataracts; medication or surgery for glaucoma	Keep clear common pathways in the home Assist in reading labels
Gangrene	Poor circulation, skin breakdown, invasion of tissue by bacteria, nerve damage	Heat in area, skin reddened, formation of ulcers that do not clear up, foul odor and spread of infection and tissue destruction	Medication; may require amputation of limb	Assist with dressing changes and maintaining clean environment
Kidney disease	Too much sugar free in urine; filtering system works inefficiently	Frequency, pain, dysuria, anuria; retention of urine	Diet modification and medication; kidney dialysis	Observe and record intake/output; color and appearance of urine
Vascular disease and nerve degeneration	Heart problems Osteoporosis Dementia Neuropathy	Blueness of fingers and toes Pain in bones; fractures Confusion Loss of feeling in legs	Medication	Give proper foot care; encourage proper diet; keep legs elevated

FIGURE 20-6   Long-term effects of diabetes.

are unable to see to check their feet. They rely on the aide to do the checking.

Foot Care. Because of nerve damage and poor circulation to the feet, the feet of a diabetic are very prone to infections. A client's feet and legs need to be examined daily for signs of dry, scaly, itching, or cracked skin; blisters; corns; infections; blueness and swelling of the ankles; and discolored nails.

Any abnormality must be reported to the case manager. Bunions and corns must be treated by a podiatrist (health care provider who specializes in foot problems).

In the older adult, the nails become thick and difficult to cut. Nail care (both fingernails and toenails) must be carefully done by a nurse or someone who has been taught to do it correctly. **NOTE:** The aide may **not** cut the diabetic client's nails. There is danger of infection from skin cuts around the nails. The following foot care guide will help reduce injury to the feet:

- Bathe the feet daily in warm, not hot, water.
- Pat the feet dry with a soft towel, especially between the toes.

- Massage the feet with a lanolin lotion to prevent dryness and to increase circulation.
- If the areas between the toes are moist due to perspiration, a very small piece of lamb's wool or cotton can be placed between the toes.
- Wear clean white cotton socks and change socks daily.
- Avoid walking barefoot.
- Always wear comfortable, well-fitting shoes.
- Do not use commercial corn pads.

Vision Impairment. Loss of vision is a common problem of clients with diabetes. A few older adults may have vision problems and be unable to read directions to do blood sugar testing or to read the numbers on the insulin syringe. Because of these vision problems, the home health aide may need to read the directions to the client and also double-check the readings. Diabetes can damage the blood vessels of the retina (diabetic retinopathy), which can lead to blindness.

Kidney Damage. The filtering system of the kidneys of diabetics does not always work correctly. This damaged filtering system can lead to kidney failure or end-stage kidney disease.

Susceptibility to Infections. Clients with diabetes are very susceptible to any type of infection. If they do get the flu or a cold, their blood sugar levels usually decrease and increase erratically. Diabetic clients need to monitor their blood sugar more closely if they have even a mild cold or fever.

Healing of Abrasions. Diabetic persons have problems with the healing of small cuts or abrasions. Special attention by the aide to keep any cut or abrasion as clean as possible will assist in the healing process. Slow healing is due in part to poor circulation. The slow healing process leaves the skin open to infection. The risk of infection is also increased because of the extra sugar in the blood. The extra sugar creates an ideal environment for bacteria to grow. Bacteria can multiply quickly before the body is able to defend itself. Poor circulation delays the transport of substances needed to fight off the bacteria.

Gangrene. When blood vessels are injured or diseased, the surrounding cells die from lack of nutrition and oxygen. A large area of dead tissue is called gangrene. Gangrene is a serious condition because it is easily infected with certain bacteria. Gangrene is a form of an infection. The bacteria causing gangrene thrive in dead tissue. The bacteria spread quickly, causing severe pain and greater tissue damage.

  The aide should monitor the client's feet and broken skin areas for signs of gangrene (Figure 20-7). The first sign is a hot and reddened skin area. This area becomes cold and bluish (cyanotic). After the tissues are dead, they turn black and flake off. Drainage from the area may be bubbly and emit a strong, foul odor.

Hypoglycemia (Low Blood Sugar) or Insulin Shock. If the blood sugar goes too low, a condition called hypoglycemia occurs. This is also called insulin shock. Normal blood sugar is between 70 mg and 110 mg. Hypoglycemia occurs when there is an imbalance between food intake and the appropriate dosage of hypoglycemic drug therapy—oral drugs, insulin, or both. Exercise, intake of alcohol, or decreased kidney or liver function can aggravate this condition. The signs of hypoglycemia are:

- Change in mental functioning
- Heart palpitations
- Sweating

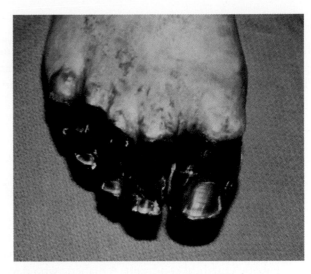

FIGURE 20-7 Gangrene of the toes and foot often requires eventual amputation.

- Hunger
- Shaking
- Seizures
- Blood sugar level below 70 mg

If it is confirmed that the blood sugar is below 50 mg, this is an emergency. If the client is alert, give some form of concentrated sugar such as hard candy, honey, or glucose tablets. If the client becomes unresponsive, call 911 and begin your emergency protocol.

Hyperglycemia (High Blood Sugar) or Diabetic Coma. If a client's blood sugar is high, this is called hyperglycemia. This condition can also be called diabetic coma or acidosis. A person's blood sugar can rise for many reasons, such as too much stress or exercise and eating too many sweets. The signs of hyperglycemia are:

- Increased thirst, hunger, and urination
- Weakness
- Dry mouth
- Generalized aches and pains
- Nausea and vomiting
- Fruity odor to breath

  This is a serious condition. Your case manager should be contacted immediately. If the person is unresponsive, you should call 911 or follow the emergency protocol. Insulin is needed as well as fluid replacement and blood tests to evaluate the client's metabolism. If either insulin reaction or acidosis is not corrected immediately, coma or death can occur.

Identification Tag

All diabetics should wear a Medic-Alert identification tag. The ID is a labeled tag worn as a bracelet or necklace (Figure 20-8). The ID tag should be worn by the diabetic individual at all times. The label indicates:

- Name
- Address
- Phone number
- Medical condition
- Health care provider's name

In emergencies, the Medic-Alert ID informs emergency personnel, police, health care providers, and others of the diabetic's medical condition. A diabetic who develops acidosis or insulin shock needs immediate help. The ID tag notifies health personnel that the person's emergency is possibly a diabetic condition. If the person is unconscious, the tag may provide information necessary to save the person's life. Medic-Alert tags are also worn by clients who have Alzheimer's disease, epilepsy, or allergies to certain drugs.

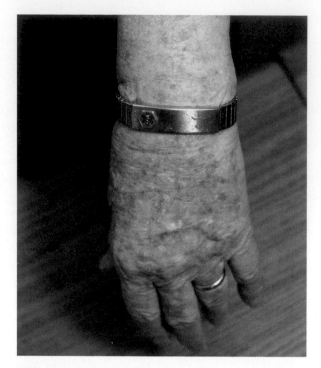

FIGURE 20-8 A Medic-Alert identification tag provides essential information in case of an emergency.

WORKBOOK REVIEW

Go to the workbook and complete the review exercises and activities for Unit 20.

REVIEW

1. List two organs of the endocrine system.

   _____

   _____

2. List two signs of hypothyroidism.

   _____

   _____

3. List five signs and symptoms of diabetes.

_____

_____

_____

_____

_____

4. If a client's blood sugar is 250 mg, the client is most likely experiencing
   a. hypoglycemia.
   b. hyperglycemia.
   c. hypotension.
   d. hypertension.

5. List three signs of hypoglycemia.

_____

_____

_____

6. List three signs of hyperglycemia.

_____

_____

_____

7. What should the home health aide do if the client's blood sugar goes below 50 mg?

8. What should the home health aide do if the client's blood sugar goes above 250 mg?

9. List three long-term effects of diabetes.

_____

_____

_____

10. Why is good foot care important when caring for a client with diabetes?

11. Why is it important to have a client with diabetes exercise on a routine basis?

12. Which of the following is *not* true regarding foot care for the diabetic client?
    a. The toenails should be cut frequently by the home health aide.
    b. The client's feet should be soaked in warm water.
    c. Have the client wear shoes.
    d. The client's feet should be rubbed with lotion to keep the skin in good condition.

13. Which of the following is *not* a common complication of diabetes?
    a. Blindness
    b. Vascular diseases
    c. High risk of infections
    d. Loss of memory

14. Diabetes can be treated by which of the following?
    a. Special diet
    b. Oral medication
    c. Insulin injections
    d. All of the above

15. In a client with diabetes, the ___ is not producing an adequate amount of the hormone insulin.
    a. thyroid
    b. pancreas
    c. adrenal gland
    d. liver

Case Studies

16. You are with your client, Mrs. Jones, who is a known diabetic. You notice that she is increasingly confused and is somewhat shaky. She is also perspiring. Is this a life-threatening situation? What would you do to assist Mrs. Jones?

17. Your client, an 87-year-old diabetic, is partially blind, and as a result is inactive. Although you know your client is on a restricted-calorie diet, she continues to ask you to provide her with high-calorie sweet snacks. What steps can you take to help your client, while being mindful of the diet restrictions? What factors might be contributing to her wanting snacks all the time?

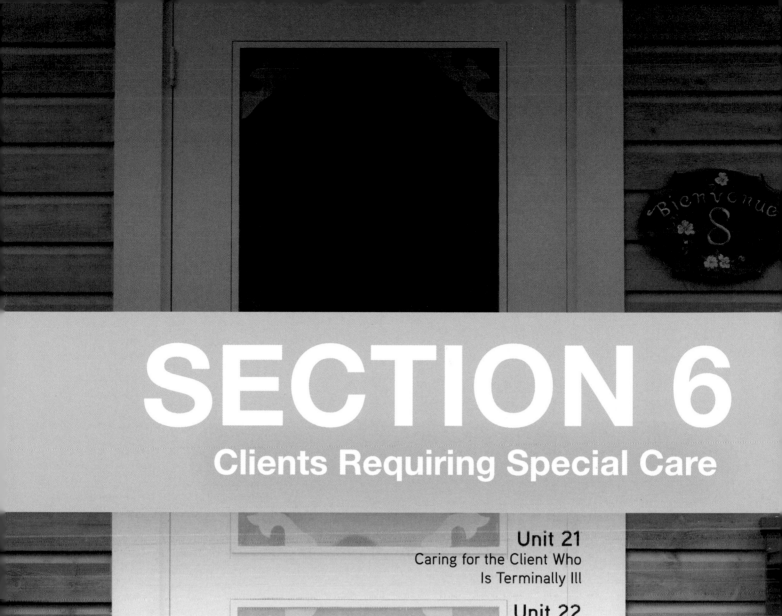

SECTION 6
Clients Requiring Special Care

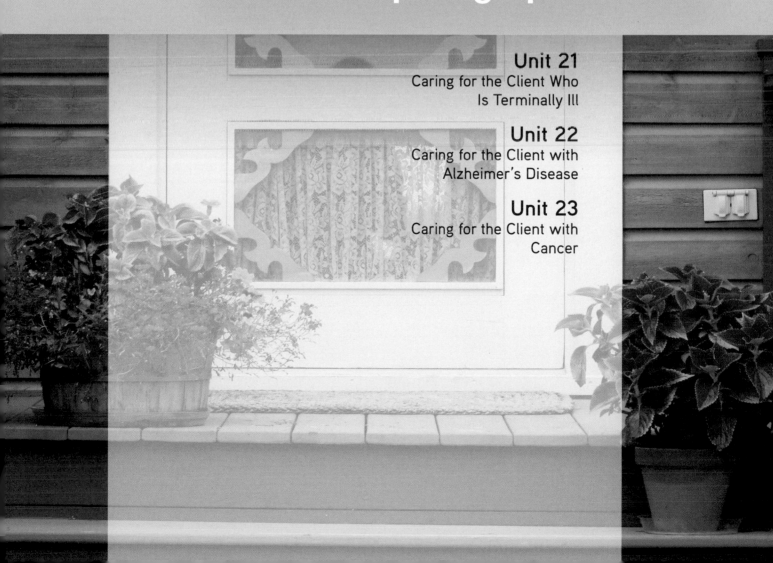

UNIT 21

Caring for the Client Who Is Terminally Ill

KEY TERMS

advance
  directives

autopsy

comatose

durable power of
  attorney

embalming

grieving

hospice

living will

mental health directives

mottling

palliative

Patient Self-
  Determination Act

terminal

LEARNING OBJECTIVES

After studying this unit, you should be able to:

- Explain the hospice program

- Discuss advanced directives

- Describe the five stages of grief

- Discuss the home health aide's responsibilities in providing supportive care and keeping the client pain-free

- List the physical signs of approaching death

- Identify ways in which a person may react to the death of a family member or friend

- Briefly describe major religious beliefs related to death and dying

- Explain the importance of grieving

Most people in our society feel uncomfortable talking or thinking about death. This is more true today than in earlier times in history. Gathering in the room of a dying relative was a custom practiced no more than 40 years ago. Death was accepted as the natural end to life. Children openly shared the final moments of life with a dying grandparent, parent, or sibling.

This is the first time in society that three or four generations of one family are living at the same time. Death experiences in some families have been rare. For many individuals, death is extremely difficult to deal with. In the 1980s, 80% of deaths occurred in the hospital setting and few people assisted their loved ones in their last days. In recent years there has been a reversal of the trend of transferring a loved one to the hospital to die. Families are now allowing their loved ones to die in their own homes in a familiar environment. This is due primarily to the expansion of the hospice program.

Hospice Program

Hospice care is a choice for clients who have been given a diagnosis that death will most likely come within the next 6 months. Hospice care involves a team of professionals such as nurses, home health aides, clergy, health care providers, social workers, and volunteers. The hospice service is available to respond to questions or crises 24 hours a day and is available to the home health aide if the aide has any questions or concerns. Hospice emphasizes comfort and relief from physical and emotional pain for both the client and the family as they work through the dying process.

Hospice offers comfort and support to relieve suffering that is often neglected—pain, fatigue, anxiety,

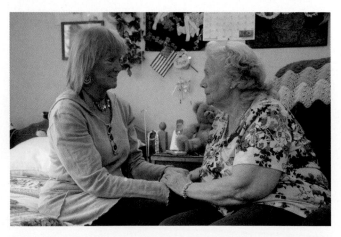

FIGURE 21-1   Daughter visiting her mother, who is terminally ill.

depression—once doctors give up on treating the client with aggressive medical treatment.

Some hospices are independent programs offering services in the client's home; others are a part of a hospital or long-term care facility. Medicare, Medicaid, and private insurance will cover a major cost of the services, if the client is enrolled in one of these programs. The criterion to enter a hospice program is that the client's life expectancy is less than 6 months due to a terminal illness. The client is in the terminal stage (final stage) of a fatal illness (Figure 21-1). The primary concern of hospice is quality of life and not prolonging the client's life.

Advance Directives

Medical science has made treatments more available and more effective. Because of these and other changes, people can expect to live for many years. Diseases once incurable have been conquered. New medicines and surgical techniques have been developed that save thousands of lives daily. Most of these medical advances improve the quality of life. However, some of the medical advances prolong life but do not always improve the quality of life. The value of life-support systems is being questioned today. At times a client is kept alive by machines but has no awareness of being alive. These machines take over the vital functions for the client. Because of problems with the making of decisions regarding use of life-support machines and other life-prolonging measures, in 1991 the Patient Self-Determination Act was passed. This law requires home health agencies receiving Medicare and Medicaid to implement procedures to increase public awareness regarding the rights of clients to make choices. The law is concerned primarily with advance directives. An advanced directive is a statement made by clients that defines care they deem acceptable if they become incapacitated. It effectively allows clients, while competent, to participate in end-of-life decisions and to choose the types of life-sustaining procedures they permit if they become unable to make their own decisions.

Advance directives can be done by a living will, durable power of attorney, and, in some states, mental health directives. A durable power of attorney allows the client to appoint a person to make health-related decision when the client is incapable of making them. A living will is a document prepared by a competent adult that provides direction regarding medical care should the person become incapacitated or otherwise unable to make decisions personally. Mental health directives provide specific directions or designate an agent to make decisions

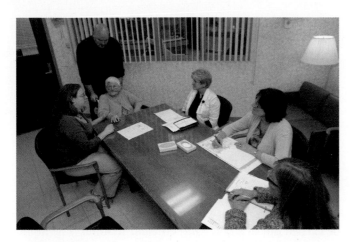

FIGURE 21-2 Client seeking advice when preparing advance directives.

concerning mental health treatment (Figure 21-2). Before you start caring for a client, decisions may already have been made by the client concerning what he or she wants done when seriously ill. One of these forms has almost certainly been completed already by the client. Your case manager will inform you of your client's wishes. You may have two clients with the same serious illness, yet one client may have mechanical life support and the other one only pain medication to keep him or her comfortable. The health care providers are just following the client's wishes. This eases the burden on the family and also the health care provider in making the decision to use or not use mechanical life support.

Changing attitudes toward death have appeared partly as a result of increased life expectancy. People seem to fear death as never before. They want to hold on to life and try not to think about death.

Stages of Grief

Dr. Elisabeth Kübler-Ross has made careful studies of dying persons and their families. She has described a general pattern common to persons facing death. The pattern may apply to both the dying person and the person's family. Dr. Kübler-Ross has noted five stages of grief. Clients may go through the five stages at different times. Sometimes the client may repeat a stage or bounce back and forth through the stages. The aide must listen and closely observe the client and try to recognize what the client is communicating. The stages are as follows:

1. Denial—This is not happening to me; perhaps someone else, but not me.

2. Anger—An extension of denial; feeling that this death is unfair; bitterness and loss of faith; fighting against death or loss of a loved one.

3. Bargaining—Starts bargaining for more time to live: "I promise to live a better life if I can just get better now."

4. Depression—Clients come to full understanding that they might die. They may display brooding, withdrawal, lack of communication, or thoughts of suicide—"I'd rather kill myself than die from this disease" (Figure 21-3).

5. Acceptance—Calmly facing what is to be or feeling a sense of peace; looking forward to release from pain and sorrow; hoping for the release of a loved one to a better world.

Home health aides who are in an environment of expected death may see these patterns develop or may find themselves experiencing these stages. The aide should be understanding, kind, and empathetic. By knowing what to expect in the way of reactions, the home health aide is better prepared to adjust to the situation.

Sometimes a client may die suddenly and unexpectedly. Other times death is preceded by a long illness. Some people are relieved that life is ending. Some clients become **comatose** (unconscious) just before death. Of the five senses (hearing, taste, touch, sight, smell), the last to

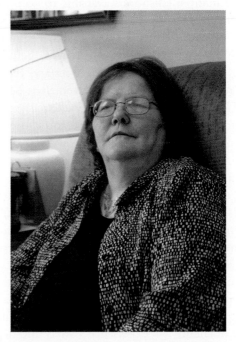

FIGURE 21-3 Depression is associated with the dying process.

be lost is hearing. For this reason, when working with an unconscious client, the home health aide should be careful of what is said in the client's presence. It would be cruel if the last words a client heard were, "Well, she's almost gone; she'll be dead by morning." The home health aide's first duty is to keep the client clean and as comfortable as possible. The client should be treated with kindness and dignity at all times. In addition, the aide should provide emotional support to the client and the family. Good communication skills are needed when dealing with the dying client and the family.

Home Health Aide Responsibilities in Caring for the Dying Client

As a home health aide, you will be working with the client more than the other members of the health team. You will see the client often, and it is important to create and maintain a trusting relationship with the client. When the client knows there is no cure for his or her illness, the care given to this client is called **palliative** care. This type of care emphasizes quality of life, not prolonging life. The goal of palliative care programs is to keep chronically ill clients out of the hospital—for example, keeping the client from ending up in the emergency room at 3 a.m. because of pain crisis. The health care team now focuses on how to manage the best quality of life for the client. The physical pain arising from a terminal illness such as cancer can be unbearable, terrifying, and dehumanizing. There are many medications available to keep the client as pain-free as possible. Encourage the client to verbalize presence of pain. When a client is first beginning pain medication, oral medications usually work better and are easier to take. As the disease progresses and the pain increases, narcotic drugs are often given. It is best for the client to keep ahead of the pain and take pain medication on a regular basis. Once the pain gets too severe, stronger pain medication may be needed. If the client is unable to take pain medication by mouth, there are other ways the medication can be given. Pain medication can be given through the rectum by means of a suppository, under the tongue (sublingually), through patches on the skin, by injection into the skin, and through intravenous injections. The home health aide needs to observe and monitor the client for pain and report when the pain medication ordered for the client is no longer effective. Another observation the aide may need to make is how the client is handling the emotional stress of the terminal illness. The majority of clients will experience anxiety and depression over their diagnosis. A little distress is normal, but if it is prolonged the aide should report this, as the client may

need some counseling or may need medication for depression. As the disease progresses in the body, other physical problems need to be addressed such as nausea, constipation, and breathing. The client may need medication for the nausea, enemas or suppositories for constipation, and oxygen to help with breathing. It is of utmost importance to keep the case manager informed on the status of the client and any changes occurring with the client. This will assist the case manager in deciding when and what to do for the client to keep the client as comfortable as possible. As death gets closer, nursing care measures become greater. The duties of the home health aide will need to be carried out in a quiet and efficient manner. The home health aide will need to pay particular attention to client comfort measures. The client will need:

- Position changed every 2 hours
- Mouth care performed every 2 hours
- Lip moisturizer applied often
- Artificial eye drops instilled in eyes because eyes may cease to blink
- Vital signs monitored
- Skin kept clean and dry
- Small sips of water given often

If the home health aide has time, the aide can just sit and hold the client's hand, or read from the Bible (Figure 21-4) or other books that might be available.

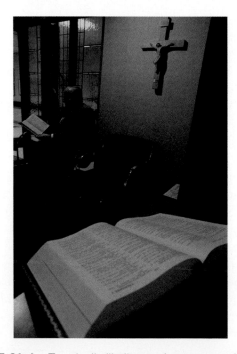

FIGURE 21-4   Terminally ill clients often request that a part of the Bible be read to them.

Another suggestion is to play soft music. Clients generally will like a quiet, softly lit room, but soft music is often welcomed.

Signs of Approaching Death

Certain signs indicate that death is approaching. These signs are:

- Respirations are moist and noisy.

- Breathing will stop (apnea) and then breathing will be labored (dyspnea), known as Cheyne-Stokes respirations.

- Pulse is irregular, rapid, and weak.

- The client is incontinent of bowel and bladder.

- Skin is cool, moist, and clammy.

- Eyes do not respond to light.

- Body relaxes and jaw drops.

- Sense of pain is diminished.

- Skin becomes pale and **mottling** (discoloration) can occur.

The dying client will normally try to hold on, even though it may bring prolonged discomfort, in order to be sure that those who survive will be all right. When a client is ready to die, allowing family members or friends to say good-bye is a final gift of love and achieves closure to life.

When death occurs, family members may be highly emotional. The home health aide must remain calm and notify the case manager if death has occurred. Death is a legal event that calls for certain formalities. Before a funeral can take place, a health care provider must complete a death certificate that states the cause of death, and formally register the death. In some cases, a death may have to be investigated by a medical examiner or a coroner, and an **autopsy** (a detailed examination of the body to determine the exact cause of death) may be ordered. An autopsy provides more information about the client's illness and may either be requested by the family or required by law in the event of an unexpected or unexplained death. Funeral directors can be helpful in making these arrangements and will come to the home to remove the body and take it to the funeral home. After a home health aide has cared for a terminally ill client for a length of time, the aide may feel grief after the client has died. It helps if the aide can attend the client's funeral and share his or her feelings with the family. Figure 21-5 lists the duties of a home health aide when the client dies.

1. Call the case manager. Write down the time the client stopped breathing and you felt no pulse. The case manager will call the health care provider, family, and funeral director. A death certificate will be completed by the health care provider.

2. Do not touch the client until the case manager states it is all right to do so.

3. Clean the client's body and remove all tubings. The funeral home will come to the home to pick up the body.

FIGURE 21-5 What to do when a client dies.

Religious and Cultural Influences

Cultural and family differences will influence the death and dying process, including the public behavior of grieving. For example, Native Americans and Inuit people followed customs that today may be thought of as uncivilized. The elderly, ill members of Inuit tribes were taken to an iceberg and left alone with a small amount of food. This was the accepted way to die. In certain Native American tribes, people who were ill and unable to do their share of work were taken to an isolated spot to await death. These customs were accepted as a natural and respectable way for life to end. Native Americans felt that it was good to allow life to end naturally. When human power to cure with herbs and medicines was not effective, it was time for death to come.

Among some Jewish families, burial occurs within 24 hours after death. Jewish religious practice forbids **embalming** (treating the body with preservatives to prevent decay) the body and requires that the casket remain closed. After the funeral the family may have a period of formal mourning. During this time, friends and relatives come to the home to comfort each other.

In other Jewish families and in Catholic or Protestant families, the body is usually taken to a funeral home. Friends and family meet at the funeral home during the day or two before the body is buried.

Religious practices differ from one group to another and even from family to family (Figure 21-6). Most people recognize the need for the sharing of grief. This is part of the final acceptance of death. Some people weep; others are angry. Some are very quiet. As people work through

Religion	Autopsy	Organ Donation	Beliefs and Practices
Judaism (Orthodox)	Only in special circumstances	With consultation of rabbi	Visits to the dying are a religious duty. Witness must be present if death occurs, to protect family and commit soul to God. Torah and Psalms may be read and prayers recited. Conversation is kept to a minimum. Someone should be with the body after death until burial, usually within 24 hours. Body must not be touched 8 to 30 minutes after death. Medical personnel should not touch or wash body unless death occurs on Jewish Sabbath; then care may be given by the health care worker wearing gloves.
Hinduism	Permitted	Permitted	Priest ties thread around neck or wrist of deceased and pours water in the mouth. Only family and friends touch the body.
Buddhism	Personal preference	Permitted	Buddhist priest is present at death. Last rites are chanted at the bedside.
Islam (Muslim)	Only for medical or legal reasons	Not permitted	Before death, read Koran and pray. Client confesses sins and asks forgiveness of family. Only family touches or washes body. After death, body is turned toward Mecca.
Roman Catholic	Permitted	Permitted	Sacraments of the Sick administered to ill client, to client in imminent danger, or shortly after death.
Christian Scientist	Unlikely	Not permitted	No ritual is performed before or after death.
Church of Christ	Permitted	Permitted	No ritual is performed before or after death.
Jehovah's Witness	Only if required by law	Not permitted	No ritual is performed before or after death.
Baptist	Permitted	Permitted	Clergy ministers through counseling and prayers.
Episcopalian	Permitted	Permitted	Last rites are optional.
Lutheran	Permitted	Permitted	Last rites are optional.
Eastern Orthodox Christian	Not encouraged	Not encouraged	Last rites are mandatory and are given by ordained priest.

FIGURE 21-6   Beliefs and practices related to dying and death for major religions.

their emotions, they come to accept the loss. Many believe that the death of an older person is less tragic than the death of a younger person. A death that is sudden is more difficult to accept than one following a long, painful illness. Mixed emotions may be felt by families when a client dies after a long illness. On the one hand, families are glad that their loved one is no longer suffering, yet on the other hand, their loved one will be missed.

The grieving process is the physical and emotional response to a loss, and the process of accepting it. The grief process can take a long time, and it is hard work. It can take from several months to a year to readjust to the loss of a loved one. Often, the first several months are the most difficult. Grief is a private journey that is different for everyone, influenced by cultural and family differences. Although life is never the same when a loved one dies, not all the changes experienced after a death are negative. Often a person grows in new ways, developing new coping styles and becoming more introspective, questioning values and lifestyles. Grieving can help a person discover inner strength and resiliency, emerging as a more caring and compassionate person. Although all people cope with grief in different ways, grief needs to be expressed, or processed, so it can be healed. If grief is not expressed, symptoms of erratic behavior or failing health may appear. Today there are special support groups for individuals to assist them in the grieving process. The hospice's chaplain can be very important in helping the client find spiritual peace before death and can also support the family after the client's death. Many hospices have bereavement coordinators to help the family at this time and follow up with the family for a year after the client's death.

WORKBOOK REVIEW

Go to the workbook and complete the review exercises and activities for Unit 21.

REVIEW

1. List the five stages of grief.

_____

_____

_____

_____

2. What is the primary goal of hospice?

3. List five signs of approaching death.

_____

_____

_____

_____

_____

4. T F   Palliative care means that the care will be directed toward curing the client.

5. T F   Two examples of advance directives are durable power of attorney and a living will.

6. T F   Hearing is the first sense to be lost in the dying process.

7. T F   The dying client needs to be kept as pain-free as possible.

8. T F   The grieving process is the physical and emotional response to a loss, and the process of accepting it.

9. As death approaches, which of the following changes occur in the body?
    a. Rapid, weak pulse
    b. Cold, clammy skin
    c. Cheyne-Stokes respirations
    d. All of the above

10 During which of the five stages of dying would a client most likely say, "If only I could live to see my oldest daughter get married"?
    a. Denial
    b. Anger
    c. Bargaining
    d. Acceptance

Case Studies

11. Mr. Jones, who was terminally ill, has just died. You informed the case manager of the client's death. The wife and daughter are in the home with you. Now what do you do?

12. Mrs. Clark, who is 87 years old, has been diagnosed with terminal cancer. As the aide gives her a bath, she states, "I want to kill myself to get it over with, as my medical bills will take all of my savings." Should the aide report this conversation to the case manager? Why or why not?

UNIT 22

Caring for the Client with Alzheimer's Disease

KEY TERMS

Alzheimer's disease

catastrophic
  behavior

dementia

habilitation

hoarding

pillaging

reality orientation

reminiscence

repetitive behaviors

shadowing

sundowning

suspiciousness

validation
  therapy

wandering

LEARNING OBJECTIVES

After studying this unit, you should be able to:

- Describe the term *dementia*

- Discuss how Alzheimer's disease is diagnosed

- List the eight warning signs of Alzheimer's disease

- Discuss the five stages of Alzheimer's disease

- Discuss the various behaviors that are characteristic of dementia

- Discuss how to work with clients who display various behaviors, such as wandering and sundowning

- Identify the benefits of using habilitation, validation therapy, and reminiscence when working with clients with dementia

- List five tips for communicating with the client with dementia

Alzheimer's Disease

Alzheimer's disease is the most common form of dementia (loss of mind). When a client has dementia of any type, the results are similar. The client will experience impaired thinking, inability to comprehend, loss of memory, loss of reasoning ability, and loss of judgment. Statistics from the Alzheimer's Association state that as the population ages, Alzheimer's disease (AD) will affect a greater percentage of people. The number of seniors over the age of 65 and older will double between now and 2050 to 88.5 million, to make up 20% of the population. The risk of Alzheimer's disease doubles every 5 years beyond 65 years of age. Remember that dementia is not a normal part of aging. Only 10% of all individuals with dementia have early-onset dementia, which is seen in individuals under the age of 65. Signs and symptoms come on gradually and include memory loss, decline in the ability to perform routine tasks, disorientation, personality changes, difficulty in learning, and loss of language skills. The time from onset of symptoms until death can range from 3 to 20 years. In the advanced stage of the disease, clients are totally dependent on others for activities of daily living.

No single clinical test can identify Alzheimer's disease. A comprehensive evaluation to establish the diagnosis will include a complete health history, physical examination, and neurological and mental health status exams. Diagnostic tests used to rule out other diseases that can cause dementia are magnetic resonance imaging (MRI) and computed tomography (CT). Documenting and recording of the client's behavior by a friend or family member over time will assist the health care provider in the diagnosis. Recently, new drugs are being used in the beginning stages of the disease, and they do help delay the progression of the disease. Examples of these drugs are:

Generic Name	Brand Name
rivastigmine	Exelon®
galantamine	Razadyne®
donepezil	Aricept®
memantine	Namenda®

Other drugs can also be given to soothe agitation, anxiety, and sleeplessness, and to enhance the client's ability to participate in activities.

Warning Signs

Memory Loss. The client will forget recent events, names, and placement of everyday items such as a toothbrush. For example, the client might remember the details of her wedding dress, but will not remember if she ate or not at noon.

Confusion About Time and Place. The client will not remember the current day or month and might easily get lost in a local grocery store. The client may drive her car around for hours before arriving at home.

Inability to Perform Activities of Daily Living. The client may put her clothes on in incorrect order and may even try to brush her teeth with her comb.

Speech Is Incoherent. The client will answers questions inappropriately or say "no" when she means "yes." The client's ability to follow directions is flawed. The client may repeat the same sentence or phrase over and over again.

Decision Making and Judgment Are Decreased. The client may cross the street with cars coming from all directions and not know it. The client may go outside in the winter without shoes or a coat.

Change in Personality and Mood. The client may accuse family members or caregivers of stealing and be very suspicious of their actions. Client may show very little interest in doing anything but sitting in a chair.

Problems with Abstract Thinking. The client is unable to balance the checkbook or pay monthly bills on time. When eating out, the bill may be $5.00 and the client will want to pay the waitress $50.00.

Stages of Dementia. No two clients with this disease are alike. One client might progress quite quickly through the various stages, whereas another client will go slowly through each stage.

The five basic stages of the progression of dementia are as follows:

1. Mild cognitive impairment—The client may experience some memory problems but is able to live independently.

2. Mild dementia—The client starts experiencing short-term memory loss and has problems with everyday thinking skills. The client will need assistance in financial matters, grooming, dressing, meal planning, and cooking. The client becomes somewhat confused when in public or around

large crowds. The client will experience problems remembering everyday events and handling money. The client will start to have problems with dressing and may need someone to pick out his or her clothing. If left alone, the client would not know how to cook a meal.

3. Moderate dementia—The client has severe memory loss and has problems talking with others and understanding what other people are saying. The client can no longer live alone and needs assistance with all activities of daily living. Behaviors such as wandering, sleeplessness, and shadowing become more evident. The client may make threats, accuse others of stealing, curse, kick, hit, bite, or grab things.

4. Severe dementia—The client experiences severe problems communicating with others. The client becomes incontinent of urine and then feces, and requires care 24 hours a day. The caregiver is required to bathe, dress, and assist the client with feeding and toileting. Often in this stage, the family seeks out long-term care arrangements for the client.

5. Profound dementia—Body functions slowly shut down. The client is able to say about six words, loses the ability to walk, then loses the ability to sit up, then loses the ability to smile, and finally is unable to hold the head up.

Support for Caregivers of Those with Alzheimer's

There are support groups for caregivers of those with Alzheimer's in many communities. Family members can meet to share common problems and learn more about how to cope with their parent or relative as well as face up to their own feelings and fears. The Alzheimer's Association can link families with resources in their community to help them cope with this disease. The national toll-free number of the Alzheimer's Association is 1-800-272-3900, and the Web address is www.alz.org. In some areas there are special day-care centers where Alzheimer's disease clients can be taken for a few hours a day. These centers provide activity, and clients will often enjoy talking, playing cards, playing the piano, or singing with others, plus an exercise area (Figure 22-1). These centers may also provide a place where the client can be given a shower or bath. Clients may have "good" days or

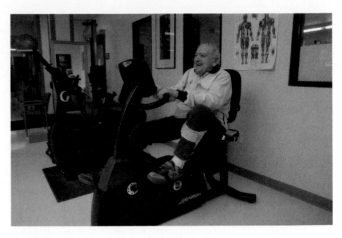

FIGURE 22-1   A client at a senior day-care center using an exercise bike.

weeks when they function reasonably well at such centers. On the other hand, if the group activities have a negative effect on the client, the family may need to seek another option for care for the client.

Caring for the Client

Taking care of a client with dementia is difficult and requires a great deal of patience, empathy, and understanding of the disease process.

The home health aide may be employed by the family to provide respite care for 2 or 3 days a week. That is, while the home health aide provides care, the family may take advantage of these breaks to take care of errands or just experience freedom from caregiving responsibilities.

Home Environment

Keeping the home environment safe is an important role for the home health aide, especially when working with a client who suffers from memory problems or who may wander away. The aide should look for safety hazards in the home and remove them. If your client smokes, urge the family to keep all smoking materials away from the client, who may forget and leave a lit cigarette unattended. If possible, restrict access into the kitchen, where there are likely to be many opportunities for danger. Remove knobs from the stove, and disconnect appliances that are not in use. Be sure that all poisons, cleaning products, lotions, shampoos, perfumes, and medications are kept in a locked cabinet. Keep the Poison Control number (1-800-222-1222) by the phone. Potential falls can be avoided by eliminating throw rugs and clutter on stairs and floors. Lighting should be improved if an area is particularly dark or full of glare. Remove excess furniture and make the environment uncluttered. It is recommended to install sturdy handrails on steps and rails in bathrooms. Mirrors should also be removed, as the client may find images in mirrors confusing and frightening. Identify bathrooms and other rooms with picture signs to help re-orient the client. Put a sign up by doors saying "stop" or "do not enter." Limit the decorations for holidays, as this may make the client more confused. Cover garbage cans to prevent the client from rummaging through the garbage. Reset the hot water heater to 120 degrees Fahrenheit to prevent burns.

Dressing

Allow the client to dress her- or himself as long as possible. As the client starts to need assistance in dressing, some helpful hints are:

- Lay out articles of clothing in the order the client should put them on. Let the client choose between a limited amount of clothing (Figure 22-2).

- Use Velcro® closures for clothing, instead of shoelaces or buckles.

- Have three sets of clothing that are alike and the same color, as the client may want to wear the same clothing every day. The client will not know the difference if you place a fresh set of clothing out instead of the soiled one.

- Have pants with elastic waistbands that are easy to get off and on. Sweat pants and tops are great.

- Give simple instructions when assisting the client to dress. Hand the client one item of clothing at a time.

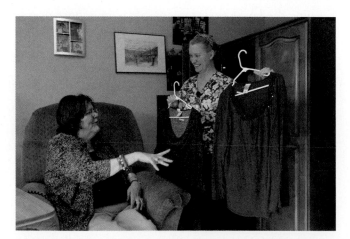

FIGURE 22-2   A client can readily choose a piece of clothing if the choices are limited to two.

- Do not allow the client to place a piece of clothing on backwards, such as a shirt.

- Keep the choices of clothing to a minimum; you may need to keep the closet door locked.

Incontinence

Urinary and fecal incontinence can occur in any stage of the disease process. In the first stage of the disease, the client may need to be reminded to go to the bathroom every 2 or 3 hours. But as the disease progresses, the client should wear loose, comfortable clothing and pants that are easy to pull down to give the client quick access to the toilet. The toilet seat should be at a good height. A colorful seat may assist the client to identify the toilet. Label the door of the bathroom—an Alzheimer's client can read until the last stages of the disease, which is why signs should be used often. Limit the client's intake of fluids after supper and give the client fruit instead of a drink before bedtime. In the late stage of the disease, the client is totally incontinent and will need to wear adult briefs.

Behavioral Considerations

A dementia client who is confused, frightened, or in pain might demonstrate behavior that would be troublesome. If possible, the aide should identify and remove the cause of the problem behavior. Keeping the environment and routine the same is very important. Any change in either the environment or routine can cause undesirable behaviors. Sometimes when behavior management does not work, medication is ordered to control the problem behavior. Almost all medications have some side effects. Occasionally the side effects may be worse than the behavior itself. Therefore, if a client is put on medication, the time, dose, and side effects of the drugs should be closely monitored.

Wandering

Wandering is the most common agitated behavior among people with Alzheimer's disease. Frustration, fear, confusion, fatigue, and discomfort of the client can increase wandering. Often, the client is looking for something, for example, the bathroom, food or drink, a remedy for pain and suffering, a place to lie down, or a familiar face. Other times the client may wander because he or she is playing out an old routine, such as leaving work for home or going to get a loved one. At times a client

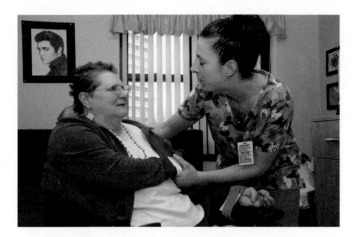

FIGURE 22-3 Never underestimate the value of touch when working with a client with dementia.

wanders to escape a task or activity or to avoid noise or tension. A safe wandering area should be provided for clients to move about freely without risk of injury. Simplify the environment to minimize confusion or distraction. Avoid the use of child safety gates because the client may climb over them or kick them down. If possible, walk with the client when he or she begins to wander, gently redirecting the client back home or to a task or activity. In fact, it may be helpful to schedule regular times for walks in or outside the home with the client, while holding onto the client's hand. Never underestimate the value of touch when working with a confused client (Figure 22-3). A wristband is now available for the client to wear to track where the client may be wandering. Be sure the client is wearing an ID bracelet and has identification in his or her jacket or pockets. Keep doors locked. It may be necessary to use a key deadbolt, or add another lock placed up high or down low on the door. An announcing service can also be installed that chimes when the door opens.

The Safe Return Home Program is a national program that a person with dementia can be registered for. In this program, if the client wanders away and gets lost, the program will assist the client with a safe return home.

Hoarding

Hoarding is collecting and putting things away in a special place. The client may take apples, sugar packets, or cookies and place them in the drawer in the bedroom, for example. The caregiver will need to make sure that food hidden by the client is removed to prevent spoilage. The caregiver needs to do this without the client's knowledge.

Pillaging

When **pillaging**, the client will take things or items that belong to someone else and think they are his or her own. For some unknown reason, shoes are items that clients often take and relocate to another part of the home. One must maintain a sense of humor and patience when working with these clients. The caregiver will need to return items to their proper place. A client who eats meals in a center dining room in an assistive living facility may try to steal food from a person sitting nearby (Figure 22-4).

Repetitive Behaviors

Repetitive behaviors are seen often in dementia. The client will ask the same question repeatedly, or may tell the same story repeatedly, or do the same activity repeatedly. One example of this is with time. The client will ask every few minutes, "What time is it?" The caregiver will tell the client the correct time, and within 2 minutes the client will ask again, "What time is it?" If the client does an activity repeatedly, let the client keep doing it, unless there is harm in the activity. This can become quite annoying for the caregiver and family to deal with, and it takes a great deal of patience on the part of the caregiver. That is why it is highly recommended that the main caregiver take time off at definite intervals to prevent "burnout."

Shadowing

The client may follow the caregiver around and mimic the behavior of others. This is called **shadowing**, and it is quite commonly seen in the client with dementia. It is recommended to just let the client follow the person around as long as the client does no harm.

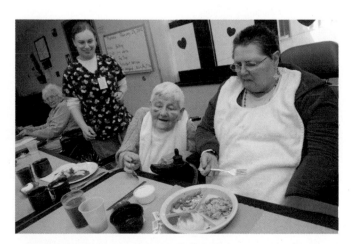

FIGURE 22-4 A client may try to steal another person's food in an assistive living facility dining room.

Sundowning

Sundowning is the term used to describe the behavior of clients with dementia in the late afternoon and evening. At that time of day, there is a definite change in behavior, such as restlessness and irritability in some clients. Something has happened previously that disrupted the body's "internal clock" for the client. One will see many undesirable behaviors occurring with the client experiencing sundowning (Figure 22-5). Evening hours are difficult for some clients and certain things can be done to avoid sundowning behaviors. Hints to avoid these behaviors are:

- Limit caffeine and sugar intake to morning hours only.
- Keep the client in a well-lighted room and have a night light on at night.
- Keep the client reasonably busy with activities during the day, with rest periods in between (Figure 22-6).
- Feed the client at frequent intervals during the day.
- Toilet the client at regular intervals during the day.
- Keep activity simple and at low levels in the afternoon.
- Try to have the client go to bed at the same time each night. Playing soft music the client likes may also help.

Suspiciousness

Because the client forgets where he or she might have placed something, the client often will accuse the caregiver or others of stealing. This behavior is called **suspiciousness**. Do not try to reason with the client; distraction works better in these scenarios.

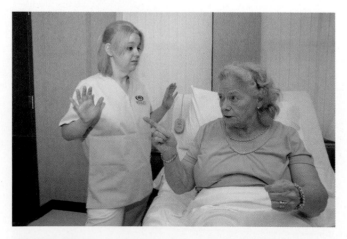

FIGURE 22-5   A client may have hallucinations—seeing things that are not there.

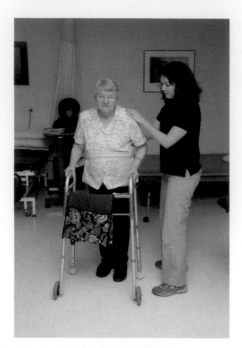

FIGURE 22-6   Keep the client walking as long as possible.

Communication

Tips for communicating with the client with Alzheimer's are:

- Ask questions that only require a "yes" or "no" answer.
- Limit the number of choices—for example, "Would you like apple juice or orange juice?" instead of "What do you want to drink?"
- Offer simple instructions—for example, tell the client to pick up the spoon, then place the spoon in the pudding; once the food is on the spoon, tell the client to place the spoon in the mouth, then to swallow the pudding.
- If the client curses, do not correct the client, just try to get the client to say another phrase.
- Do not use "baby talk" when talking with the client.
- Stand in front of the client when talking and try to get eye contact (Figure 22-7).

Figure 22-8 identifies other useful hints for communicating with a client with dementia.

Sexuality Changes

Changes may occur with the client in terms of expressing sexual desires. Sometimes, clients are overly interested in sex. The client may masturbate openly and try to lure others. These behaviors are part of the disease process and don't normally mean the client wants sex. Masturbation is satisfying to the client and is not harmful. If you see the client masturbating, provide privacy and leave that area of the house. If the client asks the aide for sex, tell the client tactfully that this behavior is not acceptable (Figure 22-9).

Catastrophic Behavior

Catastrophic behavior is a response to stimuli that is overwhelming to the client. The client will react by screaming, cursing, threatening, hitting, or biting. The cause for this type of behavior can relate to any number of physical, emotional, or environmental factors, including fear, anger, hunger, the need for attention, or feelings of hopelessness or despair. It is important to note what appears to trigger these behaviors and to take steps to involve the client in situations that are less likely to lead to catastrophic behaviors. When a client is having one of these attacks, do not try to reason with the client. One needs to protect the client so that she or he is not injured. Often the family or other caregivers will be able to give each other ideas on how to approach the client to diminish this type of behavior.

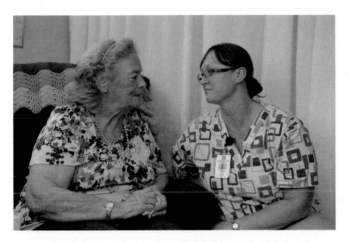

FIGURE 22-7   Maintain eye contact when talking with a client with dementia.

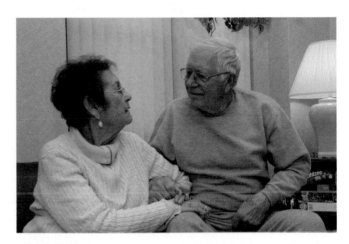

FIGURE 22-9   Provide privacy for couples to express their sexuality.

1. Make sure you have your client' attention *before* you begin to speak; make sure that she can see and hear you, and that she knows that you are talking to her.
2. Face your client when you speak to her, and speak slowly and clearly.
3. Do not talk too much! Give one instruction at a time.
4. Speak in positives instead of in negatives. Your client will respond better to "Come with me" than she will to "Come away from there!"
5. If necessary, repeat the statement or question—do not change the wording.
6. Lead the client in answering if the client cannot find the right words—point to objects to provide clues.
7. Listen carefully to what your client is saying. She may be telling you something important.
8. Respond to your client's feelings, not just to her words.
9. For clients with severe memory loss, focus on validation, not on reality orientation.
10. Be aware of body language—yours and your client's.
11. If your client is frustrated by not being able to make you understand her, then reassure her that you still care about what she feels: "I'm sorry I can't understand what you are saying. Why don't you wait a while and try to tell me later?" Then, move on to another activity.
12. *Never* ask, "Do you remember . . . ?" It may embarrass your client if she can't remember. Instead, tell your client what you want her to remember, for example: "We went to your health care provider's office on Tuesday, and he said that you need to drink more water."

FIGURE 22-8   Tips for communicating with a client with dementia.

Interventions

At the present time there is no cure for Alzheimer's disease. However, good planning, medical care, and a well-structured, calm environment can ease the burden to the client and family. Physical exercise and good nutrition will help maintain the client's health. Watch for signs of dehydration such as dry mouth, dizziness, hallucinations, and rapid heart rate. Keep things simple. Have a daily routine, so the client knows what to expect. Reassure the client that he or she is in a safe place and you are there to help. Use distraction from undesirable behavior by using music, singing, or dancing. Ask the client for help doing simple tasks such as washing dishes or dusting furniture.

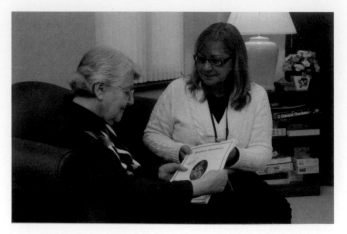

FIGURE 22-10   Reminiscing through old photos.

Validation Therapy

Validation therapy is a communication technique that is used for moderately to severely disoriented clients with diagnosed dementia. The goal of this therapy is to increase self-esteem and validate the client's feelings. The basic premise is that if the client wishes to remain in the past, that should be allowed and no attempt should be made to reorient the client. An example of this type of communication technique is as follows. Suppose an 80-year-old client with Alzheimer's disease is telling you (after her bath and shampoo) not to set her hair because her mother will be coming to do it. You know her mother died 20 years ago. Instead of telling her that her mother is dead, which might make her feel bad, you ask the client something about her mother, such as her mother's name or her mother's hobbies. This will help relay a message to the client that you are concerned with her wishes and will make her feel good about herself. Once clients have dementia, the ability to reason with them has diminished. Often, if you try to reason with them, they become more agitated and combative.

Reminiscence

From the time of diagnosis until the end of life, clients with dementia and their families are victims suffering from the pressures and strains of this disease. These clients have poor short-term memory, but long-term and deep-seated memories may remain. These memories, whether pleasurable or sad, can be recalled by reviewing past life history. **Reminiscence** helps the client with Alzheimer's disease experience being cared for with compassion.

Family involvement can be an important part of this therapy. This time for reclaiming the past creates connectedness. The present moment of a relationship increases family and client satisfaction. Sharing of information might be done by reviewing old movies, videotapes, pictures, songs, and popular radio programs, or even using scrapbooks in which to write and draw (Figure 22-10).

Habilitation

Habilitation is the term used to describe care for the client, which focuses on what the client can do, not what the client used to do. This is recommended for the middle stages of the disease. The aide or caregiver is directed to move into the client's "current world" rather than the "real world."

Reality Orientation

For those clients with mild to moderate memory loss, and particularly for those who continue to understand words, it may be helpful to provide simple memory aids to assist the client in day-to-day living. For example, a prominent calendar, lists of daily tasks, written reminders, signs, labels, and clocks can help to orient the client to the present. It is also recommended to have photos of close family members placed where the client can see them daily. This process of orienting the person to the present moment is known as **reality orientation**. This technique would not be appropriate, however, for someone with a more severe memory loss and may cause frustration, agitation, and loss of self-esteem. The home health aide must use imagination, patience, kindness, and understanding to give the client the service and care that best meets the individual's needs.

WORKBOOK REVIEW

Go to the workbook and complete the review exercises and activities for Unit 22.

REVIEW

1. T   F   Occasional forgetfulness is a sign of having Alzheimer's disease.

2. T   F   Dementia affects memory, personality, behavior, communication, and the ability to perform routine tasks.

3. T   F   Try to use distraction when the client wants to leave, such as having a snack or listening to the client's favorite music.

4. List eight warning signs of Alzheimer's disease.

    _____

    _____

    _____

    _____

    _____

    _____

    _____

    _____

5. Choose the best statement:
    a. Alzheimer's disease is a hereditary disease and results in irregular involuntary movements of the extremities.
    b. Alzheimer's disease is caused by a lack of dopamine, which is the neurotransmitter substance in the central nervous system.
    c. Alzheimer's disease is a progressive, irreversible disease that gradually affects cognitive intelligence, memory, and functional abilities.
    d. Alzheimer's disease is caused by an obstruction in the normal flow of spinal fluid, which in turn causes fluid accumulation in the brain.

6. The primary reasons for wandering include which of the following?
   a. Looking for food or drink
   b. Looking for a familiar place
   c. Trying to escape a task or an activity
   d. All of the above

7. Dementia is seen most often in what age group?
   a. Younger adults
   b. Middle-aged adults
   c. Older adults
   d. All age groups

8. _____ is a communication technique that is helpful with clients who are moderately to severely disoriented with diagnosed dementia.

9. A useful tool to increase the self-esteem of clients with dementia by sharing past events is called _____.

10. A strategy used to orient a client to the present, which is useful only if the client continues to understand words, is called _____.

Case Studies

11. You are assigned to a new client, Mrs. Stone, who has moderate dementia and likes to wander. What safety recommendations could you make to the family that would ensure a safe environment for your client?

12. You are taking care of a client with dementia. During the middle of the night, he wakes up and wants to leave the house. What steps could you take to help your client and redirect him back to his bed?

UNIT 23
Caring for the Client with Cancer

KEY TERMS

abdominal perineal
  resection
adjuvant therapy
alopecia
benign
benign prostatic
  hypertrophy (BPH)
biopsy
cachexia
cancer

carcinogen
chemotherapy
colonoscopy
encapsulated
hormone therapy
hysterectomy
laryngectomy
larynx
lobectomy
lumpectomy

malignant
mammogram
mastectomy
melanoma
metastasis
oncologist
palliative
pneumonectomy
prostate-specific antigen
  (PSA)

prosthesis
radical hysterectomy
remission
sigmoidoscopy
targeted biologic therapy
trachea
tracheostomy
transurethral resection
  of the prostate (TURP)

LEARNING OBJECTIVES

After studying this unit, you should be able to:

- Define *benign*, *malignant*, *metastasis*, and *carcinogens*

- Explain briefly the grading of cancer

- List seven warning signs of cancer

- List four screening tests for cancer

- Describe various ways cancer can be treated

- List common side effects of therapies used to treat cancer

- Describe nursing measures to minimize the side effects of cancer treatments

- Discuss breast and testicular self-examination

- Discuss, briefly, the following types of cancer: colon, lung, cervical, and larynx

- Describe the special nursing care given to a client with terminal cancer

- Describe the appearance of a cancerous skin lesion

Cancer

Cancer is the uncontrolled growth of abnormal cells. In healthy tissue, body cells grow, die, and are replaced by new cells. This is a normal process that goes on day after day. Sometimes cells do not follow the rules of the body; they begin to divide quickly, stealing nourishment from surrounding cells and pushing normal cells out of the way. They prevent normal cells from doing their regular jobs. Finally, these cells cause changes in the body, which produce signs and indicate something is wrong. Any individual experiencing one of the warning signs listed in Figure 23-1 should see his or her health care provider as soon as possible.

The exact cause of cancer is unknown. However, studies are beginning to determine some factors that lead to the formation of cancer cells. A substance or agent that produces cancer is called a carcinogen. The most common groups of carcinogens are chemicals, environmental factors, hormones, and viruses. A chemical could be ingested with food, such as red dye #2, or the chemical could be inhaled as tar or asbestos. Environmental factors include such physical agents as x-rays, sunlight, and trauma. Hormones may cause cancer if there is a hormone excess, deficiency, or imbalance. Viruses seem to upset the functions within a cell. Certain forms of cancer are inherited or have a familial tendency, such as cancer of the breast and colon.

The way that carcinogens change normal cells into cancer cells is unclear. Therefore, a cure is not yet possible. Most health care providers agree, however, that the sooner cancer is detected, the less chance it has of spreading to other parts of the body.

Benign tumors tend to be encapsulated, or confined within a capsule (Figure 23-2A). The tumors generally stay in one area, and if removed, they rarely reoccur. Malignant or cancerous tumor cells spread rapidly and infiltrate other areas of the body (Figure 23-2B). When

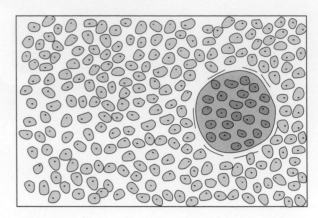

FIGURE 23-2A Growth of cancer cells. A. Benign tumor growth (with capsule around it).

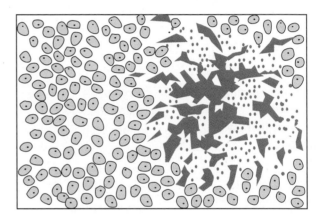

FIGURE 23-2B B. Malignant cancer growth (no capsule with random growth).

viewed under a microscope, cancer cells vary in size, are disorderly, and do not form tissues as normal cells do. These cancer cells spread to other body tissues through a process called metastasis. The cancer cells are carried to other sites by either the blood or lymph system. If the spread of cells is not controlled, the effects on the body can be cachexia (marked wasting away of the body) and death. A biopsy (sample) of the body tissue is done if the health care provider suspects the individual has cancer. This biopsy is done to confirm the diagnosis and to assist in identifying the type of cancer cell. Other tests are also done, such as body scans, imaging tests, x-rays, and blood tests, to determine what stage the cancer is in.

If the cancer is Stage I, it is in the very beginning of development, whereas Stage IV cancer is well developed in the body. Treatment is more successful in the earlier stages than in the advanced stages of the disease. When cancer is treated early and does not reappear for 5 years, the cancer is considered to be cured or in remission.

Warning Signals	
C	Change in bowel or bladder habits
A	A sore that will not heal
U	Unusual bleeding or discharge
T	Thickening or lump in the breast or elsewhere
I	Indigestion or difficulty swallowing
O	Obvious change in wart or mole
N	Nagging cough or hoarseness

FIGURE 23-1 Warning signs of cancer.

Remission means no longer growing or spreading. An oncologist is a physician who specializes in caring for people with cancer.

There are more than 100 types of cancer. Cancer is second only to heart disease as the leading cause of death each year. However, statistics also show that deaths due to cancer are increasing, whereas those due to heart conditions are decreasing.

Cancer Treatments

Several kinds of treatments may slow or stop the growth of cancer cells. Surgery, chemotherapy, radiation, hormone therapy, and targeted biologic therapy or combinations of one or more of these are used to treat cancer. A client may have a tumor surgically removed from her breast, for example, and then need to go through a series of radiation treatments; this is called adjuvant therapy (therapy that aids the surgery). Home health aides are often employed to care for a client temporarily when the client is undergoing one or multiple types of cancer treatment.

If your client is undergoing radiation therapy, the area receiving treatment is usually outlined in black ink or may even be outlined in tiny tattoos. After a few treatments the skin in the enclosed area may become dry, red, itchy, or scaly. Other side effects include fatigue, anemia, hair loss, nausea and vomiting, and mouth sores.

If your client is receiving drugs or medications to treat the cancer, this process is called chemotherapy. These drugs can be given orally, intravenously, or intramuscularly. Short-term side effects of chemotherapy include nausea and vomiting, anemia, fatigue, hair loss, change in appetite, mouth sores, and skin and nail changes.

Hormone therapy is used to slow or stop the growth of prostate cancer in men and breast cancer in women. Hormone therapy acts by decreasing the amount of hormones made naturally in the body. Common short-term side effects for women include hot flashes, vaginal discharge, joint pain, headache, and depression; side effects for men include hot flashes, constipation or diarrhea, nausea, dizziness, and headache.

Targeted biologic therapy is the use of drugs or biologic substances that stop or slow cancer growth by interfering with specific molecules in the body involved in the process of creating cancer cells. Common short-term side effects include an acne-like rash, nausea and vomiting, anorexia, fatigue, increased risk of infections, dry mouth, and increased risk of blood clots.

Regardless of which of the cancer therapies the client is receiving, the client will experience some unpleasant side effects. Some general guidelines to follow with the client relating to some of these side effects are:

- If hair loss (alopecia) occurs, protect the scalp from sun and cold exposure.
- Do not use a hard toothbrush and floss teeth gently.
- Rinse the mouth with 1 teaspoon of baking soda mixed with warm water. Have the client hold the rinse in the mouth for about a minute. Avoid commercial mouthwashes.
- Chewing gum will stimulate salvia and assist with a sore mouth.
- Use lip balm.
- When bathing, use very mild soap and pat dry the area that is under radiation treatment.
- If skin becomes dry, soften it with cream.
- Drink plenty of fluids.
- Eat bland and soft foods.
- Avoid food or juices high in acid content, such as tomato, orange, or grapefruit juice.
- Use liquid or powdered meal replacement, if unable to eat regular foods.
- Eat foods high in iron or folic acid to help with anemia (low blood count).
- For mild diarrhea, use the BRAT diet—eat bananas, rice, applesauce, and toast and drink 3 quarts per day of clear liquids.
- Use an electric razor for shaving to avoid cuts that may cause bleeding.
- Minimize contact with birds and their cages and cats and their litter boxes.
- Avoid clothing that will increase friction and rubbing in the outlined area for a client receiving radiation. It is better to wear loose cotton clothing.
- Avoid large groups of people to limit the client's exposure to other infectious diseases.
- Space activities with rest periods to avoid extreme fatigue in the client.

So-called miracle cures for cancer are sold in many forms. Most people who market these products are only interested in making a profit from the misfortune of others. Some people with cancer choose to take experimental drugs or may take natural herbs and vitamins in hope of a cure. The best treatment plans are based on sound research.

Caring for a Client With Cancer

When a cancer client becomes too weak to care for him- or herself, a home health aide is often employed to assist the client with activities of daily living. Caregiving is focused on relieving symptoms, such as pain, but is not expected to cure the disease (**palliative** care). Its main purpose is to improve the client's quality of life. For the client who has cancer in the later stages, nutrition is a main concern. The diet is designed to focus on increased protein, fluids, and calories in the diet to prevent malnutrition, weight loss, and dehydration. The food texture may need to be modified due to sores in the mouth and the inability to chew. High-fiber foods are usually eliminated from the diet. The client is advised to eat in small amounts, and to have high-calorie snacks available. The client should avoid an empty stomach, as this will prevent nausea from occurring. Sipping fluids throughout the day rather than drinking large amounts of fluids at one time is helpful. Another useful tip is to have the client suck on ice chips, popsicles, or hard candy if the client's mouth is sore. Occasionally, a client may have "upbeat" times during the day when he or she may feel like eating. The home health aide should take advantage of these times and offer the client high-calorie foods to eat.

If the client with cancer is terminal, the client will slowly become weaker and weaker. As the cancer spreads throughout the body, the client may have a distinguishing odor due to the death of body cells. In these cases, room deodorizers can be used to mask the odor.

Pain management at every stage is an important concern, and the generous use of various painkillers and noninvasive techniques that promote relaxation and distractions is encouraged (see Unit 8). The goal of care in the final stages is to keep the client as comfortable as possible. As cancer spreads throughout the body, the pain may become more severe and less tolerated by the client (Figure 23-3). It is important that the home health aide monitors the pain level in the client. If the pain medication is not working, the aide needs to inform the case manager. Sometimes, the client may choose to enter into hospice care. Hospice is designed to relieve the physical and emotional suffering of terminally ill clients. The main goal is to provide comfort, peace, and dignity to the dying client and emotional support to the family and loved ones (Figure 23-4).

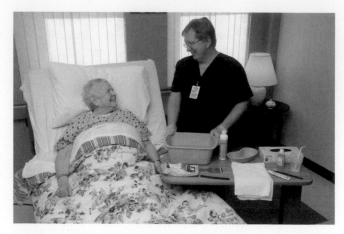

FIGURE 23-3 The goal of care in the late stages of cancer is to keep the client as comfortable as possible.

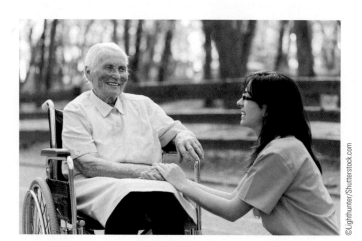

FIGURE 23-4 Touch and just being there are important for a client with cancer.

©Lighthunter/Shutterstock.com

Cancer of the Female Reproductive System

Cancer of the Uterus and Cervix

Among women in the middle years and older, problems may occur in the reproductive system. All women should have an annual physical examination, including a Pap smear. A Pap smear detects early cellular change in the cervix. A microscopic examination is made of cells scraped from the uterus. If repeated Pap smears show cellular changes, the physician takes a biopsy. A biopsy is a sample of tissue cut from the area where cellular change is present. Through a microscopic examination of the tissue, the biopsy determines the seriousness of the cell changes. Sometimes a cone-shaped section is cut out for examination. This is called a conization. The most important risk factor for cervical cancer is infection with the sexually transmitted human papillomavirus. If cancerous cells are found, a partial or complete hysterectomy may be performed. A simple hysterectomy is the removal of the uterus and cervix; if the fallopian tubes and ovaries are removed, it is called a radical hysterectomy. The majority of women would be able to care for themselves after this type of surgery. If the client is older and more fragile, a home health aide may be employed to care for the client.

Some women develop fibroid tumors in the uterus. These tumors are benign or noncancerous. They can become large or cause heavy bleeding during menstruation, or cause pain. When these problems exist, a hysterectomy may be needed. After any major surgery it may take from 9 to 12 weeks for full health to return. If the ovaries have been removed, hormones may be prescribed to replace those normally produced. Although a hysterectomy prevents further childbearing, it does not physically prevent enjoyment of sex.

Breast Cancer

Breast cancer is the second most common cancer occurring in women, after skin cancer. An excellent method of detecting breast cancer is self-examination. Each woman should self-examine her breasts monthly about 7 to 10 days after each period. She should check for changes in the shape of each breast, swelling, dimpling of the skin, or changes in the nipple. She should check for lumps while lying on her back with a pillow under her right shoulder. Using the finger pads on the three middle fingers on her left hand, she should move around the breast in a set way. If a lump is noticed, she should go to her health care provider for further examination. Not all lumps are malignant (cancerous). Many women have simple, benign breast tumors. Sometimes it is necessary to remove the benign tumors through surgery.

One diagnostic technique used in suspected breast cancer is an x-ray called a mammogram. Special x-ray studies can detect unhealthy or cancerous cells. In some cases, a biopsy is ordered if there is a suspicion of cancer of the breast. An incision (cut) is made in the breast and a microscopic examination of tissue is made at once. If cancer is diagnosed, some health care providers remove only the growth itself. This can only be done when the diagnosis is made early. This procedure is sometimes known as a lumpectomy. Sometimes it is necessary to remove the entire breast tissue, underlying muscles, and the lymph glands under the arm. This procedure is called a radical

mastectomy. If there is any sign that the cancer cells have metastasized (spread), both breasts may need to be removed. A woman's self-image is often decreased after a mastectomy. She may see the altered shape of her body as a deformity. However, an increasing number of women who have had this surgery talk about it quite openly. Because they have talked about their own surgery, other women have become more aware of the need to examine themselves. As a result, many breast cancers are discovered early enough for successful treatment.

Following a mastectomy, there is often a time of depression. It is very important for a mastectomy client to have the support of her loved ones. She must understand that her life can continue as before. Part of this is accepting that she is just as much a woman as she was before surgery. After a mastectomy client returns home, special arm exercises must be continued regularly. After the incision is healed, most clients are encouraged to have a prosthesis (artificial breast) made. In some cases, the prosthesis may be surgically fitted under a flap of skin. Other prosthetic devices shaped as cups are fitted into a special bra.

Many women who have breast surgery are helped by the American Cancer Society's Reach to Recovery Program. This is a free service to help meet the physical, emotional, and cosmetic needs of women who have had breast cancer. The Cancer Society carefully trains select volunteers who have a previous history of breast cancer and have coped well with their own breast cancer. A volunteer and the client can talk over fears arising from this disease, the impact on a client's body and self-image, and concerns for her future. The volunteer can talk about the need for exercises and how to adjust to the prosthesis that replaces her breast. This has been a successful program and has given many women the courage to accept the loss of a breast.

Cancer of the Male Reproductive System

Prostate Cancer

Prostate cancer is the most common cancer in older men. The signs of this cancer are silent at first. It is important that the male have a routine physical examination done to detect this cancer in the early stage of the disease. The tests for prostate cancer include the prostate-specific antigen (PSA) and a digital rectal examination by the health care provider. As the cancer advances, the male will experience frequency of urination, urinary retention, and decreased size and force of the urine stream. The medical term for this disorder is **benign prostatic hypertrophy (BPH)** (Figure 23-5). The surgery indicated for removal of the prostate is called **transurethral resection of the prostate (TURP)** (Figure 23-6). If the tumor is malignant, the male may need to have chemotherapy, hormone therapy, or radiation. Often it is benign and no more treatment is necessary. A common problem after surgery is that the male may have problems controlling his urine and may need to wear adult briefs until control is regained. He will need to go to the bathroom every 2 hours and will gradually increase his ability to control his urine.

Testicular Cancer

Testicular cancer is a primary cancer of young men. As in many cases of cancer, signs of this cancer are silent at first. Health care providers promote a monthly testicular self-examination for men to detect any abnormality of the testes early. The American Cancer Society recommends the following method to perform the examination. The best time to perform this examination is during or after a shower or bath when the scrotum is relaxed. The man should hold the penis out of the way and examine each testicle separately. He then holds the testicle between the thumbs and fingers with both hands and rolls it gently between the fingers. He should look and feel for any hard lumps or nodules or any change in the size, shape, or consistency of the testes. If any abnormality is felt, he should see his health care provider as soon as possible. Treatment for testicular cancer is a surgery called an orchiectomy, which is removal of the testicle, followed by radiation therapy or chemotherapy depending upon the grade of cancer.

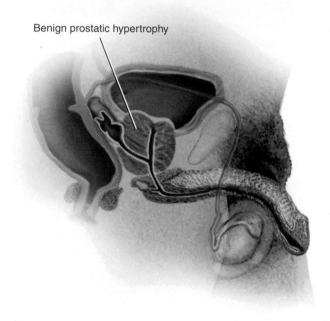

FIGURE 23-5 Benign prostatic hypertrophy.

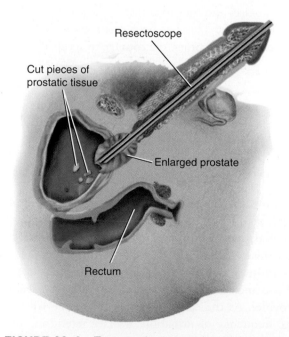

FIGURE 23-6 Transurethral resection of the prostate.

Cancer of the Respiratory System

The respiratory system is on duty 24 hours a day from birth to death. Fresh air is inhaled into the body and carried to the lungs. The oxygen from the air is carried to all parts of the body by the circulatory system. As oxygen is delivered to the cells of the body, waste gases are picked up and carried back to the lungs. Carbon dioxide is exhaled and expelled from the body.

Lung Cancer

Cancer can start to grow in the lungs. Lung cancer is the second most common cancer. The most common cause of cancer of the lungs is smoking. Signs and symptoms of lung cancer are:

- A persistent, hacking cough
- Tiredness
- Sudden weight loss
- Coughing up blood
- Recurrent bronchitis or pneumonia

- Difficulty swallowing
- Deformity of fingers and toes
- Hoarseness
- Shortness of breath
- Loss of appetite
- Swelling in the neck and face

The type of lung cancer and the stage of the disease will determine what treatment is needed. If a biopsy shows cancer cells, surgery can sometimes be done to remove all or part of a lung. Removal of part of the lung is called a lobectomy. Removal of the entire lung is called a pneumonectomy. Radiation, targeted biologic therapy, and chemotherapy are also used to treat the cancer. Most clients with lung cancer are cared for in the home setting. As the cancer progresses, the client becomes more tired and has difficulty with breathing even with oxygen therapy. The client may require oxygen therapy 24 hours a day. The client will most likely need to sit in a chair to breathe. If the client does go to bed, the bed will need many pillows because the client cannot breathe well when lying down.

Cancer of the Larynx

The larynx (voice box) is located at the top of the trachea (windpipe or airway between the nasal passages and the lungs). Cancer of the larynx occurs in men more often than in women. In addition, 75% of the people who develop cancer of the larynx have been heavy smokers and have a history of alcohol abuse. Signs and symptoms of cancer of the larynx or voice box include a sore throat or cough that does not go away, trouble swallowing, ear pain, a lump in the neck or throat, and change or hoarseness in the voice. A common treatment for cancer of the larynx is surgical removal of the larynx, called a partial laryngectomy, and the client keeps the ability to talk. Another surgery is the total laryngectomy, in which the whole larynx is removed. During this operation a hole is made in the front of the neck to allow the client to breathe. This is called a tracheostomy. The tracheostomy is an artificial airway that can be used to supply oxygen to the lungs. A tracheostomy tube is placed into the artificial airway to keep it open (Figure 23-7). Care of the tracheostomy is done by a nurse, client, or family member.

Speech therapy is needed to teach the client how to talk after a total laryngectomy. One of the methods is to gulp air in through the tracheostomy tube, swallow it, and then burp out words. It takes a great deal of practice to relearn how to speak. Another method the laryngectomy

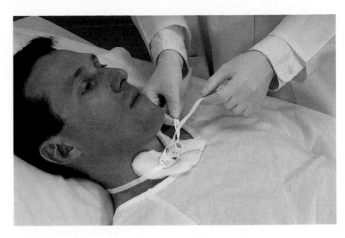

FIGURE 23-7   A tracheostomy tube provides an airway for the client.

client may use to aid speech is an electric larynx. The electric larynx makes a humming sound like the vocal cords. Some models are used in the mouth; others are placed in the neck. When wishing to speak, the client places the vibrator against the side of the neck. The vibrator vibrates the air inside the client's mouth as the client tries to make sounds. A home health aide must be tactful and patient when caring for such clients. It may be hard to understand what the client is struggling to say.

Colorectal Cancer

The death rate from this type of cancer has been declining for the past 20 years because of early detection and improvements in treatment. Colorectal cancer is the third most common cancer among men and women in the United States.

Warning signs and symptoms of colon cancer are:

- Change in bowel habits
- Blood in or on the stool
- Unexplained anemia
- Unusual stomach or gas pain
- Fatigue
- Vomiting

When a client has a physical examination, the health care provider usually has the client collect three stool specimens to be checked for hidden blood in the stool. If the test is positive for blood, the health care provider will order either a sigmoidoscopy or colonoscopy to see if there are any irregularities in the colon or rectum. A sigmoidoscopy is an examination whereby an instrument with a light attached is inserted into the client's rectum and guided up the client's colon to check for any unusual lesions. A colonoscopy is an examination whereby the entire large intestine is examined by use of a scope. If surgery is needed to remove a tumor, one type is an abdominal perineal resection. Another, less invasive type is laparoscopic colorectal surgery. If a large amount of the colon is removed, a surgeon may need to do a colostomy, which can be temporary or permanent.

Skin Cancer

Skin cancer is becoming a common type of cancer, especially among older adults. Skin cancer is caused by heredity and overexposure to sunlight, sunburn, tanning, and environmental factors in the younger years. The lesions can be either benign or malignant (Figure 23-8).

Common types of skin cancers are basal cell (Figure 23-9A) and squamous cell (Figure 23-9B). The first sign of skin cancer is a sore on the skin that does not heal. The sore may look like a lump. The lump can be smooth, shiny, waxy, red, or reddish brown. The lump

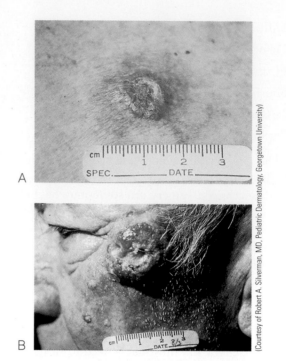

(Courtesy of Robert A. Silverman, MD, Pediatric Dermatology, Georgetown University)

FIGURE 23-9 Carcinoma: A. basal cell, B. squamous cell.

can feel rough or scaly. If removed in the first stage of the disease, it rarely reoccurs because it is usually benign. The type of skin cancer that is malignant is a melanoma, which can quickly metastasize to other areas of the body. The ABCD's of melanoma are: **a**symmetry (one half is different); **b**order (irregular); **c**olor (varies); and **d**iameter (greater than 6 mm). In men, the lesion is more often found in the area between the shoulders and hips. In women, the lesion may be found on the back or legs, or anywhere on the body. If the home health aide notices any of the signs of skin cancer while bathing or dressing a client, the aide should report the lesion to the case manager. If detected and treated early enough, the prognosis is good. Treatment options are surgery, targeted biologic therapy, and chemotherapy or radiation therapy.

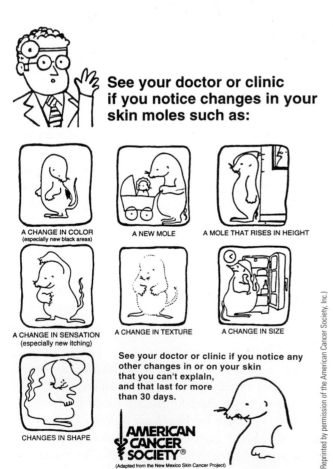

(Reprinted by permission of the American Cancer Society, Inc.)

FIGURE 23-8 Seven warning signs for skin moles.

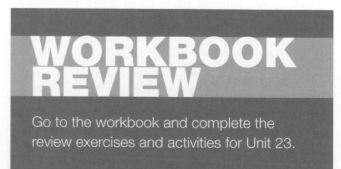

WORKBOOK REVIEW

Go to the workbook and complete the review exercises and activities for Unit 23.

REVIEW

1. List four common side effects of clients receiving cancer treatments.

    _____

    _____

    _____

    _____

2. List seven warning signs of cancer.

    _____

    _____

    _____

    _____

    _____

    _____

    _____

3. List three diagnostic tests used to diagnose cancer.

    _____

    _____

    _____

4. List four surgical procedures used in cancer therapy.

    _____

    _____

    _____

    _____

5. List three nonsurgical types of cancer treatment.

    _____

    _____

    _____

6. List three ways of increasing the food intake of a client with late-stage cancer.

    _____

    _____

    _____

7. T   F   Cancer of the lung is one of the leading causes of death from cancer in men.

8.   T   F   In the late stages of cancer, the client may become very thin. The client may also suffer from constant pain. The goal of care in this phase of the disease is to keep the client as comfortable and as pain-free as possible.

9.   T   F   A deodorizer is often used in the room of a cancer client to diminish the odor due to the client's cancerous condition.

10.   T   F   A malignant type of skin cancer is called melanoma.

11.   T   F   A client who has mouth sores should be given a diet high in spices and fiber to assist in cleansing the mouth.

12.   T   F   Stage IV cancer is the beginning stage of cancer.

13.   Match the term in Column I with the definition in Column II.

Column I

_____ 1. remission
_____ 2. benign
_____ 3. carcinogen
_____ 4. lobectomy
_____ 5. malignant
_____ 6. biopsy

Column II

a.   substance that can produce cancer
b.   no longer spreading
c.   sample of tissue cut from an area of the body
d.   removal of part of the lung
e.   noncancerous
f.   cancer

Case Studies

14.   Mr. Patterson, who is 78 years old, just returned home from having a transurethral prostatic resection. He has no control of his urine and has problems with incontinence. His wife keeps scolding him for "wetting his pants" all day. What should the home health aide do?

15.   Ms. Figgie is diagnosed with Stage IV cancer of the bone. She has taken her pain medication for weeks with good results. Today, when you arrive to assist her with her bath, she is unable to get out of bed because she is in so much pain. She just took her pain medication an hour ago, with no results. What should the home health aide do?

SECTION 7
Maternal/Infant Care

Unit 24
Maternal Care

Unit 25
Infant Care

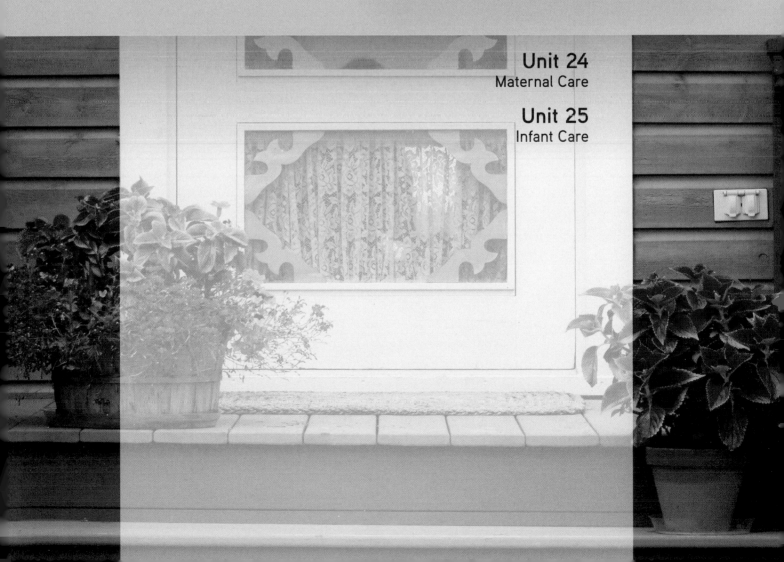

UNIT 24

Maternal Care

KEY TERMS

breast engorgement
Down
  syndrome
edema
engagement

fetal alcohol syndrome
  (FAS)
flatulence
heartburn
hemorrhoids

high-risk pregnancy
lochia
postpartum
postpartum blues

prenatal
toxemia
ultrasound
varicose veins

LEARNING OBJECTIVES

After studying this unit, you should be able to:

- List common pregnancy discomforts and their treatments

- Recognize danger signals in pregnancy

- Explain the home health aide's responsibilities in caring for an expectant mother

- List common postpartum discomforts and their treatments

The goal of the expectant mother and the professionals who care for her is the delivery of a normal, healthy baby. A key element in normal fetal development is an expectant mother in good physical and emotional health.

Discomforts of Pregnancy

Pregnancy today is regarded as a normal and natural stage of a woman's life cycle. A normal fetus will grow in a woman's uterus for approximately 280 days from the last menstrual period. At the same time, the woman must realize that extra demands are being placed on her body by the growing fetus. **Prenatal** (before birth) care should be sought as soon as a woman realizes she is pregnant and should continue throughout the pregnancy (Figures 24-1A, 24-1B). Even with regular prenatal care, often discomforts are involved with pregnancy. As the fetus grows during pregnancy, most women experience at least one of the discomforts described next (Figures 24-2 and 24-3).

Frequent Urination

Frequent urination is caused by pressure of the enlarged uterus on the bladder. This usually subsides by the second or third month of pregnancy, when the uterus rises in the abdominal cavity. However, in the last week of pregnancy, when the uterus drops into the pelvic cavity—a condition known as **engagement**—both urgency and frequency of urination are common.

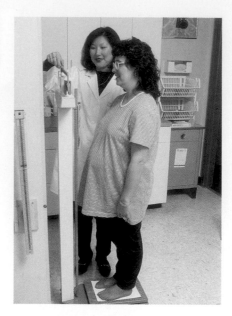

FIGURE 24-1B   Weight is measured at each prenatal visit.

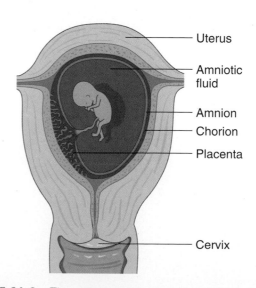

FIGURE 24-2   An ultrasound test is done to check the growth of the fetus.

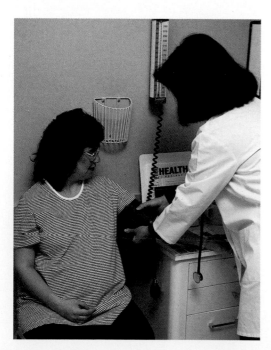

FIGURE 24-1A   Blood pressure is measured at each prenatal visit.

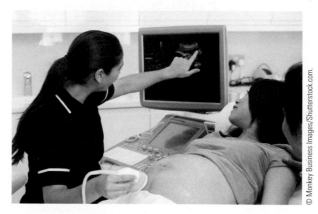

- Uterus
- Amniotic fluid
- Amnion
- Chorion
- Placenta
- Cervix

FIGURE 24-3   The uterus and the developing fetus.

Morning Sickness

Morning sickness is one of the most common symptoms of pregnancy. It is characterized by nausea and, sometimes, vomiting. Although it usually occurs in the morning, it can happen at any time of day, and most often lasts for a 4- to 12-week period during the first trimester.

Some measures for alleviating nausea include remaining in bed and resting for half an hour after awakening. During this period the expectant mother should try to eat dry toast or a cracker, or sip on soda or juice.

Heartburn/Flatulence

Diminished gastric motion during pregnancy may cause stomach contents to back up into the lower esophagus. This is commonly called **heartburn**.

Feelings of gassiness, referred to as **flatulence**, may also be present because of the action of gas-forming bacteria in the intestines. One way to alleviate flatulence is to eat slowly, chew food thoroughly, and avoid gas-forming foods, such as beans, corn, and fried foods.

Constipation/Hemorrhoids

Constipation can result from the pressure of the uterus on the intestines. Pressure exerted by the pregnant uterus can interfere with circulation in the veins. In the anal area, coupled with constipation, this can result in **hemorrhoids** (enlarged varicose veins around the anus).

Varicose Veins

Varicose veins (swollen veins) can develop during pregnancy. This can be caused by pressure on the great veins of the pelvis, a hereditary predisposition, constrictive clothing, obesity, and prolonged standing, and can affect the lower extremities. The woman should be encouraged to elevate her legs often and wear support hose (Figure 24-4).

Backache

Backache is a common complaint of pregnant women and results from adjustments in posture caused by carrying the baby's weight, the changes in the mother's center of gravity, and the relaxation of the joints at the base of the spine. Wearing flat, firmly balanced shoes and watching weight gain may help, as well as practicing good posture, using proper body mechanics, and getting adequate rest.

Leg Cramps

Leg cramps or spasms of the lower leg and foot muscles are a common and painful experience during pregnancy. The cramp may occur without warning, sometimes in the middle of the night. The calf muscles in one leg may feel

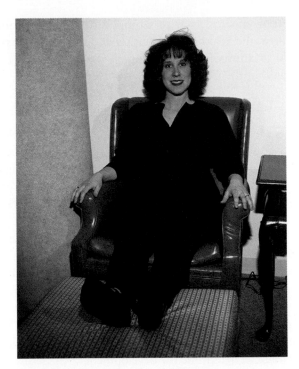

FIGURE 24-4   Elevation of the legs is a common method to reduce edema of the ankles and feet.

like a "knotted ball." The best treatment for the cramps is stretching the muscles. It is helpful to massage or knead the leg to try to relax the muscles.

Edema

Edema, or swelling, of the lower extremities can also occur, particularly in warm climates and when standing for too long. Swelling of the woman's fingers may also occur. The fingers may become stiff and rings may be too tight to wear. Rest, elevation of the legs, support hose, soaking the feet and hands in cool water, and limiting salt intake may help the edema.

Vaginal Discharge

It is normal for women to have a pale yellow, thin vaginal discharge during pregnancy. If the discharge becomes irritating, odorous, excessive, or yellow or green in color, and is accompanied by vaginal itching, the case manager should be consulted.

Complications of Pregnancy

Although the vast majority of pregnancies progress quite naturally, occasionally complications may develop. Complications of pregnancy may be the result of the age of the mother, the use of harmful substances during pregnancy, or certain medical factors. Complications of pregnancy can affect the health of the mother and the baby. For this reason it is important that women receive prenatal care throughout the pregnancy.

High-Risk Pregnancies

When physical, emotional, or environmental situations compromise the mother's well-being, a high-risk pregnancy can result. These pregnancies can cause low birth weight, premature or brain-damaged babies, and maternal complications. These complications increase the chances of infant and maternal mortality (death).

The age of the mother can have a significant influence on the outcome of the pregnancy and its identification as a high-risk event. Statistically, women over age 35 are more likely to give birth to babies with Down syndrome, a form of retardation (Figure 24-5). Prenatal (before birth) tests are offered to pregnant women in high-risk categories. These prenatal tests include ultrasound, amniocentesis, and blood tests that can determine the development of the fetus.

Mothers who are too young are also at risk. Frequently, the pregnant adolescent does not seek prenatal care or first sees a doctor late in her pregnancy due to fear, denial, or lack of knowledge. Teenage mothers often suffer from malnutrition, anemia, excessive weight gain, drug abuse, and infections. Deficiencies in the pregnant woman's diet can cause low birth weight in her baby.

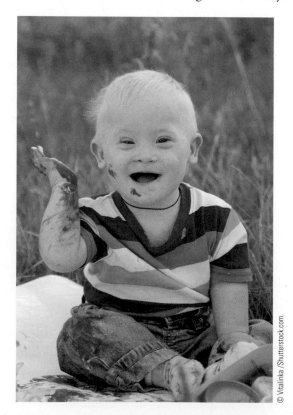

FIGURE 24-5 An infant with Down syndrome.

© Vitalinka /Shutterstock.com.

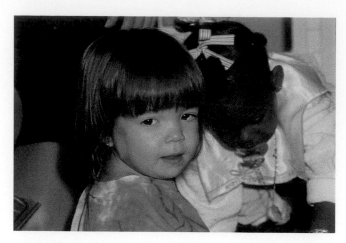

FIGURE 24-6 Facial abnormalities typical of fetal alcohol syndrome (FAS) include characteristics of the eyes, ears, and a smooth upper lip.

Pregnant women are advised against drinking alcohol during their pregnancy. Drinking alcohol during pregnancy can result in several serious complications known as fetal alcohol syndrome (FAS). This condition produces infants who are born underweight, usually mentally deficient, and with multiple deformities (Figure 24-6). Cigarette smoking can also lead to a variety of pregnancy complications. Tobacco use is one of the causes of prenatal problems such as vaginal bleeding, miscarriage, and early delivery. If the expectant mother is a substance abuser, her chances of problems during pregnancy are increased. Drug-addicted women can, and often do, give birth to drug-addicted babies.

Women also can be placed in the high-risk pregnancy group because of medical factors, such as having a history of spontaneous abortions, stillbirths, premature births, or difficult pregnancies in the past.

Disorders of Pregnancy

Many expectant mothers fear miscarriage during their first trimester of pregnancy. Some possible signs of miscarriage include bleeding associated with abdominal cramping, severe abdominal pain that does not go away, heavy vaginal bleeding or light spotting that continues for several days, and passing blood clots or grayish-pink material. Other signs include persistent vomiting, chills and fever, sudden escape of fluid from the vagina, swelling of the face or fingers, severe and continuous headaches, and blurred vision.

Toxemia is a medical condition that occurs in late pregnancy. Signs and symptoms are elevated blood pressure, edema of the hands and feet, and protein in the urine. Bed rest and a special diet are ordered for this mother-to-be.

Caring for the Expectant Mother

Home health care services for a pregnant mother can occur if a pregnancy is high risk, the mother is under unusual stress, or the mother is on limited activity.

When taking care of a pregnant woman in the home setting, some important things for the home health aide to remember are:

- Encourage a balanced prescribed diet; this is important for the mother and especially for the growth of the fetus.
- Encourage scheduled prenatal checkups.
- Follow the care plan carefully, which will include activity orders. Bed rest is sometimes ordered for high blood pressure or vaginal bleeding.
- Discourage smoking and drinking of alcohol.
- Observe the mother-to-be carefully for signs of vaginal bleeding.
- Encourage good personal hygiene.
- Try to help the mother-to-be feel as optimistic as possible; provide a calm environment to help promote a general feeling of well-being.
- Help her maintain a good fluid intake.

Caring for the Postpartum Mother

Labor and delivery are exhausting experiences, both physically and emotionally. In the past, new mothers remained in the hospital for 5 to 7 days after delivery. Today, new mothers are released to their homes within 24 to 48 hours after vaginal deliveries and in 3 to 4 days after cesarean sections. As a result of early discharge, multiple births, or being a single mother, a new mother may employ a home health aide to assist in caring for the infant the first week postpartum. The postpartum period is defined as the period after childbirth, usually lasting 6 weeks.

Postpartum Discomforts

Frequently, first-time mothers are unprepared for the discomforts of the postpartum experience. Most new mothers experience the following discomforts after the birth of an infant.

Lochia.   Lochia is the bloody, mucus-like vaginal discharge that is secreted by new mothers. Although bright red at first for several days, it should turn light pink, brown, then yellow by the end of 2 weeks. Disposable sanitary pads should be used to absorb the discharge. Excessive bleeding should be reported as well as lochia with a foul odor.

Incisional Pain.   Incisions (episiotomy or cesarean section) can be painful. Ice packs and pain medication will help.

Breast Engorgement.   A few days after delivery, breast milk comes in, causing breast engorgement. If bottle-feeding, this can be a painful experience for postpartum women. A sports bra or a tight wrap and ice packs will minimize the pain. If breast-feeding, warm showers and compresses will help the milk flow.

Abdominal Cramping.   Abdominal cramps are believed to be caused by the uterus as it contracts to its normal size. Cramping will be felt more during nursing as the sucking initiates the uterus to contract.

Difficult Urination.   Difficulty with urination is a common postpartum condition. This temporary condition should last only a short time. Encourage good fluid intake.

Depression/Mood Swings.   Postpartum blues are experienced by new mothers during the first few weeks after delivery. New mothers often feel anxious, tired, and weepy or experience mood swings.

Nutrition and Breast-Feeding

If a mother is planning to breast-feed her baby, she will need to pay close attention to her diet. The mother's diet will influence both the amount and quality of the milk she produces. Some tips to maintain the best nutrition for a breast-feeding mother are:

- Eat three regular meals and a bedtime snack.
- Additional protein in the diet is needed; eat generous servings of fish, meat, milk, eggs, or cheese.
- Choose healthy fats.
- Go easy on alcohol intake and limit coffee intake to one cup a day.
- Continue to take prenatal vitamins.
- Aim for slow and steady weight loss.
- Some drugs are passed from the mother's blood into the milk, and medication should only be taken if prescribed by a health care provider.
- Drink plenty of fluids.

WORKBOOK REVIEW

Go to the workbook and complete the review exercises and activities for Unit 24.

REVIEW

1. T F Pregnancy is a normal, natural stage of a woman's life cycle.

2. T F Regular prenatal care is not necessary during pregnancy.

3. T F Edema is a common pregnancy discomfort.

4. T F Women are advised against drinking alcohol or smoking cigarettes during pregnancy.

5. T F High blood pressure and edema of the feet and hands are signs of toxemia during the later stage of pregnancy.

6. T F Ultrasound is a diagnostic test done to monitor fetal development.

7. Match the term in Column I with the definition in Column II.

   Column I
   _____ 1. Down syndrome
   _____ 2. hemorrhoids
   _____ 3. prenatal
   _____ 4. postpartum
   _____ 5. engagement

   Column II
   a. enlarged varicose veins around the anus
   b. period of time during pregnancy
   c. period of time after childbirth
   d. a form of retardation
   e. uterus drops into the pelvic cavity

8. Backache, nausea, and leg cramps are all common symptoms of
   a. pregnancy.
   b. the postpartum period.
   c. a high-risk pregnancy.
   d. miscarriage.

9. Some possible signs of miscarriage are
   a. difficulty with urination.
   b. severe headache and blurred vision.
   c. vaginal bleeding with abdominal cramping and spotting for several days.
   d. leg cramps.

10. Common postpartum discomforts include which of the following?
    a. Depression/mood swings
    b. Abdominal cramping
    c. Breast engorgement
    d. All of the above

11. Match the term in Column I with the definition in Column II.

    Column I

    _____ 1. flatulence
    _____ 2. lochia
    _____ 3. edema
    _____ 4. blurred vision
    _____ 5. morning sickness

    Column II

    a. swelling of lower extremities
    b. danger signal during pregnancy
    c. feelings of excessive gas
    d. bloody, mucus-like vaginal discharge
    e. vomiting and nausea

Case Studies

12. You are caring for an expectant young mother who is categorized as high risk. She is on limited activity, and likes to smoke and drink alcohol. What should you do to assist her in maintaining a safe pregnancy until her due date?

13. Mrs. Smith was released from the hospital 24 hours after her first baby was born. She employs you to assist her during her first 3 weeks at home. She is tired and is depressed. What should you do?

UNIT 25
Infant Care

KEY TERMS

bottle-feeding
breast-feeding
circumcision
foreskin
glans
lactose
meconium

LEARNING OBJECTIVES

After studying this unit, you should be able to:

- Describe the different ways a mother may breast-feed her infant

- Explain the steps involved in bottle-feeding an infant

- Describe three techniques for burping an infant

- Describe the steps to bathe an infant

- Define circumcision and identify the appropriate care for the circumcised/uncircumcised penis

- Identify two safety precautions to be taken while caring for infants

- Explain how to care for the infant's umbilical cord

- Demonstrate the following:

  PROCEDURE 74 Assisting with Breast-Feeding and Breast Care

  PROCEDURE 75 Bottle-Feeding an Infant

  PROCEDURE 76 Burping an Infant

  PROCEDURE 77 Bathing an Infant

Infant Care

The birth of a baby is a time of adjustment for both the baby and the new parents. The newborn must now learn how to live in a new environment, outside the womb, where his or her needs are not automatically met, and the parents must learn how to care for their new baby. During the early years of life, the child is totally dependent on the care of others. Physical and emotional well-being are intimately related to each other. The individuals who meet the infant's primary needs significantly influence his or her physical and emotional development. Caring for a newborn baby can create anxiety for the new parents. The home health aide should try to reduce these anxieties by becoming familiar with basic infant care procedures, such as feeding, burping, bathing, and caring for the circumcised or uncircumcised penis and the umbilical cord. The majority of new mothers go home with little need for a home health aide, as they have help from either the husband or family members. The new mothers who may need assistance from a home health aide are young single mothers, mothers with emotional problems, and mothers with multiple births or premature infants.

Feeding the Infant

The newborn infant will approximately triple his or her birth weight during the first year of life. The nutritional needs during this rapid growth period are greater than at any other time in its life. Feeding the infant should be an enjoyable, relaxing time. Hold the infant close, cuddle, and make eye contact while feeding. There are two ways to feed the infant: **breast-feeding** and **bottle-feeding**. Either method can be used independently or in combination. Deciding to breast-feed or bottle-feed is a personal decision.

Breast-Feeding

Human milk is the best possible food for any infant. Its major ingredients are **lactose** (sugar), protein (whey and casein), fat, and numerous vitamins, minerals, and enzymes, all appropriately combined to suit an infant's nutritional needs. Breast milk provides important substances to fight infection.

If a mother plans on breast-feeding and does not plan to get pregnant soon, the mother may need to consider birth control options. A birth control pill called a minipill (an oral contraceptive that contains only progestin) is an effective contraceptive as long as the mother is nursing. If the mother does not want to take the minipill, there are many other options, including condoms, spermicide, or a diaphragm. Some of the newer birth control options include the vaginal ring, intrauterine device (IUD), and contraceptive patches. If the mother does not want any future pregnancies, she may consider tubal ligation or a vasectomy for her partner.

PROCEDURE 74 ASSISTING WITH BREAST-FEEDING AND BREAST CARE

Purpose

- To provide for cleanliness
- To protect the nipples from cracking or soreness
- To protect the infant from infection
- To provide for the mother's comfort
- To nourish the infant
- To promote mother–infant interaction and bonding

NOTE: Assist the mother to establish a routine, preferably in a calm environment. A rocking chair is a great place to nurse an infant, but a mother may nurse her baby wherever she wants to. While nursing, it is helpful to have a small nursing pillow to support the infant in the mother's lap, and a small stool to elevate the mother's feet to ease the strain on her back.

Procedure

1. Gather supplies:
   clean, moist washcloth
   nursing pads
   disposable towelettes
   clock or watch to time nursing period
2. Wash your hands.
3. Give the mother towelettes or a moist washcloth to wash her hands.
4. Have the mother open the front of her top.

(continued)

PROCEDURE **74**   ASSISTING WITH BREAST-FEEDING AND BREAST CARE (*continued*)

5. Have the mother sit in a comfortable position in a rocking chair with armrest and footstool to support the feet.

6. Bring the infant to the mother. Make sure the infant's nose is not pressed against the mother's breast. The nostrils must be free so the infant can breathe as it nurses. The infant should be square on the breast, the mouth facing the nipple. There are three positions for breast-feeding: side-lying, football hold, and cradle hold (Figures 25-1A–C). Rotate positions to reduce tenderness in one particular area.

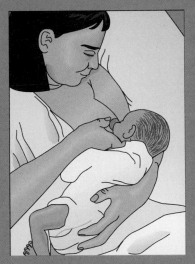

FIGURE 25-1C   Cradle-hold position for breast-feeding. The mother supports the baby with her arm on the same side as the nursing breast. The mother sits up straight and cradles her baby in her arm with the baby's head resting comfortably on her elbow. The mother places her nipple into the baby's mouth to start nursing.

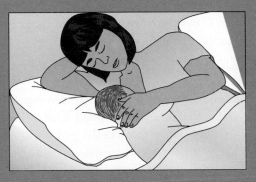

FIGURE 25-1A   The side-lying position for breast-feeding is a good choice if the mother is tired. The mother lies on her side and faces the baby toward her heart, supporting the baby with one hand.

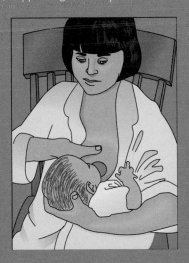

FIGURE 25-1B   Football-hold position for breast-feeding. The mother holds the baby by her side with her elbow bent. With her open hand supporting the baby's head, she lifts the baby toward her breast. The baby's back will rest on the mother's forearm.

7. The nursing period is gradually increased from just a few minutes to about 20 minutes. Some mothers prefer to let the infant nurse at both breasts (one at a time) during one feeding. Others will feed the infant only at one breast for each 20-minute feeding and alternate breasts at different feedings.

8. To remove the infant's mouth from the breast, have the mother insert a finger in the infant's mouth to break the suction.

9. Have the mother burp the infant. When the mother is finished nursing, take the infant and place the infant in the crib lying on his or her back, or in an infant seat. Check to see if the diaper needs to be changed. If the infant is getting enough breast milk, the infant should be wetting a diaper about eight times a day until the infant is 3 months old. The infant should be having at least three bowel movements each day by the time the infant is 2 weeks old. The first stools the infant will have are called meconium stools. The stools will be thick and sticky in consistency and either yellow, green, or brown in color.

(*continued*)

PROCEDURE 74   ASSISTING WITH BREAST-FEEDING AND BREAST CARE (*continued*)

10. Wash your hands.
11. Help the mother with her bra, putting fresh nursing pads over the nipples. If nipples are sore or cracked, use lanolin cream, and air-dry the nipples. Wash the mother's nipples only with water.
12. Return supplies to storage.
13. Wash your hands.

Bottle-Feeding

Infant formula used in bottle-feeding combines all the nutrients found in breast milk; however, it does not provide the antibodies found in the mother's breast milk. When preparing the infant's formula all equipment must be cleaned properly, as the infant's immune system is still immature and may be unable to fight off food-borne illnesses. The correct measurement of formula and water is also essential. Once the formula is mixed, it needs to be refrigerated and used within 48 hours. Bottle-feeding allows all members of the family to participate in the feeding process. See Procedure 75, Bottle-Feeding an Infant.

Burping the Infant

Both bottle-fed and breast-fed infants swallow air while feeding. Infants may fuss or become cranky if they need to burp. It is a good idea to burp the bottle-fed infant after the infant drinks 2 to 3 ounces. If the infant does not burp after several minutes, continue feeding and try again when the infant is finished. Refer to Procedure 76 for techniques for burping an infant.

Caring for the Newborn Infant

In addition to feeding and burping the infant, the care of an infant will include bathing, care of the penis, and care of the umbilical cord.

Bathing an Infant

The newborn infant does not require much bathing as long as the diaper area is cleaned after a diaper change. Use disposable wipes to clean the perineal areas each time you change the diaper. The wipes not only clean the perineal area but also cover the area with a protective coating, which will prevent the skin in the perineal area from breaking down. Generally, there is less chance of diaper rash with disposable diapers than with cloth diapers. Do not use powder on the perineal area or dispose of the diaper in the toilet. Disposable diapers usually work better if they are the correct size. The majority of disposable diapers have color tabs in the middle of them, which change color when the diaper needs to be changed. Sponge baths should be given until the stump of the umbilical cord has fallen off and the circumcision is healed (for males).

PROCEDURE 75   BOTTLE-FEEDING AN INFANT

Purpose

- To provide nutrition
- To give the infant the security of being held and cuddled and facilitate bonded
- To observe infant's responses, color, skin condition, and other characteristics

Procedure

1. Wash your hands.
2. Prepare formula as directed and pour into baby bottle (Figure 25-2). Put the lid on the bottle (Figure 25-3). Warm the bottle, if it is from the refrigerator. Test the temperature

(*continued*)

PROCEDURE 75   BOTTLE-FEEDING AN INFANT (*continued*)

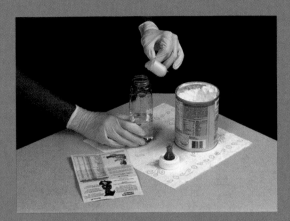

FIGURE 25-2   Prepare formula as directed. Be sure all equipment is clean before using.

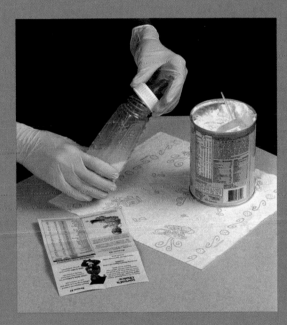

FIGURE 25-3   Put the lid on the bottle.

securely in a comfortable position for taking the nipple; start to feed the infant. Keep the nipple full of formula. Do not prop the bottle (Figures 25-5 and 25-6).

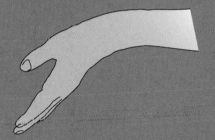

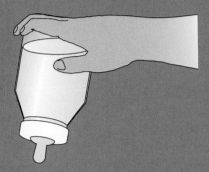

FIGURE 25-4   Test the bottle temperature by shaking a few drops on your wrist.

of the formula before feeding (Figure 25-4). Bring the bottle of formula to the baby's room.

3. Change the infant's diaper, if soiled, so the infant will be comfortable and dry while eating. Wrap the infant loosely in a clean receiving blanket. Leave the infant in the crib with the side rails up.

4. Wash your hands.

5. Support the infant's head and back when picking the infant up from the crib. Sit comfortably in the chair, holding the infant

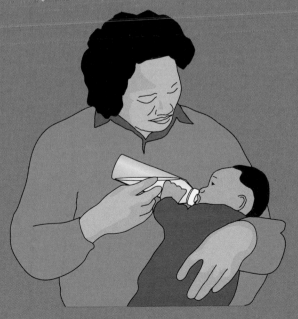

FIGURE 25-5   The infant should be held while feeding.

(*continued*)

PROCEDURE 75   BOTTLE-FEEDING AN INFANT (*continued*)

6. When the infant has had 2 to 3 ounces, burp the infant.
7. Continue feeding and burping until the infant is finished or shows no interest in eating. Do not force the infant to take more than the infant wants.
8. When the infant is finished, burp the infant once more, then place the infant in the crib, lying on the side or back. *Do not place the infant on his or her abdomen!*
   Exceptions are in the cases of:
   — Premature infants
   — Excessive spitting up or vomiting
   — Facial deformities that make the infant susceptible to airway blockage
9. Wash your hands.

Spend as much time as you can with the infant and interact with the infant (Figures 25-7, 25-8, and 25-9).

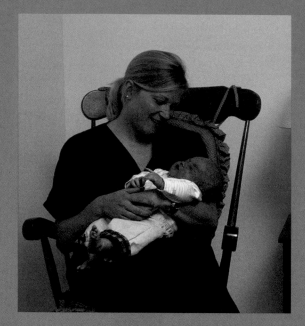

FIGURE 25-8   Infants need to be held and talked to often.

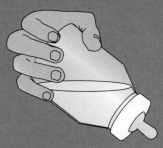

FIGURE 25-6   Be sure the neck of the bottle is covered with formula.

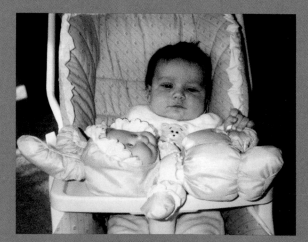

FIGURE 25-7   Place the infant in an infant seat occasionally, as it will give the infant a chance to sit up.

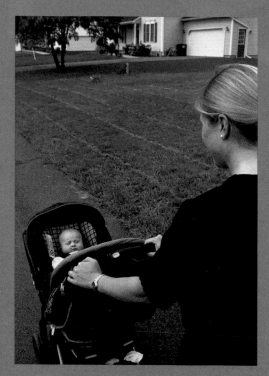

FIGURE 25-9   A stroller ride is an enjoyable occasion for both caregiver and infant.

PROCEDURE 76 BURPING AN INFANT

Technique A—Sitting Position

1. Sit the infant in your lap.
2. Support the infant's head and chest with one hand.
3. Pat or rub the infant's back gently with the other hand (Figure 25-10).

Technique B—Shoulder Position

1. Put the burp cloth or pad on your shoulder.
2. Hold the infant upright, with the head on your shoulder (your shoulder will provide support for the infant's head and neck).
3. Gently pat or rub the infant's back (Figure 25-11).

Technique C—Lap Position

1. Place the burp pad in your lap.
2. Place the infant in your lap, face down, with his or her head turned to one side.
3. Support the infant's head so that it is higher than the chest.
4. Gently pat or rub the infant's back (Figure 25-12).

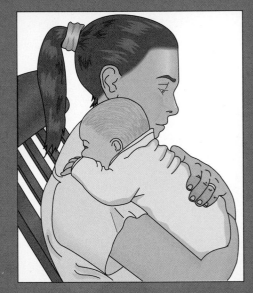

FIGURE 25-11 Hold the infant upright with the head on your shoulder, supporting the head and back, while you gently pat the back with your other hand.

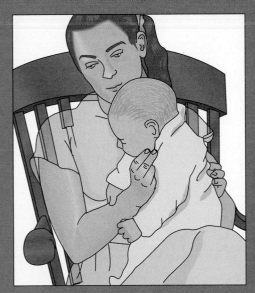

FIGURE 25-10 Sit the infant on your lap, supporting the chest and head with one hand while patting his or her back with your other hand.

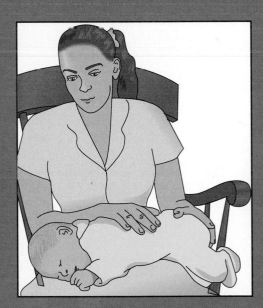

FIGURE 25-12 Lay the infant on your lap, on the infant's abdomen. Support the head so that it is higher than the chest, and gently pat or rotate your hand on the infant's back.

PROCEDURE **77** BATHING AN INFANT

Purpose

- To clean and refresh the infant
- To observe skin tone, activity, and signs of abnormality or unusual changes in behavior

Procedure

1. Gather supplies:
   warm water in basin or sink
   soft towel and washcloth
   diaper
   baby soap and shampoo
   baby lotion
   change of clothing
   disposable gloves (optional)
2. Wash your hands and apply gloves (optional).
3. Bring the infant to the bathing area.
4. Place the infant on a towel and remove clothing (Figure 25-13). Roll soiled diaper up.
5. The bathing basin should be one-third to one-half full of warm water; check the temperature of the bathwater and place the infant in the basin (Figure 25-14). If the infant does not have good head control, be sure to support the neck and head. Keep hold of the infant throughout the entire bath.
6. Carefully support the infant with one hand, and use your free hand to wash the infant's face with plain water, no soap. Pat the face dry. Clean the ears with the ends of washcloth. Do not use cotton swabs to clean the

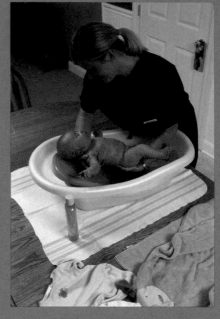

FIGURE 25-14   Slowly place the infant into a basin half-filled with warm water. Be sure to test the water before placing the infant in the basin.

inside of the ears. Pat dry. Wash and rinse the neck. Use soap very sparingly, as it dries out the infant's skin.
7. Talk or sing to the infant during the bath—make it a fun time for both you and the infant.
8. Continue to move down the body and do the hair last. You may use your hands to wash the rest of the infant's body (Figure 25-15).
9. Before washing the infant's hair, bundle him or her in a towel. To shampoo the infant's hair, hold the infant in your arms like a football. Use a warm, wet washcloth to dampen hair. Gently apply shampoo or soap and rinse carefully to avoid getting soap in the infant's eyes. Massage the scalp gently to prevent the formation of cradle cap.
10. Cover the infant's head with a towel as soon as you are done washing the hair (Figure 25-16).
11. Apply baby lotion sparingly, if needed. Dress infant and apply clean diaper (Figure 25-17).

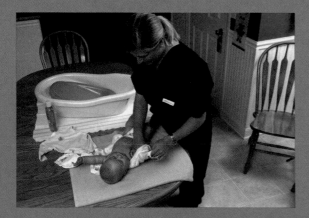

FIGURE 25-13   Undress the infant before the bath.

(continued)

PROCEDURE 77   BATHING AN INFANT (*continued*)

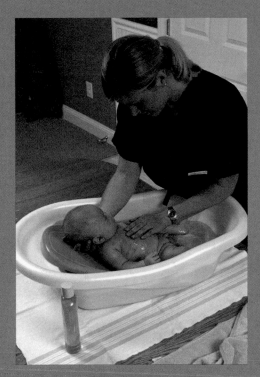

FIGURE 25-15   Wash the infant's body with your hands.

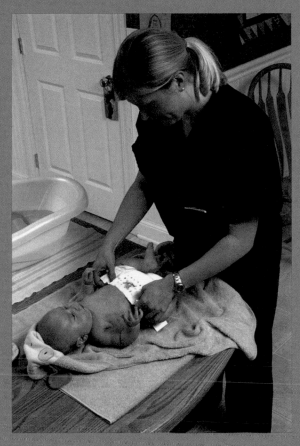

FIGURE 25-17   Apply the diaper and finish dressing the infant.

12. Place the infant in a crib or infant seat. **NOTE:** Never leave infant unattended on the bathing table.
13. Return supplies to storage area. Place soiled clothing in hamper. Dispose of diaper in proper receptacle.
14. If wearing gloves, remove the gloves and wash your hands.

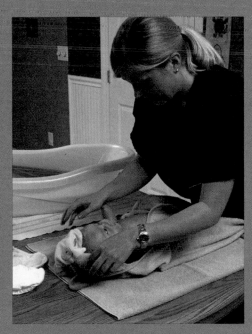

FIGURE 25-16   Cover the infant's head with a towel as soon as you are done shampooing the hair.

Care of the Penis

At birth, the boy's foreskin is attached to the glans (head) of the penis and cannot be pushed back. Urine flows through the small opening at the tip. Circumcision is a procedure in which the connections between the foreskin and the glans are separated, and the foreskin is removed, leaving the glans visible. Parents may choose to have their sons circumcised in the hospital, 1 to 2 days after birth. Some Jewish parents may have circumcision done during a religious ceremony 7 days after birth. Some parents may choose not to circumcise their sons.

Caring for the Circumcised Penis. A light gauze dressing with petroleum jelly will be placed over the glans of the penis after the circumcision procedure. At each diaper change, the dressing should be changed, as recommended by the nurse (usually for 2 to 3 days, or until healed). The area should be kept clean. The tip of the penis may appear red, and a yellow secretion may be noticed. This indicates the normal healing process. The redness and secretions should disappear within a week. If there is swelling, the redness persists, or crusted yellow sores appear, there may be an infection. The case manager should be notified. The penis requires no special care after the circumcision has healed.

Caring for the Uncircumcised Penis. During the first few months, the uncircumcised penis should be cleaned with soap and water. The foreskin is connected by tissue to the glans, so it should not be pulled back.

Once the foreskin separates naturally, the foreskin should occasionally be pulled back to cleanse the area underneath.

Care of the Umbilical Cord

During pregnancy the fetus receives its nourishment from the mother through the umbilical cord. When the baby is born, the umbilical cord is cut about 2 inches from the baby's abdomen. The remaining stump of the cord begins to dry up and then falls off within 12 to 15 days after birth, leaving the navel. Umbilical cords are not covered. Care of the umbilical cord is easy. When diapering the baby, fold the top of the diaper over so that it does not cover the navel. This will promote the healing of the site. If necessary, the baby can be sponge bathed until the cord drops off. Some health care providers may recommend swabbing delicately around the end of the stump with an alcohol swab. Gently pull on the stump and swab the base of the navel.

WORKBOOK REVIEW

Go to the workbook and complete the review exercises and activities for Unit 25.

REVIEW

1. T   F   After feeding the infant, place the infant on his or her abdomen in the crib.

2. T   F   Infants cannot be both bottle-fed and breast-fed.

3. T   F   Infants should be burped frequently.

4. T   F   Sponge baths should be given until the umbilical cord stump falls off.

5. T   F   All male infants must be circumcised.

6. Bottle-feeding
   a. allows other family members to feed the infant.
   b. provides antibodies not found in breast milk.
   c. is the only way to feed an infant.
   d. none of the above.

7. Which of the following holds can be used by the breast-feeding mother?
   a. Football hold, upside-down hold, cradle hold
   b. Side-lying hold, football hold, cradle hold
   c. Cradle hold, side-lying hold, baseball hold
   d. Only the side-lying hold

8. Match the term in Column I with the definition in Column II.

Column I	Column II
_____ 1. lactose	a. hold used for breast-feeding
_____ 2. lanolin	b. sugar
_____ 3. circumcision	c. ointment
_____ 4. cradle hold	d. a medical procedure performed on males

Case Studies

9. It is your first day at the home of a young single mother. Her infant girl is 5 days old. She is breast-feeding the infant. She complains of her nipples being sore and painful. What might she do to prevent the nipples from cracking?

10. Your client, Mrs. Jones, delivered a healthy baby boy 1 week ago. On your first visit to her home she is concerned because the tip of her son's penis is still red, and she has noticed yellow secretions. She fears that he has developed an infection from the circumcision. Are these signs of an infection, or is this part of the normal healing process? What signs should Mrs. Jones watch for that would indicate an infection?

SECTION 8

Employment

Unit 26
Job-Seeking Skills

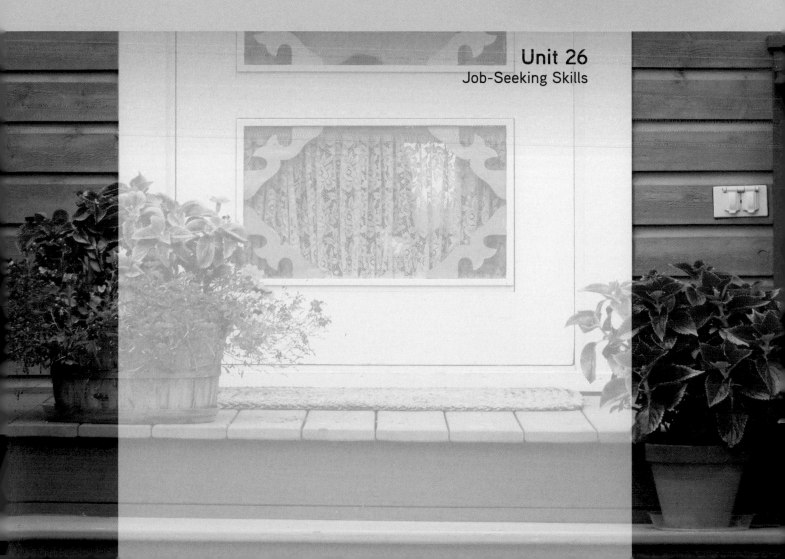

UNIT 26
Job-Seeking Skills

KEY TERMS

felony
information sheet

infractions
misconduct

personals
references

résumé

LEARNING OBJECTIVES

After studying this unit, you should be able to:

- List potential employment opportunities for homemakers/home health aides

- Prepare a personal information sheet or résumé

- Describe how to present yourself in a professional manner during an employment interview

- Practice completing an employment application accurately on paper or online

- Give five examples of misconduct on the job

One of the more challenging tasks individuals face is entering a new situation. As a student, you might have worried that you would not be able to pass the tests, recite information in class, or demonstrate a skill to the instructor in front of the other students. However, if you have passed your home health aide course, you have already met these challenges. Now, as a graduate, you are facing a new challenge—putting your newfound skills to work.

Until now, you have been guided by your instructor(s) and for the most part have worked in a team situation with your fellow students. Now you are on your own. You must "sell" yourself and your skills to an employer.

You must make your own decisions as to what kind of clients you prefer to work with. Do you want part-time or full-time work? Do you want a sleep-in job? Would you rather work with elderly clients who mainly need companionship and minimal care, or do you want to use all your skills and deal with complex medical problems? Do you prefer working with children, individuals with disabilities, or are you willing to take whatever jobs are open?

You must answer these questions so that you can conduct an effective job search that will result in employment.

Contacting Prospective Employers

Your first step in finding a job is to research your community's job market. Local and national agencies in most areas are listed in the phone directory or online. Your instructor may also be able to provide you with a list of possibilities. You can look in the employment section of your local newspaper, contact your local workforce connections agency, look online, or contact local home health agencies. You can also put an ad in the local paper for employment, advertising your availability as a home health aide, as a client or family member may be looking for a home health aide and will select an individual for the job without going through an agency.

Make a list of those places you plan to contact; then keep a record of the date you contacted each prospect and any appointments you may have set up. Remember that you may register at several agencies and you may work for more than one agency on a part-time basis. When you call for an appointment, plan ahead what you want to say, for example: "I am a graduate of the ABC home health program, and I am looking for employment. May I schedule an appointment to discuss job opportunities in your agency?"

The Job Interview, Application Form, and Job Offer

It is essential to demonstrate a professional attitude and appearance throughout the job search process. The interview provides you an opportunity to discuss your skills, and also helps you to learn more about the company providing employment and the people with whom you may be working. Completing the application form and negotiating a job offer are also important steps in the job search process, and guidelines for each step are given next.

The Interview

In preparation for an interview, research all you can about the agency. For example, check in the yellow pages to see what services the organization offers, ask employees about what type of clients they serve, and carefully read the job description for the job you are applying for. Prior to the interview, collect the following items and bring them with you to the interview: certificates of completion of programs (e.g., CPR, first aid, home health aide), skills checklist, driver's license, and Social Security card. If an automobile is required for the position, the agency may ask for verification of auto insurance. If possible, have the latest record of your immunizations, including hepatitis B and the result of a tuberculosis test.

It is also beneficial to familiarize yourself with typical interview questions and decide how you will answer them. Practice answering typical interview questions such as the following:

- Have you had previous homemaker/home health aide work experience?
- Tell me about yourself.
- Can you tell me about your previous employment?
- Explain any time gaps between jobs.
- Why did you leave your last job?
- Why are you interested in this job?
- What did you like most/least about past jobs?
- What are your strengths/weaknesses?

In addition, prepare a list of questions to ask the employer before going to the interview. The interview is the employer's chance to get to know you, but also an opportunity for you to gather more information about the company and the position. The interviewer may ask if you have questions, and having listed a few in advance shows that you prepared for the interview. Some suggested questions are:

- How far will I need to travel to and from each client? Is public transportation available or will I need to have an automobile?

- What shift or shifts will I be expected to work?

- If the position is part-time, is there a possibility of a full-time position soon?

- Is there a mechanism in place for advancement or additional training?

- Is overtime mandatory or available?

- What are the fringe benefits—are health insurance, holiday or vacation pay, sick days, or a pension plan available? (Note: Do not immediately ask about salary or benefits unless the employer brings it up first.)

- Is child care available? If so, at what times and what is the cost? Do they take infants?

- If traveling is required between clients, is mileage paid? If so, how much per mile?

After your pre-interview planning is complete, the next step in preparing for the interview is deciding what to wear. Remember that first impressions are vital. Dress neatly and conservatively—remember that you only have one chance to make a good first impression. Avoid excessive jewelry, cologne/perfume, and makeup.

It is better to go alone to the interview. Bringing someone along may give the impression that you are not able to make decisions alone. Arrive at least 15 minutes early. This will tell your prospective employer that you are prepared to arrive on time for your assignments if you are hired. Make sure you know the name of the interviewer(s) and that you know how to get to the appropriate location within the facility (Figure 26-1).

Introduce yourself to the interviewer(s) by name, with a smile, *firm* handshake, and eye contact. Always be polite, speak clearly, sit or stand with good posture, and use correct grammar—no slang. Do not chew gum or smoke during the interview. Answer all questions truthfully and avoid one-word answers such as "yes" or "no." Be ready to talk about the training and experiences you have had. Be positive about former employers and working conditions. Be honest about the kind of cases you prefer. The interview is the employer's opportunity to get to know you, and it is also the time for you to learn about the employer. Listen carefully to your interviewer. If the interviewer asks if you have any questions, select some from your previously prepared list. However, as noted, do not immediately ask about salary or benefits unless the employer

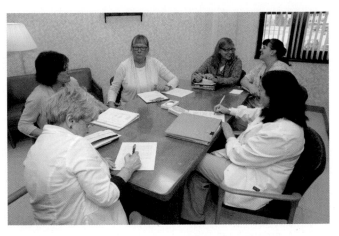

FIGURE 26-1 It is not uncommon to have a team interview you for a job position.

brings it up first. This information is usually supplied by the interviewer toward the end of the interview. If you are unclear about any aspects of the position, ask questions to clarify as needed.

You should not anticipate receiving a definite indication of a job offer or rejection at the end of the interview. The interviewer will usually let you know when you will be contacted. Remember to thank the interviewer as you leave.

After the interview, send a thank-you letter by mail or online and again express an interest in the position. Also, evaluate the interview—think about what went well and what didn't—to discover ways to improve for the next one. If you haven't heard back from the employer, it is fine to call the agency in a few days to inquire about the status of the position.

The Application Form

Prepare an **information sheet** or a current **résumé** (written summary data sheet or brief account of qualifications and progress in your career) listing some facts that usually appear on an application form, either on paper or online. This will save you time and you will not make foolish errors when you fill out the application. Some of the facts that you should have on your information sheet are listed in Figure 26-2.

If you do not have a phone, you should leave the number of a neighbor or friend who has agreed to take messages for you. **Personal references** should not be relatives, and should include your past employers, supervisors, or instructor(s). Be sure that you have permission from those people you list as references to use their names. If

TWIN OAKS ASSOCIATES
APPLICATION FOR EMPLOYMENT

EMPLOYER:

We are an equal opportunity employer. Federal and state laws prohibit discrimination in employment practices based on race, color, religion, sex, age, handicap, disability, or national origin. No question on this application is asked for the purpose of limiting or excluding any applicant's consideration for employment because of his or her race, color, religion, sex, age, handicap, disability, or national origin.

Name: Last	First	Middle	Social Security No.	Telephone No.

Address: Street	City	State	Zip Code	Licensed Nurses Only
				Mass. Reg. No. / Date Granted:

If your records may be under a name other than indicated above, please specify:

Last Renewal: / Expiration Date:

Are you a citizen of the United States? ☐ yes ☐ no

If you are not a U.S. Citizen, do you have the legal right to remain permanently in the United States? ☐ yes ☐ no   Explain

Are you between the ages of 18 and 70? ☐ yes ☐ no

Do you know of any fact that would limit or impair your ability to perform the functions of the job you are applying for? ☐ yes ☐ no   Describe

Date of last Physical Examination:

Family Physician:

I authorize my doctor to release to you the results of my pre-employment and subsequent medical examinations, and to discuss those results with you. ☐ yes ☐ no

Position desired: Hours desired: Salary expected:

Specialized training or experience not shown on other side of form:

Where now employed?   Reason for desiring change:

Have you ever pleaded guilty or been convicted of a felony? ☐ yes ☐ no   If yes to either, please explain:

or a misdemeanor other than a first conviction for drunkenness, simple assault, speeding, minor traffic violations, affray, or disturbance of the peace within the past 5 years? ☐ yes ☐ no

In case of emergency notify

name	relationship
address	telephone

*I authorize the schools, employers, and individuals listed in this application to release any information regarding my previous employment, character, general reputation and personal characteristics. ☐ yes ☐ no

I certify that the statements I have made in this application are true and hereby grant the employer permission to verify the accuracy and completeness of this information and to investigate all references and educational records. I understand that any false or misleading statements made by me on this application or in conjunction with my physical examination will be sufficient cause for the rejection of this application or for immediate dismissal if such false or misleading information is discovered after my employment. If I am accepted for employment, I agree to abide by the rules and regulations of the employer.

Signed ———————————————

Date ———————————————

E-2   "It is unlawful in Massachusetts to require or administer a lie detector test as a condition of employment or continued employment. An employer who violates this law shall be subject to criminal penalities and civil liability".

FIGURE 26-2   On application forms, answer questions to the best of your ability. Be sure the information is accurate and current.

possible, obtain letters of recommendation from these people before you go for a job interview. This will save time for the agency, and the person who is giving the recommendation only has to write one letter of reference. The agency can then make a copy of your letters of reference and confirm them by phone or online.

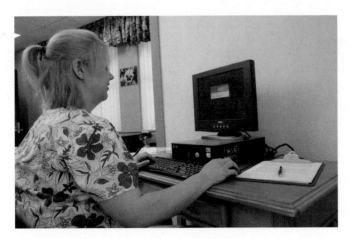

FIGURE 26-3 Applying for a job position online.

Each agency will have its own application form, but if you are prepared with the information listed in the sample in Figure 26-2, you should not have any difficulty completing the agency application form. It is always a good idea to read the application form fully and carefully before beginning. It may include special instructions, such as asking the applicant to type or print all information. Fill out each item neatly and completely. Do not leave any items blank; if the item does not apply to you, write "N.A." (not applicable). Take care to spell words correctly and to punctuate sentences carefully. Do not write in spaces marked "office use only." Review your application before submitting it to the employer.

Today, the majority of employers require the applicant to fill out the job application online. If you do not have access to a computer at home or do not have an email address, use the Internet/computer services at the public library to apply online and/or to set up an email account. The Workforce Connections Career Exploration Agency can also assist you in applying for a position online (Figure 26-3).

The Job Offer

If you are offered the job, you have the choice of accepting the agency's terms, thinking about it for a few days, or looking elsewhere for a position. Once you have accepted the position, your employer will complete a felony check or background check. Home care agencies are required by law to perform this background check, as you will be working with children, the elderly, and/or the disabled. A felony is a serious crime such as murder, larceny (theft of a large sum of money), assault, or rape. It is commonly

thought that if someone has a felony conviction, he or she may be a repeat offender and might endanger others. Your job offer is dependent on you passing this background check.

Once you have accepted the position with the agency, be realistic in your goals. As in any kind of employment, there is a system of progression in which the new employees must prove themselves and demonstrate competence. It is possible that an agency may test your attitude and availability by calling you for weekend or holiday part-time work. Many employers think it is a sign of dedication and good work ethic if you accept the assignments offered. After you have worked at the agency for some time, the employer will have a better idea of your abilities and strengths and will provide a more regular schedule.

When you are employed by an agency, you may be asked to sign a document similar to the one presented in Figure 26-4. This document will indicate the policies and rules of the agency and the consequences to employees for breaking the rules (infractions) or for incidents of misconduct (improper behavior). Read this document carefully and be willing to accept and abide by the conditions included in it.

The majority of states now require restrictive codes for agencies providing home health care services. To be qualified to operate, agencies must meet standards set by both the U.S. Department of Health and the Centers for Medicare and Medicaid. Included in the standards required by states are:

- A grievance procedure for an agency's employees
- A client's bill of rights that *must* be explained to the client (or client's family) in the presence of a witness
- Documentation of certification of all employees
- Proof of an annual physical examination by employees
- Proof of employee's attendance at a minimum number of in-service programs each year
- Proof of citizenship or verified alien registration
- Satisfactory completion of an approved home health aide program
- No legal record of client abuse or misuses of a client's property in a caregiver situation, verified through a state criminal background check
- Proof of being on the state registry for home health aides in the state in which you are applying for a position

---

TO THE EMPLOYEE

Because you are important to us, we want to help you develop a good work record. If we feel that you are violating any of our rules and policies, or that you have misunderstood the terms of employment, we will hold a conference with you. Continued *infractions* will cause your immediate dismissal. PLEASE READ THE FOLLOWING CAREFULLY.

1. *Attendance and tardiness record:*   Recurring cancellations of promised scheduled workdays may result in dismissal. Absence without call in may result in immediate termination. No pay raises will be granted if attendance and tardiness records are unsatisfactory. We must be able to depend on you. You must call in if you are unable to meet your assignment.

2. *Unbecoming conduct:*   Any of the following are considered to be gross *misconduct:* carelessness and inattention to client care; failure to perform duties; violation of safe practices; inefficiency and wasting of materials; refusal to obey direct orders; insubordination; rude, discourteous or uncivil behavior; intoxication, drinking or possession of intoxicating beverages while on duty; gambling on duty; sleeping on duty; unauthorized absence from assignment or leaving early without permission; failure to report an injury or accident concerning an employee or client; soliciting tips from clients or families; sale of services to clients or families; divulging confidential information about client and family; theft and/or dishonesty; *pilferage* of drugs or violation of any law on drug use including use or sale of same; damaging, defacing or mishandling equipment or property; interfering with work performance of another employee; falsifying client or personnel records or any form of misrepresentation.

Employee's statement:

I have read the above rules and regulations and understand my responsibilities to the agency and client. I agree to abide by these terms of employment.

_____   _____
Employee Signature   Date

_____   _____
Supervisor's Signature   Date

FIGURE 26-4   Once you have decided to accept a position with an agency, you may be asked to sign a document that states that you have read and understand the rules of the agency, such as the sample document shown here.

WORKBOOK REVIEW

Go to the workbook and complete the review exercises and activities for Unit 26.

REVIEW

1. List four records or credentials that you may need to bring for a job interview.

    _____

    _____

    _____

    _____

2. When is the best time to arrive for an interview?
    a. An hour before the scheduled interview time
    b. Five minutes late to show you are not overly eager
    c. Exactly at the scheduled interview time
    d. Fifteen minutes before the scheduled interview time

3. T   F   You should bring someone with you to the interview.

4. T   F   You should practice interviewing before you go.

5. T   F   Do not ask any questions during the interview.

6. T   F   A resume is a written summary of qualifications and progress in your career.

Use the following terms to fill in the blanks in questions 7–11.

information sheet   misconduct   personal references

infractions   newspaper

7. The employment section of the _____ is a good place to locate job leads.

8. Complete an _____ _____ before the interview so you will be prepared to complete a job application.

9. Former employers, supervisors, and instructors are considered _____ _____. Relatives are not.

10. Continued _____ could lead to immediate dismissal when employed.

11. Violation of safe work practices, carelessness, inattention to client care, failure to perform duties, and insubordination are all examples of _____.

Case Studies

12. The interviewer offers you a job with her agency as soon as you walk in the door, without asking you any questions or describing the position. What should you do?

13. You discover an ad in the newspaper for a job for which you are qualified and that is of interest to you. When you call about the position, the person states she is interested in interviewing you at her home. What questions should you ask her over the phone before going to the interview?

Appendix A
Emergency Procedures Guidelines

This appendix identifies emergency situations and the procedures that should be followed by the home health aide in emergencies.

First aid is care given to clients who suffer from accidents or sudden illnesses until more help is available. A client should be treated physically and emotionally, and may need reassurance as well as physical care. The whole environment must be evaluated to prevent further injury. First aid is **immediate care** that must be given after the **emergency medical system (EMS)** in your area has been notified.

In the home, emergency phone numbers should be posted by the phone. Include the local emergency squad, fire department, police, ambulance, poison control center (PCC), and family or friends the client wants contacted in case of an emergency. If someone needs immediate help, the home health aide may need to evaluate the situation and give emergency care according to the priority of needs.

Do not leave someone who requires immediate help. Have someone else call for help. Do not move the client unless the client is in danger. When clients need immediate help and there is no one in the home, home health aides should assess each situation and respond based on their knowledge, abilities, training, and experience. Several emergency situations and the appropriate home health aide responses will be covered in this appendix.

When a client needs help, but not immediate care to sustain life, the aide's responsibility is to prevent more injury, seek medical help, and keep the client calm.

For example, if a client's skirt caught fire and burned her legs, you would put the fire out before getting help for the burns. Good judgment is needed to give good emergency care. The whole situation must be evaluated to see what help is needed first and what further problems could arise.

Because this appendix covers only some life-threatening situations, it is advisable to take a course in cardiopulmonary resuscitation (CPR) and have current first aid books readily available for handling emergencies. Check with your agency regarding its emergency procedure policies.

Bleeding

1. Wear gloves and follow the principles of standard precautions for a client who is bleeding.
2. Cover the wound using a clean cloth, gauze, or your hand.
3. Place your hand over the bandage. Apply firm pressure for approximately 5 minutes or until bleeding slows or stops.
4. Do not lift the bandage to check bleeding. If blood soaks through, apply another bandage on top. Remember to keep firm pressure on the wound.
5. Raise the injured body part above the level of the victim's heart (unless you suspect broken bones).
6. Stay with the client until help arrives.

Burns

Burns are very painful and, in extreme cases, can be life-threatening injuries. To determine the severity of the burn, you will need to know the degree of injury involved:

1st degree—Red and painful, like a sunburn

2nd degree—Red and painful, with blistering

3rd degree—May be black or white; there may or may not be pain involved

What to Do

1. If at all possible, stop the burning if it is still in progress. This is done by removing the source of burn, for example, a hot iron.

2. Immerse the burned area in cold water. If this is not possible, apply cold water directly to the area with a cloth or sponge.

3. *Do not* apply oil, butter, or ointments to the burn (these hold heat in).

4. *Do not* break blisters.

5. Place a clean wet dressing on the area (use sterile cloth if available).

6. Call the health care provider or emergency room for further instructions. Stay with the client until help arrives.

Choking

When a client is choking, you must act quickly; seconds count and can mean the difference between life or death. Figure A-1 shows the universal sign for choking.

1. If the client can speak, wheeze, or moan, encourage him or her to cough out the object.

2. If the client is coughing, encourage him or her to keep coughing until the object is actually dislodged.

3. If the client is unable to make any noise, do abdominal thrusts:

    *   Stand directly behind the client.

    *   Reach both your arms around the client's waist.

    *   Make a fist with one hand, keeping the thumb straight (Figure A-2A). Place your fist, thumb side in, against the client's abdomen slightly above the navel.

*   Grasp your fist with your other hand (Figure A-2B); press your fist inward and upward, using short, quick movements.

*   The procedure should be repeated until the object is dislodged or the person becomes unconscious.

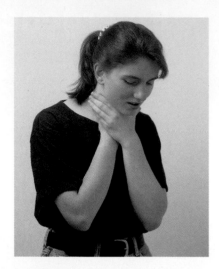

FIGURE A-1 The person is choking. She cannot speak, cough, or breathe.

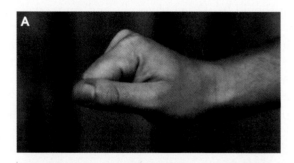

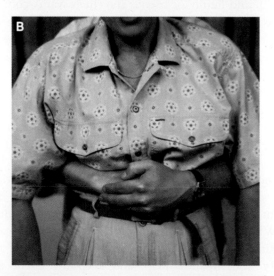

FIGURE A-2A & B Abdominal thrust.

Poisoning

Swallowed

When you suspect someone may have swallowed poison, the three most important things you can do are:

1. Find out exactly what was taken (you will need to know the name, ingredients if listed, and amount swallowed).
2. Activate EMS immediately.
3. Follow the instructions EMS gives you.

Do not give antidotes or induce vomiting unless specifically told to do so.

Inhaled

1. Get fresh air for the client—preferably outdoors.
2. Call the poison control center (PCC) or activate EMS.

Skin

1. Flush with water for at least 10 minutes.
2. Call the PCC or activate EMS.

Shock

Shock can be a life-threatening injury and requires immediate attention. Symptoms may include pale, cool, moist, or sweaty skin; restlessness or drowsiness; rapid and irregular heartbeat and breathing; nausea and chills; bluish discoloration of the lips and nail beds; and enlarged or dilated pupils.

What to Do

1. Activate EMS immediately.
2. Induce the client to lie down.
3. Elevate the client's legs (unless you suspect fracture).
4. Cover the client with a light blanket.
5. Keep the client quiet and comfortable (be reassuring).
6. Do NOT give anything by mouth.

Heart Attack/Stroke

Heart attacks and strokes are both serious medical conditions that require immediate attention.

Heart attack symptoms may include chest pain (described as pressure, or like something sitting on the chest), nausea, indigestion, vomiting, profuse sweating, or pain radiating into the arm or jaw.

Stroke symptoms may vary, but the most common symptoms are sudden weakness or numbness in the face or arm on one side of the body, loss or slurring of speech, inappropriate answers to questions, and unsteadiness.

Because stroke damage can be reversed, prompt medical treatment is necessary and should be sought immediately.

What to Do (If Victim Is Conscious)

1. Activate EMS immediately.
2. Tell EMS your exact location.
3. Stay with the client and remain calm.
4. Do not take the client to the hospital yourself or allow the client to refuse treatment.
5. If you are trained in CPR, be prepared to start the procedure immediately if symptoms require CPR.

Appendix B
Prefixes and Suffixes Commonly Used in Medical Terminology

a-, an-: without, not
ab-: from, away
ad-: to, toward
adeno-, aden-: gland, glandular
-algia: pain
ambi-: both
angio-: vessel, duct
ante-, pre-: before
anti-, contra-: against
arthro: joint
audio-: sound, hearing, dealing with the ear
auto-: self
bi-, bis-: twice, double
bio-: life
brady-: slow
bronch-, bronchi-: air tubes in the lungs, bronchi
cardi-, cardia-, cardio-: pertaining to the heart
-cide: causing death
crani-, cranio-: pertaining to the skull
cyst-, cysto-, cysti-: bladder, bag
-cyte, cyt-: cell
derm-, derma-, dermo-, dermat-: pertaining to skin
dia-: through, between, apart
dorsi-, dorso-: to the back, back
dys-: difficult, painful
ecto-, ex-, exo-: outside of, external
-ectomy: surgical removal of
endo-: within, innermost
entero-: intestine, pertaining to the intestine
gastro-, gasti-: stomach

-genetic, -genic: origin, producing
genito-: organs of reproduction
glyco-, gly-: sugar
gyn-, gyno-: women, female
hemi-: half
hema-, hem-, hemo-, hemato-: blood
hepato-: liver
hetero-: other, unlike, different
homo-, homeo-: same, like
hydro-: water
hyper-: over, increased, high
hypo-: under, decreased, low
hystero-, hyster-: uterus
inter-: between, among
intra-: within, into
-itis: inflammation, inflammation of
leuko-, leuco-: white
-logy, -ology: study of, science of
mal-: abnormal, disordered
mast-, masto-: breast
micro-: small
mono-: one, single
multi-: many, much, a large amount
myo-: muscle
neph-, nephro-, ren-: kidney
neuro-, neur-: nerve or nervous system
-ology: study of a science
ophthalm-, ophthalmo-: eye
-ostomy: creation of an opening by surgery
ot-, oto-: ear

-otomy: cutting into

path-, patho-, pathy, -pathia: disease, abnormal condition

ped-, pedia-: child

peri-: around

plasty: surgical replacement

-plegia: paralysis

pnea-: respiration/breathing

pneum-: lung, pertaining to the lungs

post-: after

proct-, procto-: rectum, rectal

pseudo-: false

psych-, psycho-: pertaining to the mind

sclerosis: hardening

scopy: visual examination

sep-, septic-: poison, rot

sub-: less, under, below

super-, supra-: above, upon, over

tachy: fast

therm-, thermo-: heat

-toxic, -tox: poison

tracho-: trachea, windpipe

-uria: urine

Glossary

A

abandonment being left without care or support by family or agency.

abdominal perineal resection abdominal surgery done on the large intestine, primarily to remove cancerous tumors.

abduction movement away from midline or center.

abuse mistreatment or improper treatment, including physical abuse, sexual abuse, emotional abuse, and seclusion.

accommodation adjustment of eye to focus on objects close-up then objects at a distance.

acidosis a condition in which the balance of acids and bases in the body is disturbed because of loss of salts, sodium and potassium, or the accumulation of acids.

acquired immunodeficiency syndrome (AIDS) progressive disease of the immune system caused by the human immunodeficiency virus, a retrovirus that destroys the body's ability to fight infection. As the disease progresses, the individual becomes overcome by disorders, including cancers and opportunistic infections.

active listening a tool that allows total involvement in the communication process; techniques include paraphrasing, reflecting the speaker's feelings, asking for more information, and using nonverbal communication.

active range-of-motion exercises the client does the exercise without the assistance of another person.

activities pursuits or pastimes that help a person who is disabled relearn skills that were lost due to illness or accident.

activities of daily living (ADLs) the activities necessary for the client to fulfill basic human needs, such as dressing, eating, and toileting.

acute illness is an illness that arises quickly, requires immediate care, and can be expected to go away quickly.

adduction moving a part toward the midline of the body.

adjustment changes a person makes in his or her behavior to deal with a situation.

adjuvant therapy assisting or aiding other therapies.

adolescence the period of physical and emotional development from early teens to young adulthood (usually between the ages of 13 to 18).

adult day-care center facility that provides care for adults who need minimal care or supervision during the day.

advance directive document specifying the type of treatment individuals want or do not want under serious medical conditions in which they may be unable to communicate their wishes. Three common forms: living will or durable power of attorney and mental health directives.

afebrile without a fever.

Affordable Care Act this act put consumers in charge of their care. This law requires that nearly everyone have health insurance.

aiding and abetting not reporting dishonest acts that one observed.

airborne carried through the air.

alopecia loss of hair.

Alzheimer's disease type of dementia characterized by loss of memory and confusion.

ambulate to walk.

amyotrophic lateral sclerosis (ALS) a progressive degeneration of the nerve cells in the brain and spinal cord that control the voluntary muscles. Commonly known as Lou Gehrig's disease after the famous baseball player who died from this disease.

analgesic drug used for relief of pain.

anemia deficiency of quality or quantity of red blood cells in the blood.

aneurysm localized enlargement or ballooning out of a blood vessel; may be due to a congenital defect or weakness of the vessel's wall.

angina pectoris mild heart condition that may cause pain in the chest region. Pain is usually relieved with a drug called nitroglycerin.

angiogram a heart test to see inside of the arteries around the heart.

antibiotic-resistant diseases such as MRSA and VRE that are resistant to antibiotic therapy.

antibodies   proteins formed in the body that protect a person against specific organisms.

anti-inflammatory   drug used to decrease pain and swelling in joints and muscles.

anxiety disorder   a type of mental disease whereby the client is always worrying about something.

aphasia   impaired or lost ability to communicate through speech due to dysfunction of brain centers. There can be a loss of verbal understanding, word blindness, inability to understand the meaning of spoken or written words, or speech in meaningless phrases.

apical   heartbeat.

apnea   absence of breathing or respirations.

arrhythmias   irregular heartbeats.

arterial insufficiency   a narrowing of the arteries that deliver blood to the lower extremities.

arteriogram   series of x-ray pictures that show the flow of blood in the arteries after the injection of a dye or contrast substance into the arteries.

arteriosclerosis   a condition in which the arteries become hard and lose the elasticity needed for good blood circulation.

artery   vessel that carries oxygenated blood from the heart to various parts of the body.

arthritis   inflammation of the joints causing pain, swelling, and enlargement of the joints.

arthroplasty   replacement of a joint.

arthroscopy   minor surgery done on the knee using a scope.

aspirate   drawing foreign material by suction into the respiratory tract.

assault   an intentional attempt or threat to touch a person without the person's consent.

assisted-living center   facility that provides supervised medication programs, cleaning and laundering services, meals, and minor assistance in activities of daily living. Clients pay only for services they elect to have.

asthma   a disorder of the respiratory system. Symptoms may include labored breathing, wheezing, and coughing. There may be secretion of fluid from the bronchials.

atrophy   wasting away of the muscle tissue.

auditory   relating to hearing.

autism spectrum disorder   developmental disorder of infants and children.

autopsy   a detailed examination of the body to determine the exact cause of death.

B

Background Information Disclosure Form   a form that is completed by a potential employee to show that there is no evidence of caregiver abuse after the age of 18 in his or her legal record.

bacteria   one-celled germs that are round, rod-shaped, or spiral in form. They can cause infections in the body or in the environment.

bariatric   refers to the causes, prevention, and treatment of obesity.

base of support   the area in which an object rests.

battery   the actual touching of a person's body without that person's consent.

bedbugs   parasites that bite and cause painful rash-type area on the skin. Infests beds, furniture, and other items and is active mainly at night.

benign   noncancerous.

benign prostatic hypertrophy (BPH)   tumor of the prostate gland, which can cause urinary problems.

biohazard   waste items or laboratory specimens or materials, and their containers, contaminated by body fluids; these have the potential to transmit disease. Discarded items must be labeled. Special precautions are taken to handle and contain this waste.

biopsy   removal and examination of a piece of tissue from a living body.

bipolar disorder   a mental disorder whereby the person swings with no reason from being overly depressed to overly elated.

bladder   a muscular organ for storing urine.

bland diet   diet in which foods that are irritating to the digestive system are restricted such as highly seasoned, fried food, raw vegetables, and fruit

blood lancet   small, pointed surgical instrument used to pierce the skin to obtain a blood sample.

blood pressure   the force exerted by the blood on the walls of the blood vessels.

blood tests   human blood is analyze for different components.

body language   a form of communication that uses gestures and facial expressions instead of words.

body mechanics   the techniques used to get the most effective and least taxing body movements.

bonding   a process of attachment of mother, father, and infant, happening immediately after birth. Infant is placed on mother's abdomen and father feels and touches infant.

bone density test   a diagnostic test to detect the thickness or density of the bones.

bony prominences   areas of the body where bones protrude, such as the elbows, wrists, knees, pelvic bones, spinal column. Such bones have little natural padding and are areas where pressure sores can easily form.

bottle-feeding   to feed a baby with a bottle.

brachial   artery in the arm that is used for taking blood pressure.

bradycardia   an extremely slow heartbeat.

breast engorgement   swollen, hard, and painful breasts resulting from the milk let-down process after birth.

breast-feeding   to feed a baby mother's milk from the breast.

bursitis   condition in which the bursa becomes inflamed and the joint becomes quite painful.

C

cachexia   wasting away of the body due to malnutrition; often seen in cancer clients.

cancer   a disease characterized by rapid growth of abnormal cells that form a tumor; it often spreads to other sites.

carcinogen   a substance or agent that produces cancer; may be related to environment or heredity.

career   is an occupation or profession for which one has been specially educated.

carotid arteries   arteries found on both sides of the neck.

carotid ultrasound   test used to diagnose a stroke.

cartilage   a hard coating on the end of bones that allows bones to slide over each other.

case manager   a professional member of the health care team who coordinates all the services the client may require in the home. Commonly a social worker or registered nurse.

cataract   opacity of the lens of the eye causing loss of vision.

catastrophic behavior   severe and unpredictable violent behavior of a person with dementia.

catheterization   procedure in which a thin tube is introduced into an artery or vein and passed through the heart or when a tube is passed through the urethra to the bladder to drain urine.

Celsius/centigrade scale   a temperature scale where 0° is freezing and 100° is boiling.

cerebral palsy   condition in which there is impaired muscular power and coordination due to lack of oxygen to the brain before or during birth.

cerebrovascular accident (CVA)   a disorder of the blood vessels of the brain due to a blockage caused by an embolus or hemorrhage.

certified home health aide   a caregiver who has completed a formalized education program and passed the certification examination for home health aide.

certified nursing assistant (CNA)   a caregiver who has completed a formalized education program and passed the certification examination.

cerumen   earwax.

cervix   the mouth of the womb.

chaplain   a member of the health care team who tends to the religious needs of the client.

chemotherapy   a treatment for cancer in which chemicals are used to destroy or slow the growth of cancerous cells.

Cheyne-Stokes   term used to describe breathing in which periods of apnea are followed by periods of dyspnea.

child abuse   emotional or physical abuse of an individual under the age of 18 by an adult.

chlamydia   one of the most common sexually transmitted infectious diseases caused by bacteria.

cholesterol level   diagnostic blood test to check the blood cholesterol level.

chronic bronchitis   inflammation of the bronchi, causing symptoms of low-grade fever, productive cough, lethargy, and malaise.

chronic illness   a long-term condition.

chronic obstructive pulmonary disease (COPD)   any condition such as asthma, emphysema, or bronchitis that interferes with normal respiration or breathing over a long period of time.

chronological age   how long a person has lived.

circumcision   the removal of the foreskin of a male.

clean-catch specimen   a procedure for obtaining a urine specimen for a diagnostic test; the specimen collected this way is as free of contamination as possible.

clear-liquid diet   diet in which all the foods are liquid and are clear such as soda, tea and plain gelatin.

clichés   a trite remark or saying.

closed bed   a bed made completely with top covers on.

closed fracture   break in the bone with the skin enclosed.

Clostridium difficile (C-diff)   germs that multiplies and produces toxins that can damage the colon.

cognitive   being able to reason and make judgments.

collateral circulation   when small blood vessels take over the circulation from nearby damaged or scarred blood vessels; the small vessels enlarge themselves to carry the blood to the body parts.

colon   large intestine.

colonoscopy   diagnostic examination of the entire colon by use of a scope.

colostomy   the removal of a diseased area of the large intestines and the creation of an external opening on the abdomen called a stoma; may be a temporary solution in cases in which the intestine can be reattached to the bowel later, or may be permanent.

comatose   unconscious.

communication   the sending and receiving of messages; may be verbal or nonverbal.

companion   a person hired to keep a client company or maintain safety. Usually does not provide personal or homemaking services.

compulsion   act that corresponds with the person's obsession.

computerized tomography (CT)   a specialized exam where a dye is injected into the vein and x-ray beams create a 3-D image of the blood vessels in the brain and neck.

conception   formation of a viable zygote by the union of the male sperm and the female ovum.

condom catheter   external male catheter applied to drain urine into a drainage unit.

confidentiality   keeping a client's personal affairs private. A home health aide must not give out information about the client except to the case manager or health care provider.

congestive heart failure (CHF)   a condition in which the heart cannot pump enough blood to the body; characterized by shortness of breath, edema of the ankles, and abnormal retention of fluid in the body.

conjunctiva   membrane that lines the eyelids.

conjunctivitis   infectious pinkeye.

constipation   difficulty in emptying the bowels.

contact precautions   practices used to prevent the spread of disease by direct or indirect contact.

contaminated   dirty, containing pathogens that may cause infection.

contracture   the abnormal shortening of muscle tissue.

copious   large amount.

corporal punishment   use of painful treatment to change or correct behavior.

cultural diversity   mixture of individuals from different cultures.

culture   the behavior patterns, arts, beliefs, institutions, and all other products of human work and thought as expressed in a particular community or period.

cyanosis   lack of oxygen in the blood, causing the client to appear bluish; indicates improper heart/lung function.

cyanotic   a bluish skin tone due to some problem of the respiratory system preventing proper inspiration and exhalation; the result of lack of oxygen to the blood cells.

cystic fibrosis   an inherited condition that affects children's sweat glands, pancreas, and respiratory system.

cystitis   inflammation of the urinary bladder.

D

dangle   client is sitting on edge of bed with legs over the side of the bed.

defamation   stating untrue statements about a person, which would injure that person's name and reputation.

defecation   term for having a bowel movement.

delusion   false belief.

dementia   loss of cognitive function such as thinking, remembering, and reasoning.

depression   a mental state characterized by loss of hope, feelings of rejection, generalized sadness, and, in severe cases, the inability to function.

dermis   the inner layer of the skin.

developmental disability   a mental and/or physical impairment, usually apparent at birth, that is likely to continue indefinitely and may result in substantial functional limitations and require lifelong or extended care.

developmentally disabled   the person has a severe, chronic emotional or physical disability that occurs before the age of 22.

diabetes   a chronic disorder related to carbohydrate metabolism; caused by the inadequate functioning of the islets of Langerhans in the pancreas, which produce insulin.

diabetic coma   serious condition where the blood sugar is too high.

diabetic diet   a measured carbohydrate and low- or no-sugar diet for diabetics.

diarrhea   frequent stools.

diastolic   measurement of blood pressure when the heart is relaxing.

dietitian   health professional that plans meals and therapeutic diets for the client.

digital thermometer   small plastic thermometer.

disability   a physical or mental impairment that impedes normal functioning or achievement.

disinfection   process of eliminating germs from equipment and instruments.

diuretic   a drug used to reduce fluid accumulation in the body. Persons taking diuretics urinate frequently.

diversity   the quality of being diverse, different; referring to variety, having many shapes and forms.

Division of Vocational Rehabilitation (DVR)   federal agency that can set up training programs for individuals with special needs.

documentation   to record on the proper form your observations and actions.

dorsiflexion   flex foot toward ankle.

Down syndrome   a birth defect caused by the presence of an extra 21st chromosome; the affected person has mild to moderate retardation, short stature, and a flattened facial profile.

droplet precautions   procedures used to prevent the spread of disease by droplets in the air.

duct   a tube-like structure that transports fluid or air from one part of the body to another.

durable power of attorney   legal document that designates another person to act as an "agent" or a "proxy" in making medical decisions if the individual becomes unable to do so.

dysmenorrhea   painful menstruation.

dyspnea   difficult or labored respiration.

dysuria   painful urination.

E

early adulthood   period between 20 and 39 years of age.

echocardiogram   a diagnostic test whereby sound waves of the heart are recorded.

ectopic pregnancy   implantation and subsequent development of a fertilized ovum outside the uterus.

edema   the swelling of legs or arms or other body parts when water is being retained in the tissues.

electrocardiogram (ECG/EKG)   record of the electrical activity of the heart; used to detect any abnormalities of the heart.

ELISA   diagnostic blood test for HIV.

embalming   the process of removing blood and fluid from a dead body and replacing the fluids with a chemical preservative, to keep the body from decomposing before burial.

embolus   floating blood clot.

emergency medical technician (EMT)   specially trained health care professional for emergency care.

emesis   vomiting.

emotions   basic feelings common to all, such as love, fear, anger, sorrow, and anxiety.

emphysema   an abnormal condition of the lung tissue in which the lungs lose their normal spongy and elastic character; causes poor exchange of the gases needed for normal respiration.

empty calories   foods high in carbohydrates and fats and low in proteins, minerals, and vitamins; "junk" food.

empty nest syndrome   the stage in a person's life when children leave home, often characterized by feelings of sadness and worthlessness.

encapsulated   enclosed within a capsule.

endocrine glands   ductless glands that secrete hormones directly into the blood and lymph system.

enema   a procedure whereby fluid is introduce into the rectum to remove feces and flatus (gas) from the rectum and colon.

engagement   the state of pregnancy when the uterus drops into the pelvic cavity.

enterostomal therapist (RN, ET) or Wound, Ostomy, Continent Nurse (WOCN)   a professional who works with clients who have ostomies.

enzymes   proteins produced by the body that break down organic matter (food) within the body; necessary for digestion and metabolism.

epidermis   the outer layer of the skin.

epilepsy   disorder of the brain, which can cause various types of seizures.

estrogen   any of several hormones produced chiefly by the ovaries and responsible for promoting the development and maintenance of female secondary sex characteristics.

ethical standards   guides to moral behavior.

ethics   a code of behavior. Medical ethics is the standard of professional conduct for health care team members.

evacuate   to empty or remove the contents from.

evaluation   a determination of how well a given duty or demonstration of skill is performed.

exhalation   act of breathing out.

expectorate   to spit.

expressive aphasia   unable to correctly express oneself verbally.

extension   straighten out a joint.

external rotation   to turn a joint away from the center.

external stimulus   a message or impulse sent to the nervous system from outside the body that causes a mental or physical response.

F

Fahrenheit scale   temperature scale where 32° is freezing and 212° is boiling.

fallopian tubes   either of a pair of slender ducts through which ova pass from the ovaries to the uterus in human beings and higher mammals.

false imprisonment   is the unlawful restriction of a person's freedom of movement.

fanfold   fold in pleats (top sheet).

febrile   have a fever.

felony   a serious crime such as murder, larceny (theft of large sums of money), assault, and rape.

fetal alcohol syndrome (FAS)   condition seen in infants and children due to mother's intake of alcohol during pregnancy.

fetus   the unborn young from the end of the eighth week after conception to birth.

fiber   indigestible plant matter consisting of cellulose; stimulates intestinal peristalsis.

fire extinguisher   portable apparatus containing chemicals that can be discharged to put out a small fire.

flatulence   feelings of gassiness in the abdomen.

flatus   medical term for rectal gas.

flexible   the ability to adapt to new situations or conditions; pliant.

flexion   bend a joint.

floaters   floating parts of fluid that have broken off and are floating around the eye.

fluid balance   balance between fluid intake and fluid output.

food allergy   any negative reaction to a food, or a food component, that involves the immune system.

foreskin   the loose fold of skin that covers the glans of the penis.

Fowler's position   position in which the client lies on the back with backrest elevated 45° to 60°.

fracture   a break in continuity of the bone.

frequency   urinating more than usual.

friction   rubbing of the skin against another surface, such as bed linens.

full-liquid diet   a diet where all the foods are liquid such as eggnog, milk, and cream soups.

functional age   how well an individual is able to accomplish tasks of daily living.

functional incontinence   involuntary urination because of inability to reach a bathroom because of a specific disability.

fungi   two groups of microorganisms that can cause diseases such as athlete's foot and vaginitis.

G

gait belt   see *transfer belt*.

gangrene   death of body tissue brought on by lack of adequate blood supply.

gastrostomy   an opening into the stomach that can be used for feeding.

genital herpes   a highly contagious, sexually transmitted viral infection of the genital and anal regions caused by herpes simplex and characterized by small clusters of painful lesions.

genital warts   small red or pink lesions found around the genital areas, which are contagious.

genitalia   the genitals.

germs   microorganisms capable of causing disease.

gestation   development of a fetus in the uterus.

gestation period   the time required from conception until birth; in humans, the gestation period is 9 months.

gestational   refers to a type of diabetes that occurs only during pregnancy.

glans   the head of the penis.

glaucoma   an eye disease characterized by abnormally high intraocular fluid pressure, hardening of the eyeball, and partial to complete loss of vision.

glucometer   instrument used to measure the level of blood sugar.

glucose   a form of simple sugar.

gluten-free diet   a diet that excludes the protein gluten. Gluten is found in grains such as wheat, rye ad tricale.

gonorrhea   a sexual transmitted disease that develops within 48 hours after sexual contact with an infected person. Causes painful burning sensation during urination in males; females have urinary burning and vaginal discomfort. Complications can lead to reproductive disorders, liver involvement, and blindness.

gout   form of arthritis caused by an increased amount of uric acid in the body.

grieving   the physical and emotional response to a severe loss, and the process of accepting the loss.

guided imagery   visualization of mental images of places or situations that you find relaxing.

gynecologist   a health care provider who specializes in delivering health care to women, especially the diagnosis and treatment of disorders affecting the female reproductive system.

H

habilitation   focusing on what a client can do, not what the client used to do.

hallucinations   hearing voices or seeing bugs or other things that are not really there.

hazard   that which is dangerous or could cause a serious accident.

health care provider   a general term for an agency, institution, or member of the health care team who provides medical care for the consum.

Health Insurance Portability and Accountability Act (HIPAA)   law that mandates strict confidentiality of a person's health records.

heartburn   a burning sensation near the sternum, caused by the reflux of acidic stomach fluids into the lower end of the esophagus.

hematuria   blood in the urine.

hemiplegia   a weakness or paralysis confined to one side of the body.

hemodialysis   a form of kidney dialysis.

hemophilia   a hereditary blood disease characterized by spontaneous hemorrhages due to deficiency of a clotting factor in the blood.

hemorrhage   abnormal bleeding.

hemorrhoids   varicose veins of the rectum.

hepatitis A, B, C   three different types of viruses that can cause inflammation of the liver.

hernia   a protrusion or projection of an organ or part of an organ through the wall of the cavity that normally contains it.

herpes zoster (shingles)   an acute viral infection characterized by a rash and itching.

hesitancy   a delay in starting urination.

hiatal hernia   a condition that occurs when the upper part of the stomach protrudes through the esophageal opening of the diaphragm of the lung cavity.

hierarchy   group arranged according to rank—ladder.

high-calorie diet   Diet high in high calories foods like milk shakes, steak, fried foods.

high-fiber diet   a diet which includes a high amount of fiber foods such as apples and whole grains.

high-risk pregnancy   a pregnancy marked by physical, emotional, or environmental situations that could potentially effect the well-being of the mother and the fetus.

hoarding   collecting items or things.

home care aide   caregiver who works with a client with the goal of assisting the client with independent living under professional supervision.

home health aide   person who performs personal and nursing care skills, such as bathing the client, under the supervision of a registered nurse.

home health care agencies   agencies, some of which are hospital-affiliated, that focus on providing medical aspects of care in the home.

homemaker   person who performs household duties such as laundry and cooking.

homemaker/home health aide   person who assists with general household tasks, personal care, and simple nursing duties, such as feeding and bathing the client.

hormones   products of endocrine glands that assist in healthy body function.

hormone therapy   form of therapy that fights cancer by changing the amounts of hormones in the body.

hospice   group that provides specialized care for dying clients and their families. The primary concern of hospice care is the quality of life, not prolonging the length of life. The goal is to keep the client as pain-free and as comfortable as possible.

human immunodeficiency virus (HIV)   a virus that causes AIDS; lives in the blood, semen, and body fluids of an infected person.

hygiene   personal cleanliness of the human body.

hyperglycemia   high blood sugar.

hypertension   sustained, elevated blood pressure.

hyperthermia   abnormally high body temperature (heat stroke).

hyperthyroidism   condition resulting from excessive activity of the thyroid gland; symptoms may include rapid heartbeat, restlessness, and irritability.

hypoglycemia   low blood sugar.

hypostatic   inactivity.

hypotension   blood pressure that is lower than normal.

hypothermia   abnormally low body temperature.

hypothyroidism   a condition resulting from severe thyroid insufficiency; characterized by sluggishness and fatigue, cold hands and feet, constipation, pale and dry skin, and puffiness in the face.

hysterectomy   a surgical procedure in which the uterus is removed.

I

ileostomy   the surgical removal of a diseased portion of the small intestine and the preparation of an external abdominal stoma (usually permanent) from which a liquid stool is expelled.

immune system   body system that helps fight off infections.

immunization   a process of making a person more resistant to an infectious agent.

impaction   in reference to the stool, a condition in which the feces become hardened and lodged in the lower colon or rectum.

incident report   a type of report that describes an accident or something undesirable that happened while delivering health care (e.g., a client falls in the kitchen).

incontinent   unable to control urinating of the bladder.

incubation period   the time between entry of germs into the body and the appearance of the first signs of the disease.

infection   invasion of germs causing inflammation, discomfort, or illness.

infectious disease   a disease that is readily passed from one person to another.

inflammation   protective response to the body due to an injury; classic signs are redness, swelling, heat, and pain.

information sheet   a list of key facts and information that may be needed or requested for completion of a job application, including references, job history, names, and phone numbers.

infraction   violation of a rule or law.

inguinal   type of hernia near the groin area.

inhalation   act of breathing in.

insulin   a hormone produced by the pancreas; essential for the maintenance of proper blood sugar levels.

insulin shock   condition where the blood sugar is below 50 mg.

integumentary system   body system composed of skin, nails, and hair.

interaction   the reciprocating actions between two people or between members of a group.

internal rotation   to turn a joint in toward the center.

internal stimulus   a message or impulse from within the body that is transmitted through the nervous system and causes a mental or physical response.

interpersonal relationships   the feelings and understanding that result from the interactions between two or more persons.

intraocular pressure   pressure inside the eye.

invalidate   to negate; to make unjustified.

invasion of privacy   wrongful intrusion into one's private activities

iris   membrane surrounding the pupil of the eye.

iron deficiency anemia   low hemoglobin due to lack of iron, which causes shrinkage of the red blood cells.

ischemia   lack of blood supply.

isolation   procedure whereby the client is kept away from others to prevent the spread of a contagious disease.

J

jaundice   a condition in which there is a yellowish color to the skin, mucous membranes, and eyes. It is associated with liver failure when excessive amounts of bilirubin enter the blood.

jet nebulizer   device that is used to turn drugs into a fine mist so that the lungs can absorb the drugs more effectively.

joint capsule   the joint membrane that encloses the joint's parts.

K

Kaposi's sarcoma   rare form of skin cancer seen in individuals infected with HIV.

Kegel exercises   special exercises done to strengthen the muscles around the urinary meatus.

kidneys   primary organ of the urinary system; its function is to filter waste material from the bloodstream.

kidney dialysis   artificial way of removing waste from the body.

kidney stones   buildup of calculi in the kidneys, caused by an excess of calcium.

kyphosis   forward curvature of the upper spine.

L

labia   lip of the skin outside the vaginal opening.

lactose   sugar found in milk.

laryngectomy   the surgical removal of the larynx (voice box) because of disease.

larynx   the voice box.

learning disorder   an abnormal condition that affects the person's ability to either interpret what is seen or heard or link information from different parts of the brain.

legal standards   guides to lawful behavior.

leukemia   a condition in which too many immature white blood cells are produced, blocking the normal transport of oxygen to body tissues; also called cancer of the blood.

liability   something for which a person has a responsibility or duty.

libel   false written statement about another person.

licensed practical nurse (LPN) or licensed vocational nurse (LVN)   a professional who provides direct care to clients; may supervise home care workers.

ligaments   the tough elastic fibers that hold the joints in place.

listening   hearing with thoughtful attention.

lithotripsy   a procedure whereby kidney stones are dissolved by sound waves.

living will   legal document that outlines the medical care an individual wants or does not want if he or she becomes unable to make decisions.

lobectomy   partial removal of a lung.

lochia   the normal uterine discharge of blood, tissue, and mucus from the vagina following childbirth.

long-term care insurance   form of insurance that pays for services in a long-term care facility, assisted-living facility, or home, depending on the policy.

low-birth-weight   weight of less than 3 pounds for a full-term infant.

low-calorie diet   a diet consisting of a minimum amount of calories in a day.

low-sodium diet   diet containing foods with low salt content; no extra salt is to be added.

lumpectomy   surgical excision of a tumor from the breast with the removal of a minimal amount of surrounding tissue.

M

magnetic resonance imaging (MRI)   diagnostic test used to pinpoint the area of the brain where a stroke occurred.

malignant   cancerous growth.

malnutrition   a condition resulting from a poor diet that lacks the needed nutrients to maintain health; early signs include muscle weakness.

malpractice   the failure to exercise reasonable judgment in the application of professional knowledge.

mammogram   x-rays of the female breasts used to determine if a tumor is present in the breasts.

managed care   a method of health care delivery that attempts to cut costs by controlling access to and use of health care providers, hospitals, nursing facilities, and other forms of care.

mastectomy   a surgical removal of the female breast(s); may be total or partial.

Meals on Wheels   program that prepares and delivers meals to homebound clients or to senior citizens' centers to help assure that the disadvantaged, handicapped, ill, or elderly have at least one meal a day that is nutritionally sound.

meatus   opening in the body where urine is expelled.

meconium   infant's first stool, which is thick and sticky in consistency; can be yellow, green, or brown.

Medicaid   federally and state-funded program that pays medical costs for those whose income is below a certain level.

Medicare   federal program that assists persons over 65 years of age with hospital and medical costs.

melanoma   malignant type of skin cancer.

menopause   cessation of the monthly menstrual cycle; normally occurs during a woman's middle years (late 40s to late 50s).

menstruation   the process, or an instance of, discharging the menses.

mental disorder   a disorder of the mind, characterized by difficulty in functioning satisfactorily in society as a result of changes in thoughts, behavior, personality, or emotion.

mental health directive   a type of advance directive that provides specific direction or designates an agent to make decisions concerning mental health treatment.

metabolism   the complex of physical and chemical processes occurring within a living cell or organism that are necessary for the maintenance of life.

metastasis   spreading of cancer cells away from the primary site of the cancer tumor.

methicillin-resistant *Staphylococcus aureus* (MRSA)   pathogenic organism (germ) that is resistant to treatment with antibiotics.

microorganism   germ that is not visible with the naked eye, such as bacterium or protozoan.

middle adulthood   period of time during which an individual is between 40 and 65 years of age.

millimeter   unit of measurement; 1 ounce = 30 millimeters or mL.

misconduct   improper behavior; mismanagement of responsibilities.

mitered corner   special corner made on beds to keep linens in place and give a neat appearance to the bed; often called a hospital corner.

mottling   discoloration or deformity.

multiple sclerosis (MS)   a progressive disease involving the nerves of the brain and spinal cord. It may start slowly and become worse throughout life, or there may be periods of remission when the condition seems to stay about the same.

muscular dystrophy   a progressive degenerative disease of the muscles surrounding the skeleton; characterized by loss of strength, physical disability, and deformity.

musculoskeletal disorder (MSD)   an injury or disorder of the muscles, nerves, or joints due to prolonged exposure to physical factors such as repetition, force, or vibrations.

myocardial infarction   an acute coronary occlusion; commonly called a heart attack.

myocardium   heart muscle.

MyPlate   government dietary guidelines recommending that a person's diet be approximately 30% grains, 30% vegetables, 20% fruits, and 20% protein, plus dairy products.

N

neglect   refusal or failure to fulfill any part of an obligation or duties to other persons.

negligence   failure to give care that is reasonably expected of a home health aide.

neurologist   a physician who specializes in diseases and conditions dealing with the nervous system.

neuropathy   term usually used in relation to diabetic clients, but generally means any disease of the nerves.

nitroglycerin   drug used in treatment of heart conditions.

nocturia   urinating at night.

nongonococcal urethritis   a urethral inflammation caused by an infection other than gonorrhea.

nonjudgmental   the quality of refraining from forming or expressing personal opinions, or otherwise determining the worth or quality of something; open and accepting.

nonverbal communication   a way of communicating without words, using gestures, facial expressions, or other body language.

nosocomial infection   infection acquired while being hospitalized.

Nurse Aide Registry   each state has a registry where all home health aides and nursing assistants are placed once they have completed their training and testing requirements.

nurse practitioner (RN, NP)   nurse with advanced specialized training in physical examination and assessment who works under a health care provider's supervision. Areas of specialization are with children, infants, pregnancy, the elderly, and cancer clients.

nutrition   the sum of those processes using food for growth, development, and body maintenance.

O

objective   what you actually saw, smelled, felt, or tasted.

observation   gathering of information about any change in the client's condition or behavior by using any of your five senses.

obsession   thoughts, images, or ideas that repeatedly go through a person's mind.

obstetrician   a physician who specializes in prenatal care, delivery of infants, and postnatal care.

Occupational Safety and Health Administration (OSHA)   federal agency that regulates worker's safety.

occupational therapist (OT)   a professional who evaluates a client's ability to perform skills necessary to independent living (such as bathing, dressing, cooking, etc.) and who works with clients to improve these abilities.

occupied bed   bed made with the client in the bed.

oliguria   urinating in scant amounts.

ombudsman   a person who investigates complaints and mediates problems regarding the complaint.

Omnibus Budget Reconciliation Act (OBRA)   law that regulates the education and certification of home health aides' work in home health agencies and certified hospices.

oncologist   physician who specializes in cancer clients.

open bed   bed is made with top linens fanfolded to the foot of the bed.

open fracture   break in the bones whereby the skin is broken open.

opposition   touching fingers with the thumb of same hand.

optimist   one who expects a positive outcome to a situation.

oral hygiene   care of the gums, lips, mouth, teeth, and tongue.

orchiectomy   surgical removal of a testicle.

orthopedic   dealing with bones.

orthostatic hypotension   blood pressure drops when changing from a supine position to an erect position.

osteoarthritis   degenerative joint disease caused by disintegration of the cartilage that covers the ends of the bones.

osteoporosis   loss of bone density and strength; the bones become increasingly porous and brittle, which may lead to fractures.

ostomy   surgical construction of an artificial excretory opening.

ostomy bag (stoma bag)   a sack or bag placed over the stoma (opening) to collect wastes for clients who have had a colostomy or ileostomy.

otosclerosis   hardening of the inner bones of the ear.

Outcome and Assessment Information Set (OASIS)   represents a comprehensive assessment tool used to measure the child's outcome and improve the quality of home health care.

ovaries   the paired female reproductive organ that produces ova, and in vertebrates estrogen and progesterone.

overflow incontinence   continuous or periodic dribbling of urine because of an atonic bladder.

P

palliative   relieving symptoms, but not curing the disease.

palpate   to feel.

Pap smear   a medical procedure whereby a sample of the vaginal cells are tested for cancer.

paraphrasing   restating a text, passage, or communication in another form or in other words, often to clarify meaning.

paraplegia   paralysis of the lower body involving both legs.

Parkinson's disease   a progressive degeneration of nerve cells in the area of the brain that controls muscle movement.

P-A-S-S   four steps to do when using a fire extinguisher—pull, aim, squeeze, sweep.

passive listening   listening without seeming interested in what a speaker has said and without checking to confirm the speaker's meaning.

passive range-of-motion exercises   exercises done to a client by another person.

pathogens   germs causing disease or infection in the body.

Patient Self-Determination Act   law that gives each individual the right to make choices regarding specific types and kinds of medical care before he or she becomes seriously ill.

pelvic   the bony structure formed by the sacrum, coocyx, and the ligaments that unite them.

pelvic inflammatory disease (PID)   inflammation of the female genital tract, especially of the fallopian tubes, caused by any of several types of germs, chiefly chlamydia and gonococci, and marked by abdominal pain, fever, and vaginal discharge.

pendulous   hanging downward.

penis   the male organ of copulation and male organ of urinary excretion.

perineum   in the male, the area between the anus and scrotum; in the female, the area between the anus and vagina.

peripheral vision   the outer boundaries of vision; side vision.

peristalsis   the progressive, wavelike movements that occur involuntarily to move food through the digestive system.

peritoneal dialysis   type of kidney dialysis done through the abdomen.

pernicious anemia   type of anemia that is due to lack of vitamin B_{12} in the body.

personal care worker   person who assists with a minimal level of daily living activities, such as companionship and meal preparation.

personal health information (PHI)   any information contained in automated records that is transmitted or maintained in any form or medium, including verbal discussions and electronic communications regarding the client.

personal protective equipment (PPE)   equipment such as waterproof gowns, masks, gloves, goggles, and other equipment needed to protect a person from infectious material.

personal reference a person, other than a member of the individual's family, who can give a prospective employer a recommendation concerning the character and ability of an individual seeking employment.

pessimist one who expects a negative or bad outcome to a situation, or who looks on the gloomy side of life.

phantom pain pain that a client may have in an extremity that has been amputated—a real pain.

phlebitis inflammation of a vein.

physical therapist (PT) a professional who evaluates a client's ability to stand, walk, climb stairs, transfer, and do other activities related to strength and endurance, and who works with clients to improve these abilities.

physician assistant (PA) a professional who takes medical histories, examines and treats clients, orders and interprets laboratory tests and x-rays, and make diagnoses.

physiologic relating to food and shelter.

pillaging behavior of clients with dementia in which they will take things or items that belong to someone else and think they are their own.

pivot turn or rotate the entire body, rather than twisting at the waist.

pivot disc a device used to transfer clients who can stand, but have difficulty in moving their legs.

plantar flexion flex ankle to make toes point downward.

Pneumocystis carinii **pneumonia** rare form of pneumonia that affects individuals infected with HIV.

pneumonectomy removal of the entire lung.

pneumonia an acute inflammation of the lungs.

pneumonia vaccine vaccine given to prevent pneumococcal pneumonia.

podiatrist health care provider who specializes in foot and toe problems.

portal of entry place that germs enter the body.

postpartum after childbirth.

postpartum blues feelings of anxiety, fatigue, mood swings, or sadness following childbirth.

post-traumatic stress disorder mental condition that occurs after traumatic events (e.g., soldiers often have this disorder after fighting in a war).

premature born before full term (37 weeks gestation is considered full term for humans).

prenatal before birth of infant.

presbycusis gradual loss of hearing.

pressure sore dermal ulcer or bedsore.

preventive health measures use of inoculations, special diets, or other techniques to avoid illness before it starts.

procedure the steps taken to accomplish a particular task; a course or plan of action.

progesterone a steroid hormone, secreted by the ovary and the placenta.

prognosis the probable outcome of an illness.

pronation turn hand so palm is facing downward.

prone position lying on one's abdomen.

Prospective Payment System (PPS) Medicare reimburses a home health agency for a predetermined base payment for each 60-day episode of care.

prostate male gland surrounding the neck of the bladder and the urethra.

prostate-specific antigen (PSA) blood test to detect cancer of the prostate gland.

prosthesis artificial replacement for a body part.

protozoa tiny, one-celled microscopic organisms.

psychologist mental health specialist.

psychology the study or science concerned with the mental processes and behavior of an individual; the study concerned with mental health.

psychosis a serious mental condition in which the thinking process is distorted by hallucinations, delusions, or both.

puberty the time period following childhood, when the body matures and reproduction becomes possible.

pulmonary embolus a blood clot that has broken away and travels to the lungs.

pulse the measurement of the number of heartbeats per minute.

punctuality on time, prompt.

pupil center part of the iris of the eye; this part can expand or contract (e.g., pupil as small as a pinpoint).

pureed diet food prepared by processing through a blender or strainer.

pyuria pus in the urine.

Q

quadriplegia paralysis of four extremities (arms and legs).

R

RACE steps to do in case of fire—remove client, activate the alarm, contain fire, extinguish fire.

radical hysterectomy a surgical procedure where the fallopian tubes, ovaries, and uterus are removed.

range-of-motion exercises series of exercises specifically designed to move each joint through its full movement.

reality orientation techniques used to keep clients in touch with reality.

receptive aphasia communication problem whereby a person does not understand the words someone else says.

referred pain   pain felt in another part of the body other than the part that is injured or diseased.

reflux   abnormal backward flow of fluid.

registered dietitian (RD)   a professional who provides information regarding the dietary needs of the client. Assists in meal planning for the client.

registered nurse (RN)   a graduate trained nurse who has passed a state registration examination and has been licensed to practice nursing.

rehabilitation   the restoring of physical or mental abilities following an accident or illness.

reliability   dependable, trustworthy.

reminiscence   the act or process of recalling the past.

remission   a period in an illness when the symptoms cease or become less severe.

renal diet   special diet for clients with renal failure. Restricted foods are foods high in sodium, potassium and phosphorus. Fluids are also kept at a minimum.

renal failure   kidneys stop functioning and waste products no longer can be excreted by the body.

renal function   kidney function, ability of the kidneys to produce urine.

repetitive behaviors   the client will repeat the same sentence, question, or behavior repeatedly; often seen in the middle stage of dementia.

report   a written record or oral summary of care given to a client.

reservoir   place where germs can grow.

respiration   the sum total of the processes by which the body exchanges oxygen and carbon dioxide in the respiratory system.

respiratory system   the nose, pharynx, larynx, trachea, bronchi, and lungs; system that helps maintain a constant balance in the body through effective air distribution and gas exchange.

respiratory therapist (RT)   a professional who assists the client with breathing problems and oxygen equipment.

respite care   short-term care for a client when the main caregiver needs a break to do errands or rest.

restricted fluids   a client's fluids are limited to a certain amount.

résumé   written summary data sheet or brief account of qualifications and progress in your chosen career.

rheumatoid arthritis   autoimmune response that results in inflammation of the joints.

rickettsiae   a type of germ that can cause disease; they live on lice, ticks, fleas, and mites.

rotation   the act of turning about the axis of the center of the body, as in rotation of the joint.

S

Safe Patient Handling and Mobility (SPHM) standards   a formal program for reducing the risk of injuries and muscular skeletal disorders (MSD) for health care workers, promoting a culture of safety and improving quality of care.

schizophrenia   mental disorder characterized by bizarre behaviors such as delusions and hallucinations.

scrotum   the external sac of skin enclosing the testes in most mammals.

seizure   a sudden attack; a convulsion.

self-actualization   when an individual reaches the highest level of his or her potential.

sexually transmitted disease (STD)   any of various diseases contracted through intimate sexual contact.

shadowing   the client with dementia follows the caregiver or another person around.

shearing   force on skin over bone when the skin remains at the point of contact while the bone moves, causing skin damage.

sibling rivalry   the normal jealousy and competition found between brothers and sisters in the family setting.

sickle cell anemia   a hereditary and chronic blood anemia in which the red blood cells are crescent-shaped and look like a sickle; occurs mainly in African Americans.

sigmoidoscopy   direct examination of the interior of the sigmoid colon.

sign   in medicine, a change in the client that can be observed or measured.

skilled long-term care facility   a care center that offers skilled nursing care.

slander   making a false oral statement about another person.

sleep   a natural, regularly recurring condition of rest for the body and mind.

social worker (MSW, BSW)   a professional who treat individuals, families, or groups with social and emotional problems.

source   a person, place, or thing by which something is supplied (such as a beginning of an infection).

Special Olympics   sporting event for people with disabilities.

speech therapist (ST)   a professional who assesses a client's ability to speak, hear, understand, write, and swallow, and works with clients to improve these abilities.

sphygmomanometer   the instrument used to measure blood pressure.

sprain   injury to ligament, resulting in pain and swelling.

stand lift   mechanical lift used to stand clients; can also be used to walk a client.

standard precautions   infectious disease control measures that assume that every direct contact with body fluids is infectious and requires every health care worker exposed to direct contact with body fluids or body substances to be protected.

sterile   free of germs.

steroids   hormonal drugs used to treat many conditions. Major side effects are edema, weight gain, susceptibility to infections, and elevated blood pressure.

stertorous   snoring-type breathing.

stoma   the surgically formed opening between a body cavity or passage and the body's surface.

stress   a mentally or emotionally disruptive or upsetting condition that occurs in response to adverse external stimuli.

stress incontinence   involuntary loss of small amount of urine during activities such as coughing, running, or laughing.

subcutaneously   beneath the skin; usually used in reference to an injection.

subjective   your opinion of a situation.

sublingually   under the tongue.

substance abuse   the use of alcohol or drugs that results in poor treatment of the body.

sudden infant death syndrome (SIDS)   the unexpected and sudden death of a healthy infant; occurs while the infant is sleeping.

sundowning   clients with dementia become more agitated, confused, and disoriented as evening approaches.

supination   to turn the palms upward.

suppository   a small plug of medication designed to melt within a body cavity other than the mouth.

susceptible host   a person who develops an infection.

suspiciousness   a client with dementia may forget where he or she placed something and blame others for stealing the item.

symptoms   those changes reported by the client, such as feeling pain, that may not be visible.

synchronize   cause to occur at the same time.

synovium   thin membrane of the joint that lubricates the fluid of the joints.

syphilis   an infectious, chronic sexually transmitted disease characterized by open lesions that can spread to the entire body and affect the nervous system.

systolic   measurement of blood pressure when the heart is contracting.

T

tachycardia   a very rapid heartbeat.

targeted biologic therapy   cancer treatment that targets faulty genes or proteins that contribute to cancer growth and development.

temporal artery   artery located on the forehead.

temporal artery thermometer (TAT)   an infrared thermometer designed for measuring the temperature of the skin surface over the temporal artery.

tendon   band that connects bone to muscle.

terminal   final; life-ending stage.

terminal illness   a fatal illness.

testes, testicle   the reproductive gland in a male vertebrate; the source of sperm and androgens.

testosterone   a crystalline steroid hormone, produced in the testes and responsible for male secondary sex characteristics.

theory   the practical and necessary information one must learn about a particular topic or subject.

thrombophlebitis   a condition in which a vein becomes inflamed in the lower extremities.

thrombus   blood clot that forms inside an artery.

thyroid-stimulating hormone (TSH) test   diagnostic test to detect if the thyroid is producing too little or too much thyroxine (hormone).

tophi   outpouches or protruding lesions that contain abnormal amounts of uric acid. Seen in individuals with gout.

total hip replacement (arthroplasty)   surgery whereby the orthopedic surgeon replaces a degenerated hip with a new artificial hip.

total incontinence   no control of urination.

total knee replacement (arthroplasty)   surgery whereby the orthopedic surgeon replaces a degenerated knee with a new artificial knee.

total parenteral nutrition (TPN)   high-dextrose solution that contains all essential nutrients and is fed to a client through a catheter into the blood vessels.

toxemia   high blood pressure during pregnancy.

trachea   the main tube running from the throat to the lungs to bring air in and out of the body; the windpipe.

tracheostomy   a surgical procedure to create an opening in the trachea; an emergency operation in cases where the trachea is obstructed and the person cannot breathe.

transfer belt   a sturdy cloth strap, about 3 inches wide and 3 feet long, tied around the client's waist and used by a care provider to assist in lifting a client in and out of a chair, or as added support when ambulating an unsteady client.

transient ischemic attack (TIA)   temporary reduction of flow of blood to the brain.

transmission-based precautions   special precautions taken in addition to standard precautions with clients who are known to have a contagious disease, to prevent transmission to others.

transurethral resection of the prostate (TURP) surgery done to reduce the size of the prostate gland.

tuberculosis   lung disease caused by a microorganism, easily transmitted to others by sneezing and coughing.

tympanic ear thermometer   a type of thermometer that measures the temperature in a client's eardrum.

U

ulcer   local defect (e.g., stomach or on skin).

ultrasound   diagnostic test done using sound waves; used to monitor fetal development.

umbilical   hernia near the navel.

unoccupied bed   bed made without the client in the bed.

ureter   one of the two long narrow ducts that transfer urine from the kidney to the bladder.

urethra   mucus-lined tube conveying urine from the urinary bladder to the exterior of the body; in the male, the urethra also conveys semen.

urge incontinence   involuntary loss of urine because of the inability to reach the bathroom in time.

urgency   the need to urinate right away.

urinary catheter   a tube inserted into the bladder to drain urine.

U.S. Centers for Disease Control and Prevention (CDC)   federal agency that keeps track of all diseases in the United States and issues guidelines for caring for clients with infectious diseases.

uterus   an organ of the female reproductive system; contains and nourishes the embryo and fetus from the time the fertilized egg is implanted to the time of birth of the fetus.

V

vagina   the passage leading from the opening of the vulva to the cervix of the uterus in females.

vaginitis   inflammation of the vagina.

validation therapy   a communication technique designed to foster positive self-esteem by confirming the feelings of another.

vancomycin-resistant enterococcus (VRE) pathogenic organism (germ) that is very resistant to treatment with antibiotics.

varicose veins   abnormally swollen or knotted veins.

vegetarian   one who does not eat meat or meat products.

venous insufficiency   damage to the veins that return blood to the heart, which causes pain and discoloration of the lower extremities.

vertebrae   small bones of the spinal column.

virus   germs that live and grow by feeding on living cells.

vital signs   measurements of temperature, pulse, respiration, and blood pressure.

vomitus   material the client vomits.

vulva   external female genitalia, including the labia, clitoris, and vestibule of the vagina.

W

wandering   moving around purposelessly; often seen in clients with dementia.

whooping cough   an acute infectious disease, usually affecting children, characterized by a whooping cough.

Index